STRENGTH TRAINING BIBLE

THE COMPLETE GUIDE TO LIFTING WEIGHTS FOR POWER, STRENGTH & PERFORMANCE

DAVID KIRSCHEN & WILLIAM SMITH

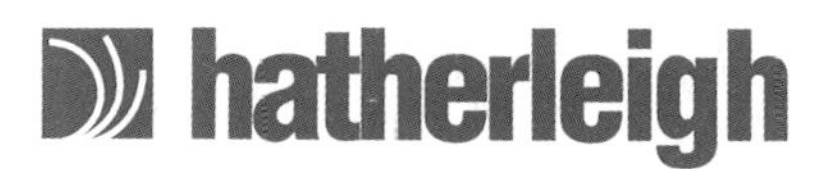

hatherleigh

Hatherleigh Press is committed to preserving and protecting the natural resources of the earth. Environmentally responsible and sustainable practices are embraced within the company's mission statement.

Visit us at www.hatherleighpress.com and register online for free offers, discounts, special events, and more.

Strength Training Bible

Library of Congress Cataloging-in-Publication Data is available upon request.

ISBN: 978-1-57826-552-7

Cover and Interior Design by Heather Magnan
Photos on pages iv, vi, 3, 13, 19, 21, and 80 by Ken Hicks, on location at EliteFTS (www.elitefts.net).

Printed in the United States

10 9 8 7 6 5 4 3 2 1

CONTENTS

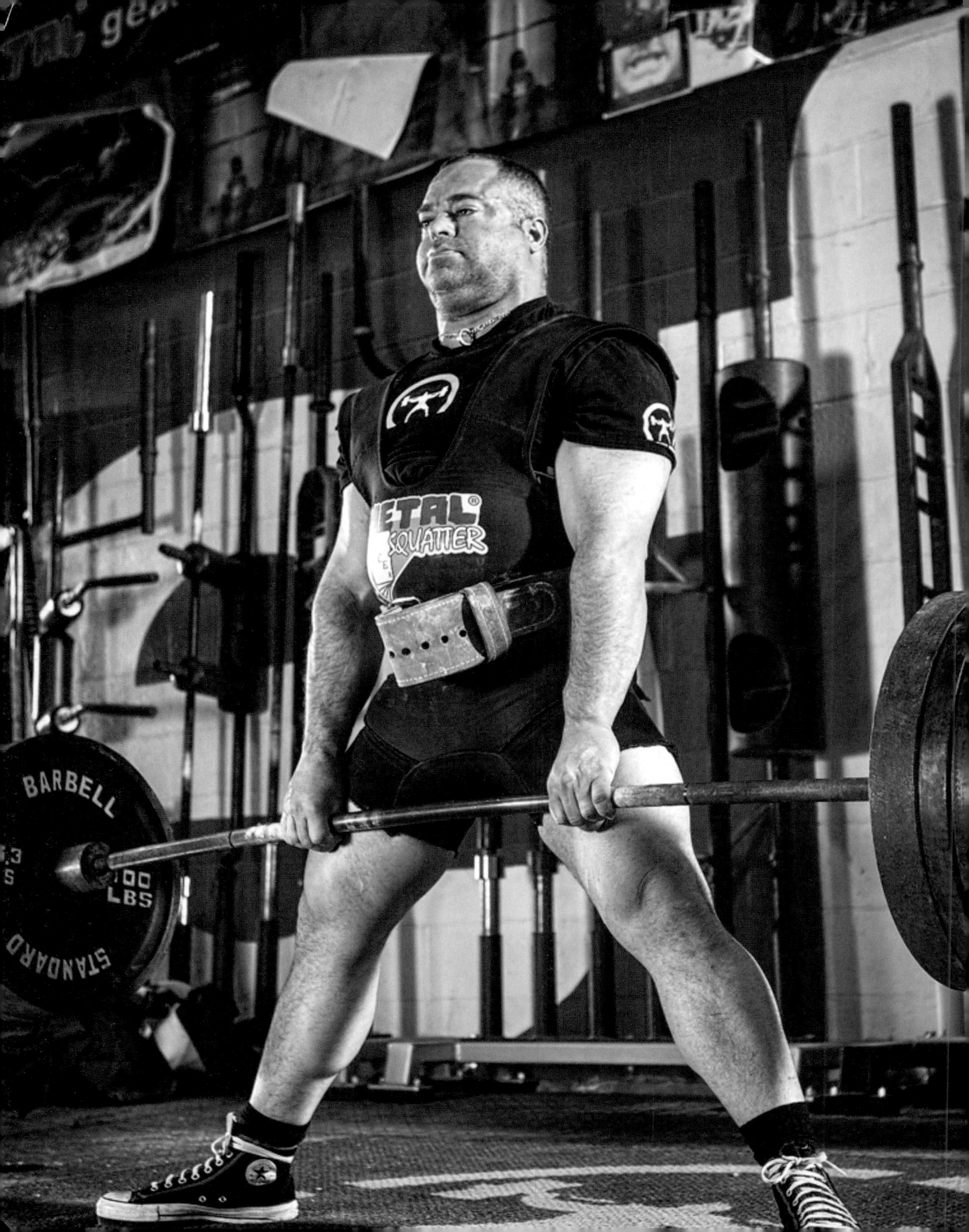

BARBELL
STANDARD
LBS
SQUATTER

INTRODUCTION

For as long as I can remember, I've always wanted to be strong.

From the time I bought my first set of adjustable dumbbells when I was 13, my life has been dedicated to the never-ending process of pushing my body to be as strong as humanly possible.

Much to the surprise of lifelong meatheads like myself, basic strength training has enjoyed somewhat of a renaissance in recent years. Back in the early 90s when I first got into the fitness business, most workouts were based on bodybuilding, still riding the popularity of Arnold Schwarzenegger and the "Golden Era" of the sport a decade prior. In most gyms, you could see a clear division in the clientele, with the serious patrons utilizing the free weights and the "soccer mom" crowd occupying the machines and cardio equipment and taking group classes. By around 2000 or so, the pendulum had swung in the direction of "functional training."

On one hand, this was a good shift, because it stressed the importance of real-life performance over appearance. The execution however, was lacking. For some reason, "functional" usually meant lifting light weights while standing on a wobble board, inflatable disk or some other oddball implement that would never be encountered in real life.

Throughout each of these eras, aficionados of the traditional barbell lifts were off in the distance of the fitness landscape, usually relegated to some dark corner of the gym where the one remaining squat rack still stood, waiting to be replaced by a Smith machine. At best, serious lifters were barely tolerated. At worst, we were handed back our membership dues and asked never to return.

Fast forward to today, and it looks like the pendulum has finally swung the other way. Barbells are the belle of the ball once again. Lifting heavy weights is back, although it never *really* went away.

While everyday fitness-minded folks used to demand amenities like rows of treadmills, complex-looking machines, and juice bars, many now flock to minimalist gyms with little more than racks, barbells, and weights (yet they often cost three times what the full service places do).

For "lifers" in this business like myself, the trend is both gratifying and a little perplexing. On one hand, it's exciting to see the general public finally exposed to these effective lifts. On the other hand, the quality of execution by both gym goers and coaches can often leave much to be desired.

Despite some liberal interpretations of what strength training is, this particular trend is a good one. Interest in strength sports like Olympic lifting and powerlifting is on an upswing, creating serious opportunities for those interested in learning, and capable of teaching the lifts. Rather than be critical of where these coaches and gym goers often fall short, I'd rather build off of the positives and do my part to increase the knowledge pool.

—Dave Kirschen

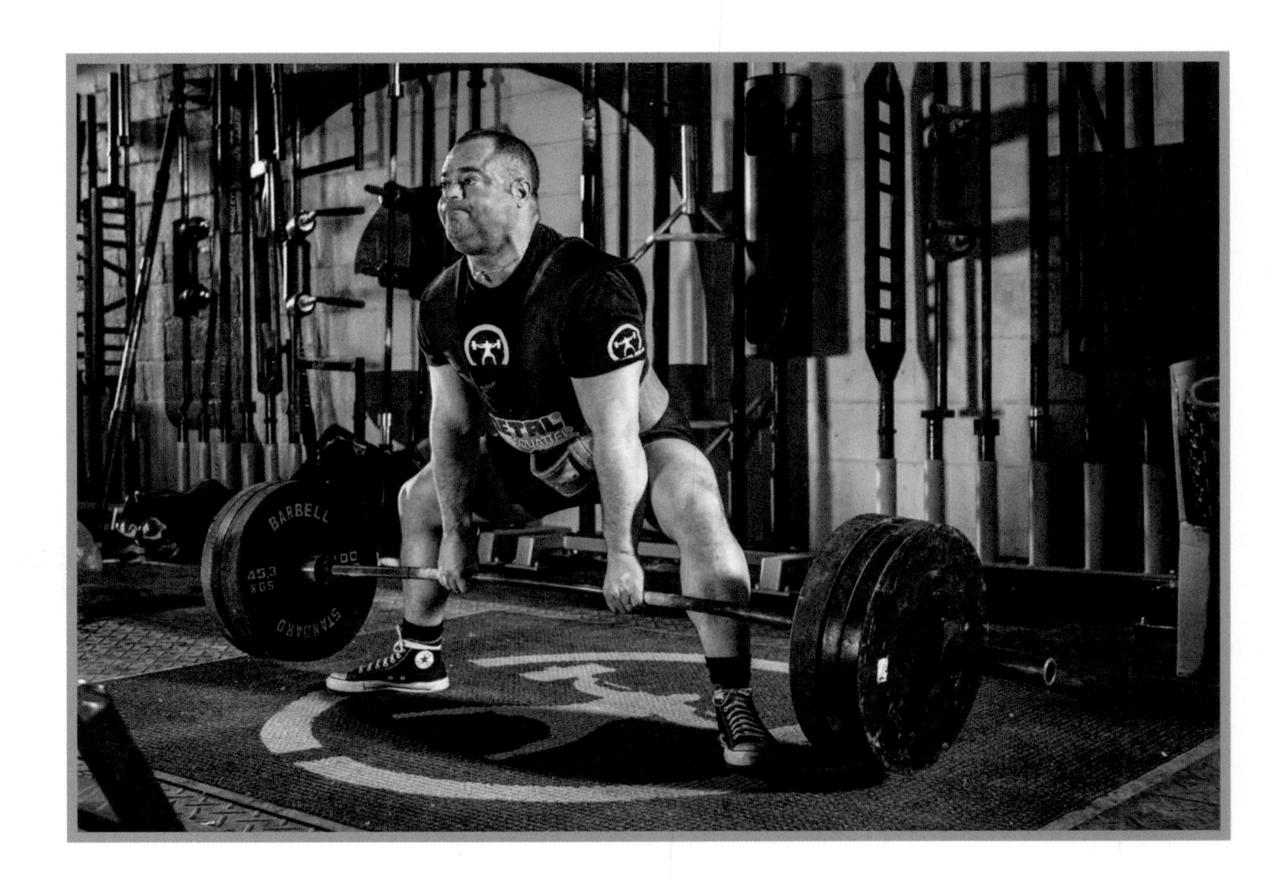

ABOUT THE EXPERTS

ABOUT DAVE KIRSCHEN

I began lifting weights in junior high school, with a set of adjustable dumbbells that I had bought at the local sporting goods store.

Like most 13-year-olds, I had no idea what I was doing. I had no clue what programming was, I made up the exercises as I went along, and didn't even buy the correct sized plates for my dumbbells, so they rattled around precariously while I lifted them. Without any practical knowledge, or anyone to guide me, I relied mostly on bodybuilding magazines and my few equally clueless friends to learn as much as I could about my new obsession.

Needless to say, my first few years of training were not nearly as productive as they could have been. However, being young and dedicated, I did get better over time, and learned a ton along the way. By the time I was 17, I knew that I would have a career in strength training and fitness, and made the decision to pursue my degree in Physical Education at SUNY Cortland, one of the best programs in the country. I also began working as a trainer at the West Side YMCA in New York City.

By age 19, I had begun competing in bodybuilding shows. While this was fun, it wasn't long before I became more interested in what I was capable of performance-wise, as opposed to how I looked aesthetically. By the time I was 21, I made the switch to powerlifting and never looked back. I am currently competing as a pro, sharing the competitive platform with some of the strongest athletes in the world.

As of this writing, I have been lifting weights in one form or another for 25 years, and have been teaching others for nearly 20 years. Now, with *The Strength Training Bible*, I have the opportunity to share my quarter century's worth of experience.

ABOUT WILLIAM SMITH

In addition to the strength programming featured in this book, you will also find robust sections on injury prevention. Since I do not claim any expertise in injury management, these sections were contributed by my friend and colleague, William Smith.

In many ways, Will and I represent opposite ends of the fitness/strength spectrum.

Will boasts an impressive academic pedigree, having worked as an Assistant Strength Coach for St. John's University while finishing his master's degree, before starting a successful personal training business in northern New Jersey. He is a frequent lecturer and consultant on the role of exercise in injury prevention and management.

Candidly speaking, Will is one of the smartest people I know, and someone whom I often turn to for advice on both the business and technical sides of the fitness industry. We've collaborated many times before, and I was thrilled at the opportunity to work with him on this project.

What makes our relationship interesting, is that despite our seemingly disparate backgrounds, our various collaborations have always come surprisingly easily, and we agree far more than we disagree on almost any topic that comes up.

The more you learn, however you go about learning it, the more you tend to come back to basics. Whether your goal is to gain muscle size and strength, improve at a particular sport, or prevent or rehab from injuries, you simply cannot go wrong with the strength training exercises found in this book.

WHY BE STRONG?

Why would you want to be strong? It's an interesting question, and one that only you can answer for yourself. Strength means different things to different people, and the reasons for pursuing it will vary from one person to the next. A quick scan of the Internet will show you countless reasons why you should want to strength train, spanning the spectrum from practical to ridiculous.

One of the more popular trends at the moment is to idealize periods of time in human history with little relevance to today, some going as far back as the Paleolithic era with frequent references to cavemen and early man. This approach to strength training depicts the caveman as something of a badass, and argues that they are the physical ideal which we should all aspire to. This all sounds well and good, but remember that early humans lived a vastly different life from us, and their (assumed) superior physiques reflected their struggle to survive in an infinitely harsher environment than we need to. Personally, I like living in a more modern age, and I would rather train to live an optimal life in this day and age, than in some romanticized imagining of a long gone era.

Another trend in strength training cites the supposed death of masculinity and the softening of America (or wherever else the target audience resides). This may be a great pitch for the services and products they inevitably are trying to sell you, but I've been in a lot of truly hardcore gyms and I've found that the toughest, most masculine guys typically don't spend much time pontificating about what it means to be a man. They just lift stuff because they like it.

Strangely, I tend to see the "lifting weights will make a man out of you" approach in *bodybuilding* resources just as much as (if not more than) in strength training literature. I personally find this curious because (as indicated later in this chapter), the sport of bodybuilding is judged exclusively on aesthetics, rather than performance. In reality, bodybuilding will not define you as a man any more than any other hobby will. Nothing against bodybuilding—it takes an insane amount of drive and discipline to become good at it—but it's interesting to see an event that in many ways amounts to a beauty contest is now being held up as the pinnacle of masculinity. Being big and strong will certainly make you feel more masculine, but in my opinion, it's your attitude, actions, and responsibilities that will ultimately define you as a man.

On the opposite end of the spectrum, there's a growing trend toward women interested in strength training. I think this feminine approach to the iron game is great. Women who avoid or overlook strength training are selling themselves short, and these resources do a great job of minimizing the intimidation factor and casting strong women in a positive light. One criticism I do have, however, is that some of the coaches who cater to women seem to do a better job of making women feel good about strength training than actually teaching them how to train optimally.

As you can see, there are lots of trends in the world of strength training, each with its own approach to training and its own justifications for being strong. But trends come and go, and in order to truly stay motivated and reach your goals, you'll need to examine your own personal reasons for wanting to strength train.

For most of the athletes and clients I've worked with, strength training comes along with plenty of ancillary benefits, including improved health, peace of mind, and better self-esteem.

Aside from improvements in physical strength and appearance, people who strength train regularly tend to notice a reduction in stress across other areas of their lives. Every day I'm in the gym, I see people start their training sessions stressed and on edge. Within an hour, they are feeling relaxed and refreshed, ready to take on whatever challenge comes next. There's just something about physical exertion that seems to act as a "release valve" when the pressures of daily life start to build up.

Strength training is also one of the best confidence builders you'll ever experience. Unlike most pursuits in life, which tend to be subjective, lifting weights is the ultimate meritocracy. Either you can lift the weight or you can't, and any improvement in a lift, even if it's only 5 pounds, represents a goal that you accomplished by yourself.

Lifting a weight that may have seemed immovable just months ago is a feeling that you have to experience to really understand. After breaking a milestone personal record, especially one that you previously thought would be out of reach, you will feel like you can do anything.

But for me, I strength train because *I like it.* I train because it's what I do, and I can't imagine not doing it. For me, it's the process, not just the result, that keeps me in it year after year. One of the more popular expressions in strength sports is that lifting is a marathon, not a sprint, meaning if you're going to get involved, be prepared to be in it for the long haul. Not everyone who picks up a barbell will get bitten by the strength bug, but those who do rarely ever look back.

Strength training has been the single most constant entity in my life since I was in junior high school. My training has out-lasted countless relationships, career changes, and friendships. It's been my consolation through the darkest times of my life, and has been the focal point of some of my fondest memories.

Now that I have a family to take care of, lifting weights is no longer the center of my universe as it was when I was a teenager, but I would argue that my training is now even more important than it's ever been. I no longer train with the sole purpose of getting bigger and stronger. Today, I train and compete because it's the one thing I do just for me. I no longer look at my goals as my reason for training, I look at them as my excuse.

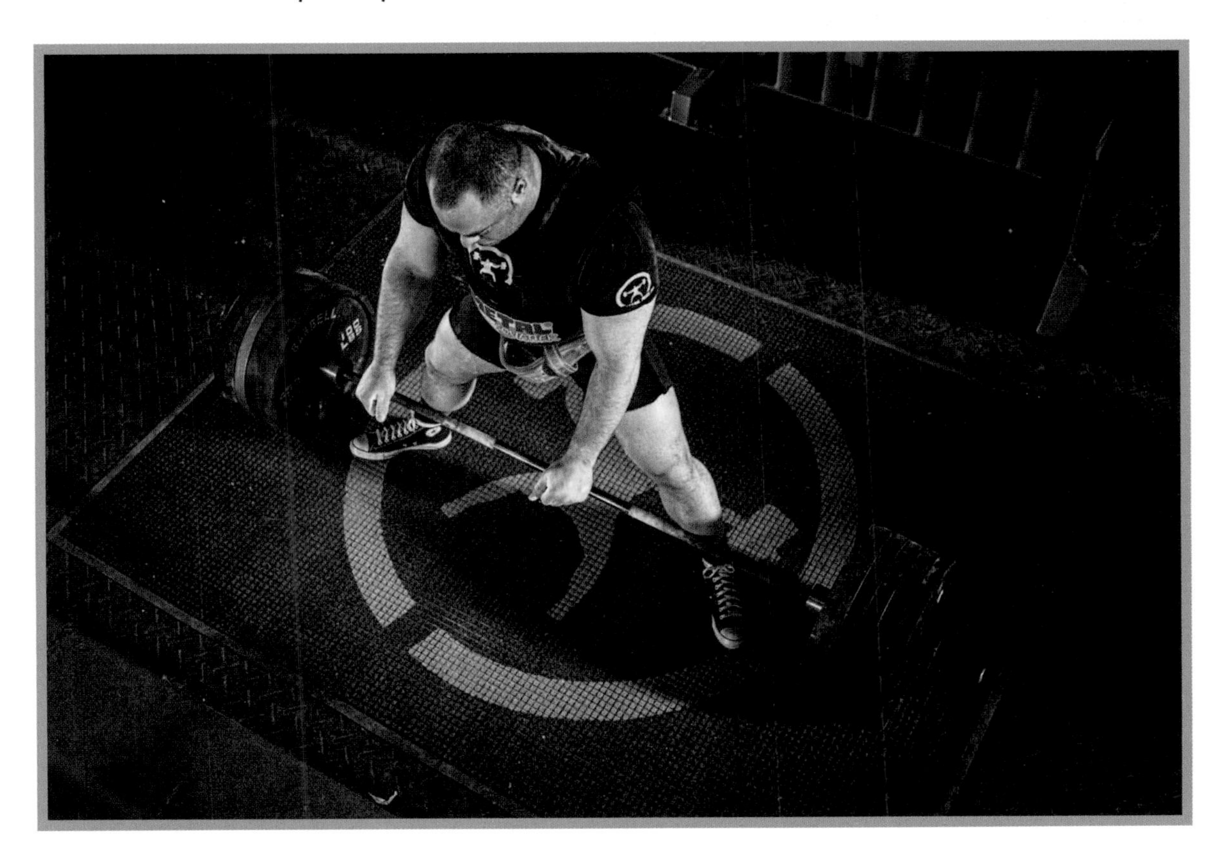

STRENGTH TRAINING VERSUS BODYBUILDING

For those of you who have never weight trained seriously before, terms like bodybuilding, weight lifting, strength training, strongman, powerlifting, and working out tend to be used interchangeably. While all of these disciplines use resistance training to achieve the desired result, they actually have very different definitions.

For example, **powerlifting** and **weight lifting** are similar, but unique sports, where the athletes compete to lift the most weight in their respective barbell lifts. **Strongman** is also a unique sport, where the lifts are more varied and tend to involve odd implements, like kegs, cars, logs, and stones.

Bodybuilding is a competitive sport as well, but there is no athletic component to the actual competition. While bodybuilders do lift weights to achieve the desired results, the actual bodybuilding competition is closer to a pageant than a sporting competition. Bodybuilders are judged on their balance of muscle size, symmetry, and definition. The difference between bodybuilding and other strength sports could be likened to the difference between an auto race and a car show.

The primary focus of bodybuilding training is to build as much muscle a possible, while maintaining an aesthetically pleasing physique. Without going into unnecessary detail, bodybuilding training works primarily by exhausting the muscles, which forces them to grow larger and more resistant to short-term fatigue.

Strength training, as the name implies, places strength gain as the primary goal. Weight lifting, powerlifting, and strongman, while different sports, all use strength training as their main form of preparation. While details of the programs will differ, especially with regard to the lifts, the overriding philosophy will be the same.

Strength training is less about building more muscle than it is about teaching your body to recruit existing muscle cells as efficiently as possible. The main desired adaptations from strength training happen at the neuromuscular level. Effective strength training allows athletes to gain strength without necessarily adding a significant amount of body weight. Gaining muscle is still important, but simply getting bigger is not the primary goal.

STRENGTH TRAINING TERMINOLOGY

Just like any hobby or sport, strength training has its own unique terminology, which acts as a shorthand between participants. In any new endeavor, one of the struggles that many beginners face is learning to decode the sometimes foreign-sounding language used by the more advanced practitioners. In this chapter, we take the guesswork out so that you can focus on your training and getting strong.

The following is an introductory list of some of the more widely used terms in strength training.

COMPOUND EXERCISE: A compound exercise refers to an exercise or lift that utilizes multiple joints and muscles. Squats, deadlifts, bench presses, and overhead presses are all examples of compound exercises.

CYCLES: How training programs are segmented. Strength training, when performed properly, tends to be cyclical in structure. This is to avoid stagnation, and to keep the athlete progressing while avoiding burnout. For more details on this topic, see Chapter 10: Creating Your Own Program.

DELOAD: A deload is a period of lower training volume or intensity with the goal of improving recovery. A deload can last anywhere from a single workout to several months, depending on the goal and the level of the athlete. Deloads tend to become more important the stronger you get, because heavier training takes a greater toll on your body.

EXERCISE: A movement performed to obtain a desired training effect.

INTENSITY: Perhaps one of the most misunderstood terms in training, intensity refers to the resistance of an exercise, and is expressed as a percentage of your 1 rep max (1rm). This term is often misused because the scientific term can be confused with the common vernacular understanding of the word. For example, a set of 20 squats wouldn't be very intense by definition, because the weight would only be around 50 percent to 55 percent of the lifter's max (any more and 20 repetitions would generally not be attainable).

While not intense by an exercise physiologist's understanding of the term, a 20 rep set of squats is often described as "intense" because it is painful and difficult.

For our purpose, "intensity" is a measure of the workload, not a description of how a training session makes you feel.

ISOLATION EXERCISES: Also called "single joint exercises," isolation exercises require the use of one joint or muscle at a time. Examples would be biceps curls, triceps extensions, and shoulder raises.

While isolation exercises focus on just one joint or muscle, the name is a bit misleading because you can never truly isolate a single muscle. Nevertheless, it's a pretty common term that you should be familiar with.

LIFT: A lift generally refers to a competitive form of an exercise. For example, the squat bench press and deadlift are competitive lifts in the sport of powerlifting, while the snatch and the clean and jerk are competitive lifts in Olympic weight lifting. Even within the context of a general strength program, it is common to refer to these exercises and their variations as lifts. While all lifts can be considered exercises, not all exercises would be considered lifts.

The first exercise in a strength program will generally be a lift, such as the squat, bench press, or deadlift.

MACRO-CYCLE: The largest cycle, the macro-cycle includes all of the training from the starting point to the goal. For most athletes, a macro-cycle will last anywhere from 2 to 4 months, although it can be longer.

MESO-CYCLE: Usually including about 1 to 2 months worth of programming, the meso-cycle generally describes unique phases of a program, often with different objectives contributing to the ultimate goal. For example, a strength program may include a meso-cycle geared toward muscle gain, followed by one geared toward strength or power.

MICRO-CYCLE: Also referred to as a "training week," a micro-cycle generally includes 1 to 2 weeks worth of workouts, usually just enough to include each lift or body part. Micro-cycles generally last from 7 to 14 days.

PERSONAL RECORD: Commonly referred to as a "pr," a personal record is your best performance of an athletic skill. In the case of strength training, a personal record usually refers to your 1 1 rep max (1rm) on a given exercise. Some lifters will also track prs in other rep ranges (like sets of 3 or 5), but in strength training, the 1rm pr reigns supreme.

Other sports or exercise modalities might quantify prs differently, such as a sprinter recording their best time in a 100 meter sprint.

Prs are also sometimes referred to as personal bests, or "pbs."

PROGRAM: Your program describes the overall structure of your training. Much like a computer program serves as a sequence of instructions for the computer's software to perform a desired task, your strength program is a sequence of instructions to help you reach a desired goal.

REP: Short for repetition, a rep is a single performance of a lift or exercise. While this may seem pretty self-explanatory, it's a term that will show up over and over in various other terms and abbreviations. For example, a "1 rep max" would be the most weight you can perform for one repetition in a given lift.

SET: A set is a group of repetitions performed as a group, usually without rest. A "set of 5" would mean 5 repetitions of a lift or exercise. Usually, when an exercise is prescribed in a written program, it will be expressed like an equation, with the weight first, followed by the number of sets, followed by the number of repetitions in each set. So 3 sets of 5 repetitions with 135 pounds, would be expressed as "135 x 3 x 5."

VOLUME: Volume refers to the total workload of a training session or program, usually with regard to number of sets, reps, exercises, and training sessions.

WORKOUT: Often confused with the term "program," a workout includes all of your training in a single session. You can even have multiple workouts in a day, provided you have a significant break in between.

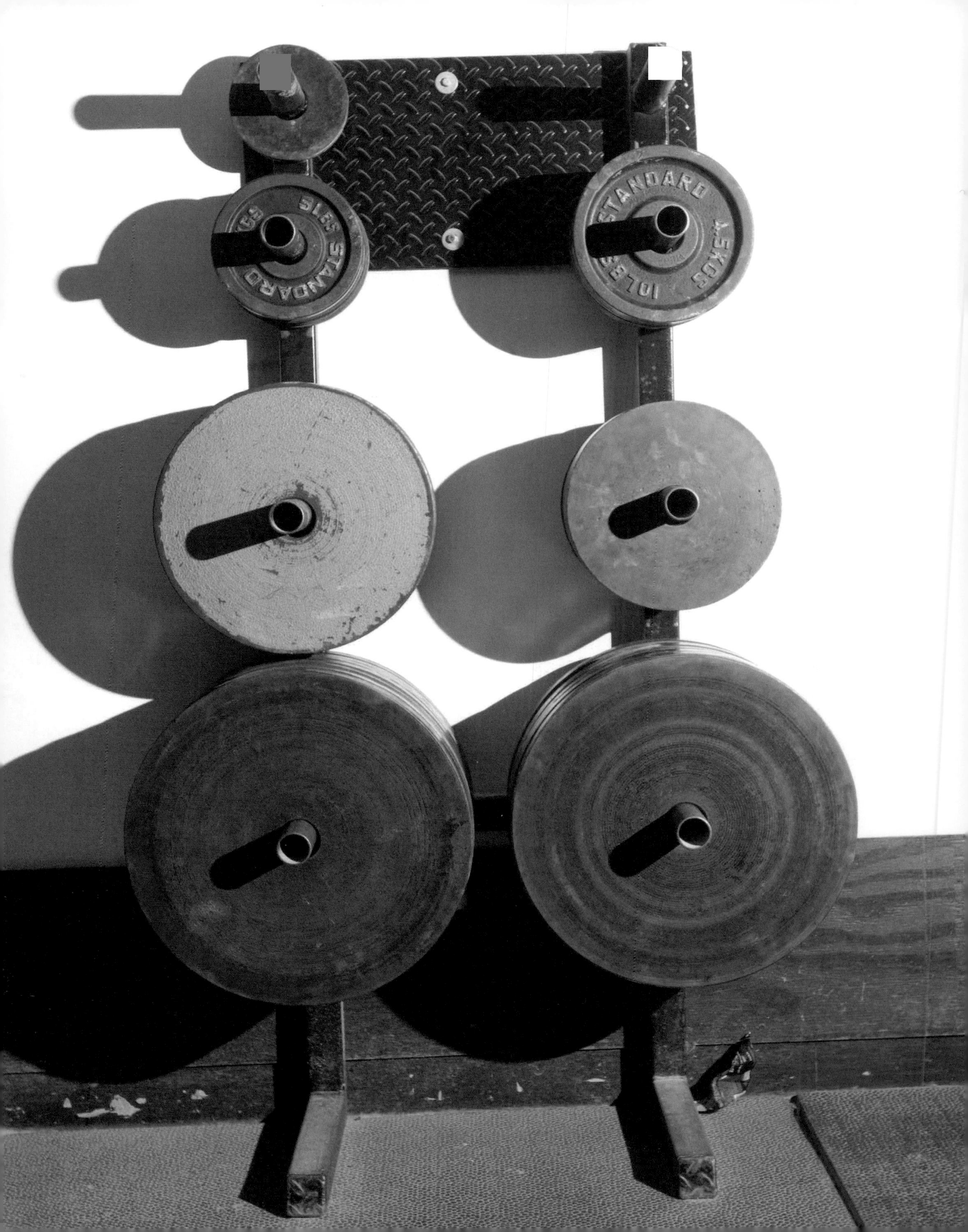
STANDARD
5LBS
STANDARD
10LBS
4.5KGS

PROGRAMMING BASICS

In training, your program (regardless of what kind of program it is) serves one single purpose: to facilitate consistent progress.

This might seem simple, but it's not. The human body is a phenomenal machine, not only for what it can do on a daily basis, but also for what it can *learn* to do, given the right stimulus. In fact, the body is *so* good at this learning, it's a challenge to modify the stimulus enough to keep the progress continuous.

If the stimulus (in this case, training) is not challenging or varied enough, there will be no reason for the body to improve. On the other hand, if it is too challenging, the body will be overwhelmed, leading to stagnation, and eventually, injury. Maintaining the correct balance is what programming is all about.

Here are two scenarios that are all too common in gyms across the country:

Lifter A, (or more accurately *exerciser A*), goes to the gym 3 days per week. He's been doing the same exercises, in the same order, with the same weights for 3 years. He may add a new exercise here and there, if the gym buys a new machine, or he learns a new one in a fitness magazine, but for the most part, it's the same workout, week after week.

He made some initial progress the first few months, but otherwise his strength, appearance, and work capacity have remained unchanged since he began.

Lifter B has also been training for 3 years. She goes to her gym at least six times per week, sometimes twice per day.

She doesn't really have a set routine, but whatever she does, she will go all out to the point of exhaustion. She keeps a personal record of every lift, and tries to break a pr in something each time she trains.

She has made a lot of progress in a short period of time, but has recently had to slow down due to some recurring injuries and has recently noticed that many of her lifts have started to backslide.

Lifter A describes the majority of members sleepwalking their way through the average fitness center. He's probably approaching his training with the best of intentions, but has no idea what hard work really feels like. His program lacks the intensity or variety needed to force his body to adapt. Aside from a few short-term adaptations in the beginning, he's spent most of his time doing just enough to maintain his initial few gains.

Lifter B is an example of a small, but growing population in the fitness industry. She has more than enough work ethic, but her lack of focus and recovery will ultimately cut her progress short.

In either case, these lifters are missing the "sweet spot" of exercise intensity and volume that smart programming should provide. Ideally, a sensible strength program should provide just enough variety and intensity to force your body to improve, without crossing over into overtraining and injury.

For the first year or so, follow the recommendations in this book as closely as possible. They are the result of decades of experience, and will hit the "sweet spot" for the vast majority of users. As time progresses, you may find some workarounds that make the programming more effective for your own needs and abilities, and that's great (optimal, in fact). But until you've gained a solid base of experience, hold off on making any major changes to the programs in this book.

"The human body is a phenomenal machine, not only for what it can do on a daily basis, but also for what it can learn to do, given the right stimulus."

THE TRUTH ABOUT STRENGTH TRAINING

THE "PERFECT PROGRAM" MYTH

Although it might make me sound old, I cannot understate the influence that the Internet has had on the world of strength training. When I was first starting out, programs were distributed primarily through books, videos (VHS), and a handful of strength-related periodicals, many of which are now defunct. Since all of these distribution methods demanded production costs of some sort, very few coaches had a strong enough reputation to command the necessary readership to turn a profit (or even break even).

Today, strength programs are cranked out almost daily by scores of "coaches" from around the world. While just a few decades ago, lifters were limited to a few basic templates, today's lifters have an enormous number of options to sift through before getting started.

The result is the phenomenon of "program hopping." Today's novices will often try out two or three (and sometimes more) programs within their first year of training, in an attempt to find the "perfect" program. What they typically get is nothing more than wasted time and mediocre results.

So the question is, for the novice trainee, how do you figure out where to start?

Here's a secret . . . The program itself doesn't matter as much as you think. Your effort level, consistency, and analytical skills are the foundation of your success. While it is important to find a solid, reliable program, the program itself won't make you stronger on its own. You'll need to make it work. And when programs fail (assuming they are well written in the first place), it's usually the fault of the follower. If you want your program to work, you need to stick with it long enough to actually let it work.

What veteran lifters know and novices often overlook is that sticking with a single program year in and year out, teaches you much more about training than switching at the first sign of a stall. Sticking with your program teaches you to make small adjustments according to your needs. Over time, these adjustments add up and the result is a program totally unique to your needs, which will work better than any pre-designed collection of sets and reps you might want to download.

The key to succeeding with a strength program is to stick with it long enough to make it your own.

Additionally, learning to make adjustments within a program teaches you how strength programming actually works, versus blindly following the latest and greatest program making the rounds on the Internet at the moment.

As much as I'd love to tell you that our program is the game-changer of the decade, the truth is that our program, just like any other, is really just a guide. The success of *any* program has much more to do with the application, year in and year out, than what's written on the page.

While we would put our programming up against anyone's, the *real* lesson to be learned is to be patient, and allow whichever program you choose to do its job.

OLYMPIC LIFTS—OVERRATED OR UNDERAPPRECIATED?

In recent years, the Olympic lifts and their variations have enjoyed a resurgence in popularity unlike any in recent memory. Due to the rise of competitively structured fitness classes, the Olympic lifts have gone from an underappreciated sport, shown at 3 AM during the Olympic Games, to a staple in the commercial fitness market.

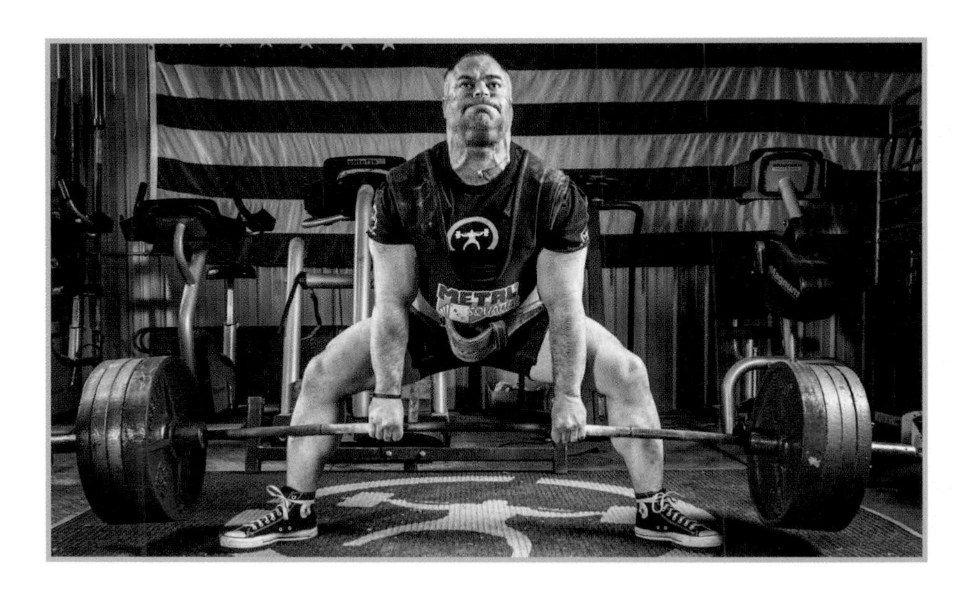

However, all of this sudden interest in these lifts has been a double-edged sword. On one hand, the surge in popularity has rekindled interest in the sport of Olympic weight lifting (typically a fringe sport in the United States). On the other hand, the sudden rise in demand has resulted in a shortage of qualified coaches, who have been replaced by trainers who lack the ability to teach these complex movements.

Unfortunately, as of this writing, most of the current instruction regarding the Olympic lifts borders on worthless. Not only are many coaches unable to effectively teach these lifts, but their typical place in group-led fitness classes ensures they will *never* be performed correctly. In the group fitness setting, the Olympic lifts are usually performed for multiple rep sets, with moderate weights, past the point of fatigue-induced breakdown. Basically, the trainees get plenty of practice performing the lifts incorrectly.

In this case, the old adage "practice makes perfect" is unfortunately inaccurate. A more appropriate term would be "practice makes *permanent*." All these reps performed with shoddy form is nothing more than a great way to practice . . . you guessed it, shoddy form. By contrast, an elite weight lifter will train with much lower rep-ranges with sufficient rest, in order to practice the most efficient form possible.

Obviously it's unfair to judge the merit of a lift based on the *incorrect* teaching of it, but I would go so far as to say that even with excellent coaching, the average novice would be better served by relying on the basic compound exercises found in this book like the squat, press, and deadlift. While the Olympic lifts are a phenomenal way to *demonstrate* explosive power, they are not always the best way to *build* explosive power, especially in novice athletes.

If anything, you should already be fairly powerful in order to even benefit from these Olympic lifts. Unless you are specifically trying to compete in Olympic lifting (or at least an exercise-based sport which includes the lifts in their competitions), you are probably better off sticking with the basic lifts until you are a little stronger, and better able to benefit from them.

How strong should you be? For men, when you can squat and deadlift twice your body weight would probably a good time to start working the Olympic lifts into your programming. For women, the mark should be around 1.5 times your body weight in the squat and deadlift.

If you don't really have any interest in Olympic lifts, or don't have access to quality coaching, that's fine too. Competitive powerlifters manage to get big and strong, and very few of them use the Olympic lifts to any significant degree.

While flipping through this book, you may have noticed that we did not include the Olympic lifts in our programming. This is not because I do not appreciate them. Quite the contrary, it's out of respect for these advanced movements that I have left them out. The Olympic lifts take *years* to even become proficient, let alone actually excel, at.

CHOOSING A COACH

At some point, if you really start taking strength training seriously, you may become interested in working with a coach. Being a coach myself, I certainly support working with a professional. Having been around the block, however, I do need to mention that you should choose very carefully.

In the last few years, strength coaching has become a big business, and the industry has been flooded with self-described "experts," all claiming to have the key to muscle gain and fat loss, not to mention any athletic goal you can think of.

Basically any "coach" can generate videos, e-books and websites, practically for free (and believe me, they do). Now don't get me wrong, some of these people are excellent, but you'll need to do your research to establish some sort of credibility before handing over your hard-earned cash.

Below are a few basic qualifications you should look for before following someone's programming:

ARE THEY STRONG THEMSELVES? It may seem simplistic, but before I look to someone for a service, I want to know that said service provider is able to demonstrate the skills they're being paid to teach. They do not necessarily need to be a pro strength athlete or bodybuilder, because talent is not always a good indicator of proficiency as a teacher. All things being equal though, it helps immensely if they are objectively considered to be *good* at the skill set you are hiring them to improve.

WHO HAVE THEY COACHED? Even more important than being able to demonstrate a skill, is to be able to teach that skill to others. There are plenty of elite-level athletes out there who I wouldn't trust to train my dog, just as there are plenty of coaches with relatively modest personal stats that can churn out one champion after another. A coach's athletes are their calling card, and if yours is unable to produce results in others, what is the likelihood they will be able to produce results for you?

WHAT IS THEIR LEVEL OF EDUCATION?

Not every great coach will have an advanced degree, or even any degree at all. I even know of one hugely successful coach that didn't finish high school. However, in most cases, a formal education in exercise science is all but mandatory. Not only does it suggest a certain level of knowledge, but it's also an indication that they take the profession seriously enough to have dedicated the time and money to get the degree in the first place. Certifications are great, but there isn't a certification out there that can compare to a relevant 4-year degree.

MACHINES VERSUS FREE WEIGHTS

For as long as weight machines have been a part of the fitness landscape, there has been debate as to their usefulness.

As is typically the case with any exercise modality, there has long been a pendulum swing with regard to machine use in strength training. When they were first introduced on a wide scale (in the late 70s), machines became immensely popular, with numerous training programs and even entire facilities dedicated to their use. Over the years, the pendulum began to swing the other way, with most gyms and programs making use of both machines and free weights, usually with beginners and women steered toward machine training, and advanced men leaning toward free weights.

Today, we've seen the pendulum swing almost all the way back, with the current trend being bare-bones facilities with few machines and an emphasis on basic barbell lifting.

As has always been the case, the optimal balance of machines and free weights has always been a matter of context.

Free weights are generally accepted as being more effective for building strength, and if you could only choose one tool, the barbell would most certainly be the wise choice. Fortunately, we don't have to choose. Most serious lifters rely on free weights, but also make use of machines for certain purposes, like rehab, or for lighter workouts geared toward recovery. Machines are also a useful tool for beginners who might lack the coordination necessary to train exclusively on free weights.

There's no such thing as a "bad" exercise or training modality, just ones that are inappropriate for that particular trainee or for their fitness goals.

While the majority of the programming in this book relies on free weights, there is a one-month introductory cycle that is almost exclusively machine training. This cycle, while not mandatory, takes advantage of the relative user friendliness of machines for those of you who are still uneasy about starting a barbell-based program right from the get-go.

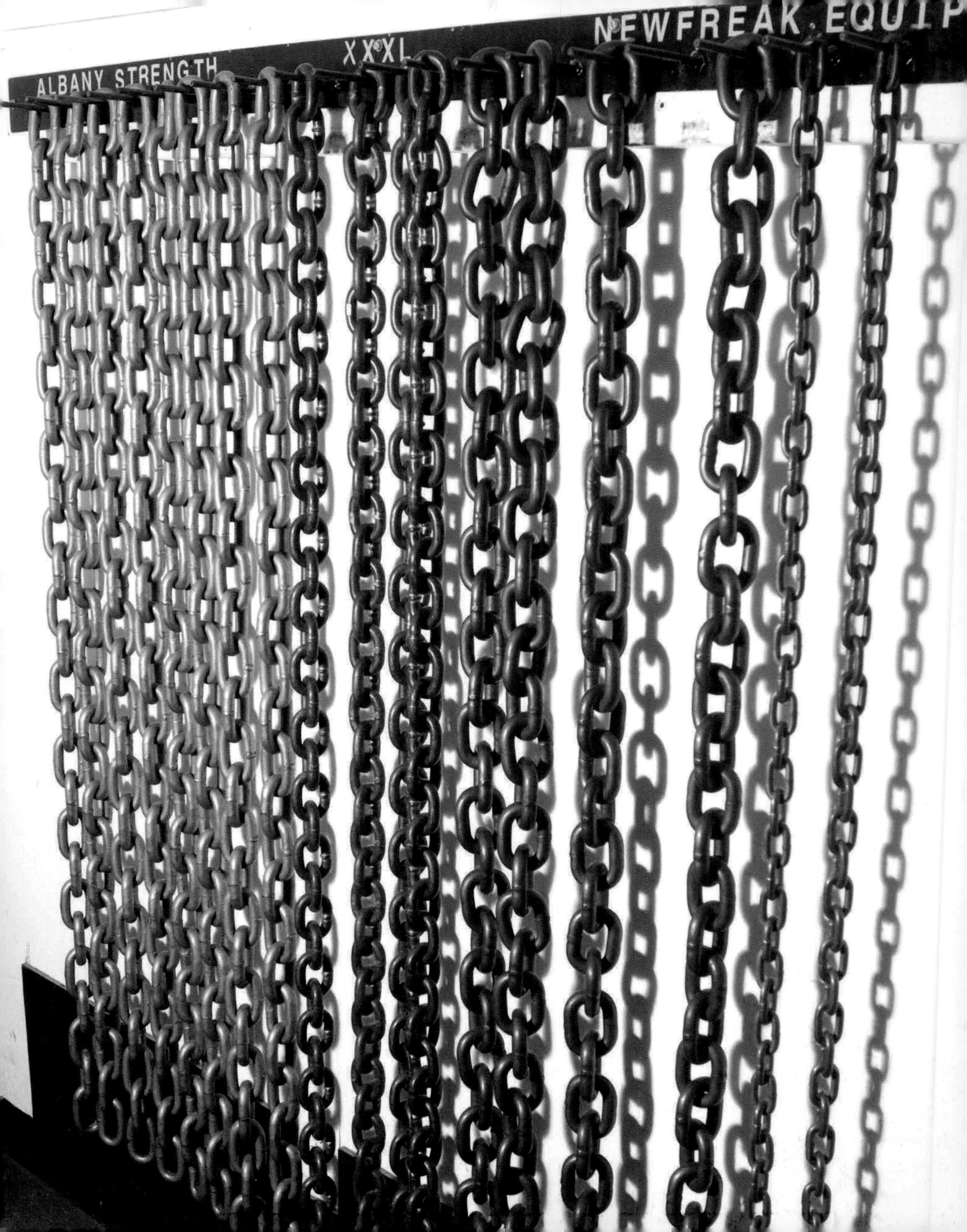

ALBANY STRENGTH
XXXL
NEWFREAK EQUIP

BASIC MUSCULAR ANATOMY

Unlike bodybuilders, who must program their training based on the aesthetic effect on their muscles, someone embarking on a strength program must always consider function over form when prioritizing muscle groups in their training. The two most important factors when considering muscle groups are:

- Which muscle groups are most important to the particular lift you're training?
- Which muscle groups are lagging, and serving as the weak link in your training?

Getting the most out of your training requires at least a basic understanding of the major muscle groups, including their location, function, and relevant exercises. This is by no means an in-depth chapter on musculoskeletal anatomy, but a quick rundown of the major muscle groups to get you started. In order to help connect the dots between muscular anatomy and your training, we have arranged the muscle groups by the types of lifts they are most relevant to.

THE SQUAT/ DEADLIFT

Posterior Chain

The posterior chain is made up primarily of the spinal erectors (which run up and down your back, parallel to the spine), the gluteus maximus (a large hip extensor that gives your buttocks their rounded shape), and the hamstrings. The term "posterior" refers to the location of these muscles, on the back side of the body. "Chain" references the relationship these several muscles have with each other, acting together like links in a chain to produce hip/back extension. Your strength in this movement will be limited to your weakest muscle group, much like the weakest link of a chain.

Typical signs of posterior chain weakness include:

- When a squatter pitches forward and rounds out, this is often due to weak hamstrings and glutes. The pitching forward is often the body trying to take stress off of the hips and load it onto the lower back.
- Squatting too upright, to the point that the knees track forward indicates lower back weakness. Generally lifters remain too far upright because they lack strength to hold a lower back arch during a heavy squat.
- Lacking drive out of the bottom of a squat can indicate weakness in the glutes.
- For the deadlift, lifters are most often limited by lower back strength, which tends to show up as a rounding of the low back.
- When a lifter's hips shoot straight up at the start of the deadlift, causing their legs to straighten prematurely, it generally means that their hips are weak, and they're lifting with their lower back almost exclusively.
- When lifters are unable to finish a deadlift at the top, the problem is most likely an inability to contract their glutes to lock the weight out.

To strengthen the posterior chain, you can use any variation of the squat, box squat, deadlift or goodmorning. Also, assistance exercises such as glute-ham raises, back extensions, reverse hypers, and cable pull-throughs can be very helpful.

Upper Back

Your upper back comprises primarily the trapezius, a triangular-shaped muscle that spans from your middle back to the base of the skull, the rear deltoids (which are located on the backs of your shoulders), and the rhomboids (which lay beneath your trapezius and retract the shoulder blades). Your upper back plays a huge role in the squat because these muscles create the shelf that you rest the bar on. In the deadlift, your upper back muscles literally connect the bar to your torso.

Typical signs of upper back weakness in the squat include:

- Rounding of the upper back.

- Inability to hold the elbows stationary during the lift.
- The bar rolling down the back during the lift.
- Holding the bar too high/inability to hold the bar across the upper back.
- Excessive rounding of the upper back during deadlifts.

Strengthen these muscles with shrugs, dumbbell cleans, dumbbell rear delt raises, face pulls, upright rows, and bent-over rows. Strong lats (latissimus dorsi) are also critical to holding your position in the squat. They are addressed more thoroughly in the bench press section.

Abdominals

In order to be able to transfer power from your legs, up through your body, into the bar, strong abs are critically important. In fact, the midsection is one of the most common weaknesses in the squat/deadlift. The abdominal muscles include the rectus abdominis (which runs the length of the front of your abdomen and has the sectioned "six pack" appearance), the obliques (which can be found on the sides of your abdomen), and the transverse abdominis (a deep corset-like abdominal muscle which plays a major role in stabilizing the spine).

Unlike more fitness-related training, you should not be pulling your abs in when you train them.

In order to make your midsection as strong as possible, you need to train the ability to breathe into your belly and push them out while you strain. The strong abs pushed against a powerlifting belt create a bulletproof midsection during a heavy squat.

To train your abs for powerlifting, don't bother with endless reps of crunches on the floor. Hit them hard with sit-ups over the glute ham bench, standing crunches with the pulldown machine or a band, spread-eagle sit-ups, side-bends with a dumbbell or band, and leg lifts. Keep the reps in the 8- to 15-rep range.

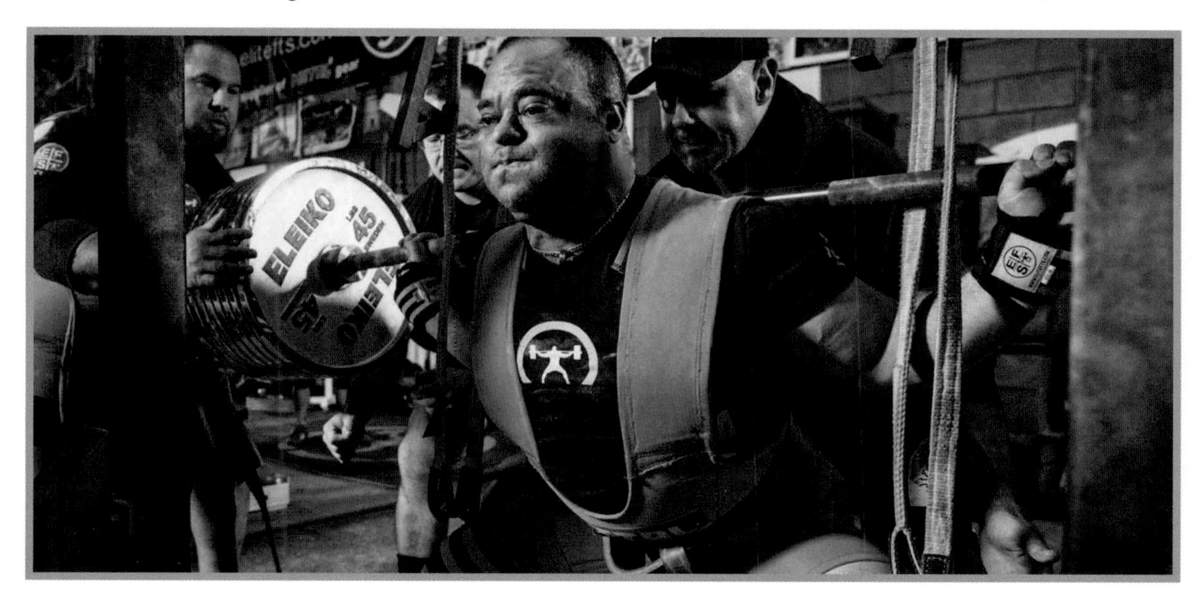

Belly Breathing

Belly breathing is an important part of setting up for and executing the power lifts. This breathing technique is just what it sounds like. Instead of breathing into your chest, take air into your belly, inflating it like a basketball. This will stabilize your entire midsection.

To belly breathe, take a deep breath while forcefully pushing your belly out. This should help you use your diaphragm to draw air into your belly. During the lift, try to exhale forcefully against your closed throat. This action, called the valsalva maneuver, will help you build up enough pressure to stabilize yourself under big weights.

Quadriceps

The quadriceps, which produce knee extension, are also an important muscle for the squat.

Good exercise choices are full-range compound movements like close stance, low box squats, leg presses, and hack squats.

BENCH PRESS

Triceps

While the bench press is usually thought of as a chest exercise, triceps strength is often a much more limiting factor in the lift. Strengthening your triceps will allow you to adapt an elbows-in style of benching that will protect your pecs and shoulders, as well as put you into a more efficient pressing position.

Signs of triceps weakness:

- The most noticeable sign of triceps weakness is the inability to completely straighten your elbows in the bench press. If your sticking point is halfway up or above, it's time to hit your triceps hard.
- An elbows-out style of benching, with the upper arms perpendicular to the body, is also an indication that the triceps are weak. Great benchers are usually able to keep their upper arms in closer to the body. Think of your arm position when trying to push open a heavy door.

Upper/Middle Back

The back is by far the most underrated muscle group for developing an impressive bench press. While your upper back muscles do not actively move the weight, during a big bench, your back serves as your foundation, literally connecting you to the bench and stabilizing you.

Strong rhomboids, traps, and rear deltoids help you keep your shoulder blades together, locking you into position. Strong lats help you lower the bar under control.

Signs of a weak back include:

- A long bench stroke. Even a long-armed bencher can take inches off their stroke by learning to pull and keep their shoulder blades together during the bench press.
- Instability during the bench press. Shaking or extraneous movement during the lift indicate that the lifter is not locked into the bench.

- Inability to touch in a shirt. Shirted benchers need a strong back to literally pull the bar to their chests (or bellies). Beefing up your rowing exercises can often fix this in a matter of weeks.

Shoulders

Shoulder strength is a necessity to get the bar moving off your chest, especially for raw benchers. With the elbows tucked at the sides, the shoulders take much of the load off the pecs so that you are less vulnerable to pec tears.

Signs of weak shoulders include:

- Failing in the bench press right off the chest.
- Another telltale sign of shoulder weakness is the elbows flaring out, forcing more stress on the pecs.

Pectorals

The pectoralis muscles, or "pecs" are located on top of the breastbone, and span from the sternum to the top of the humerus (upper arm bone). In women, the pectoral muscles lay beneath the breast tissue.

While the pecs receive a lot of direct work in bodybuilding programs, due to the distinctive shape they give the chest, they are not prioritized nearly as much in most powerlifting-based programs, because correct pressing mechanics tend to place the load on the triceps, upper back, and shoulders. While the pecs are a prime mover in the bench press, most lifters do little or no direct pec work aside from the various bench press variations.

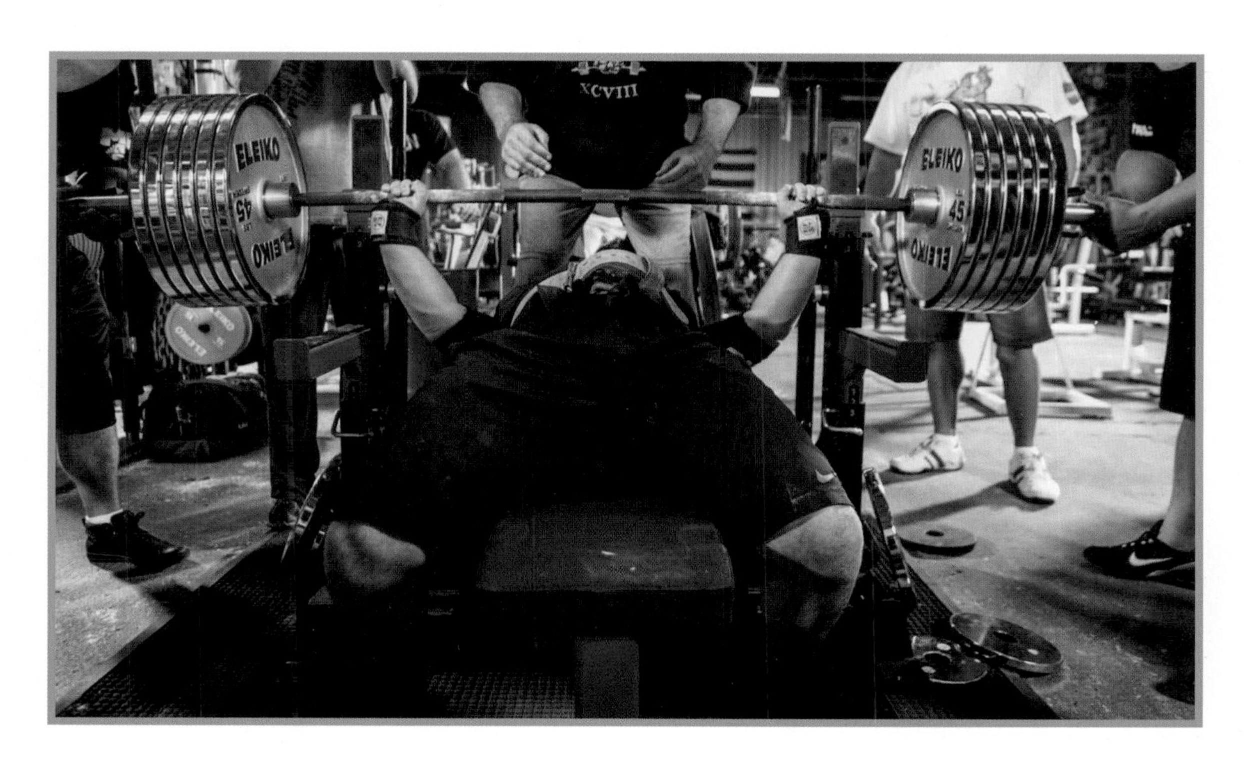

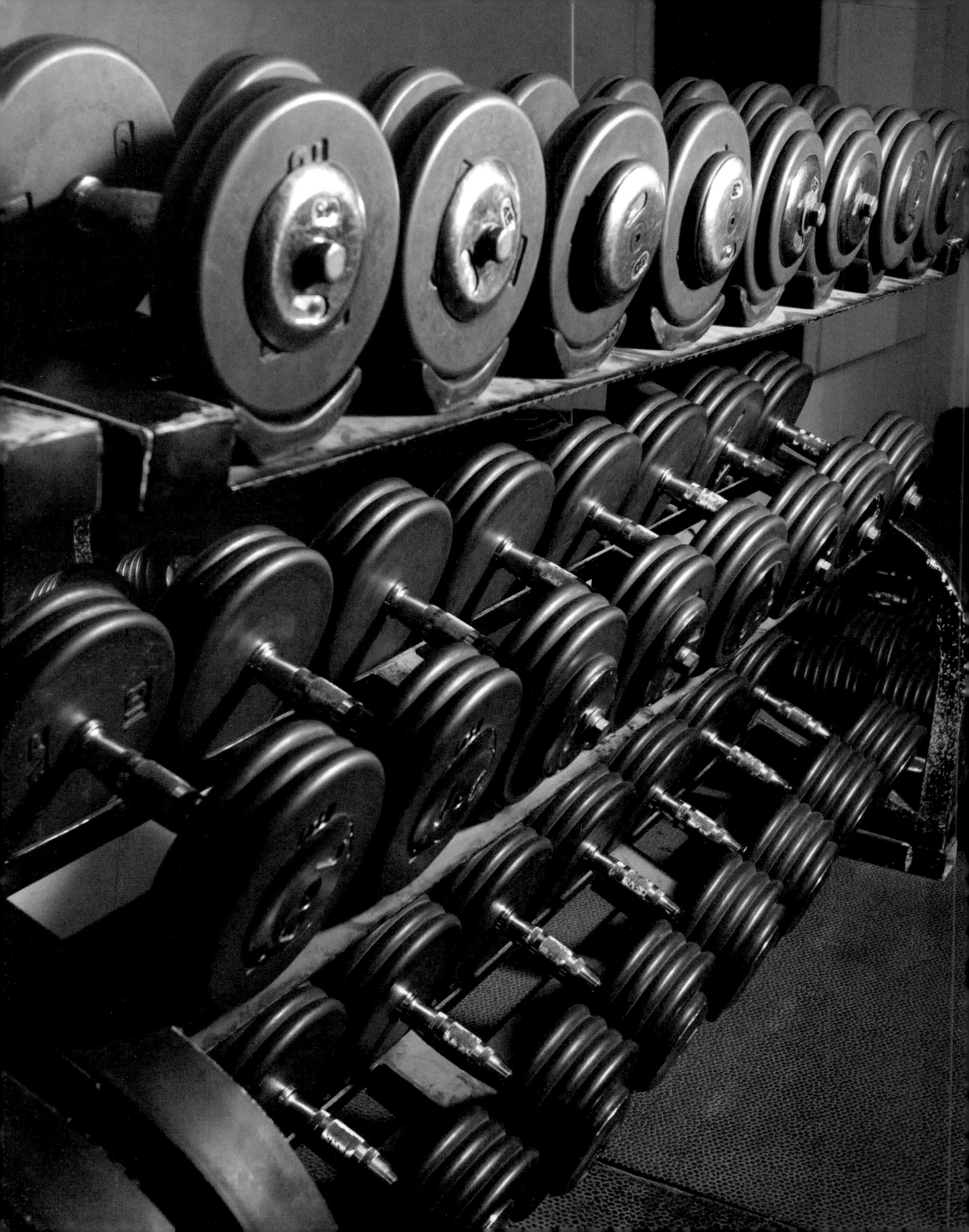

EQUIPMENT AND GEAR

SERIOUS STRENGTH EQUIPMENT

There's just no getting around it—much like a carpenter needs quality tools, a lifter has certain basic equipment requirements for productive training to take place. The following pieces are what I (and most other serious strength athletes) consider to be must-haves.

Don't let the following sections scare you and make you think that you need to buy thousands of dollars' worth of equipment just to get started. You can probably find a commercial club in your area with at least most of what you need.

Since we want to be sensitive to the cost issue for those who are interested in building their own facility, we have refrained from turning this chapter into our own personal wish list. Instead we have tried really hard to narrow it down to the bare minimum. Buy (or join a gym with) the following pieces before you even consider purchasing any other piece of equipment.

THE POWER RACK

A quality power rack should be the centerpiece of any serious gym. If you think of a gym as a church, the power rack would be the altar. If you have a good quality power rack, you'll honestly need little else to get strong. Have you ever seen those infomercials for cheesy home exercise equipment, where the spokesperson keeps repeating "it's like an entire gym in one!"? A good power rack is about as close as it gets to actually meeting this claim.

With a good rack, you can do multiple variations of the squat, bench press, goodmorning, deadlift, floor press, overhead press, and pull-up, not to mention the countless exercise variations you can make up. Combined with a good quality adjustable bench, a quality power rack should take care of the majority of your training lifts.

And by the way, although the terms are often confused, a "squat rack" and a "power rack" are not the same thing. A power rack is a multipurpose piece of equipment while a squat rack is designed primarily for squatting and will not offer the same flexibility. Although a power rack can be used as a squat rack, the opposite is not true.

What to Look for in a Power Rack

If you're joining a gym, you'll obviously be limited to whatever equipment your gym currently has. If you're considering buying your own, be selective, and don't jump at the first hunk of junk you see on Craigslist. As with just about anything you can buy, not all racks are created equal, and you generally get what you pay for. You do not need to get a $3,000 professional weight-room quality rack to get a productive workout in. You can definitely find a great piece that will outlast you for under $1,000. However, even an affordable rack should meet the following requirements:

CLOSE HOLE SPACING

The holes that the pins fit through should never be more than 3 inches apart. If the holes are spaced further than this, you will not have enough variation for partial range movements like pin pulls and pin presses. The best racks have hole spacing between 1 and 2 inches.

Sumo Base

Most racks have horizontal support beams on the sides that are too close to the bottom of the rack, limiting how far you can place your feet. In the event you want to perform a sumo deadlift (explained in Chapter 8), you will want a rack that has a few inches of clearance between this beam and the floor, so that your stance width is not limited.

Safety Pins

The "pins" are the heavy duty pipes or beams that are attached from one side of the rack to the other, to catch the barbell in the event of a drop or failed lift. Not only are the pins protective, they are also a valuable training tool. By setting the bar on the pins at various heights, you can use exercises like pin presses and pin pulls (explained in Chapter 8: The Exercises) to focus on different points in exercises like the squat and deadlift.

ADJUSTABLE BENCH

The adjustable bench is a money-saving and space-saving piece of equipment for the home gym owner because combined with a quality power rack, it eliminates the need for a large, costly dedicated bench press or overhead press bench. Just set the bench in the middle of the rack and you can use it to perform bench presses, incline bench presses, overhead presses, and pin presses.

Even without the rack, the adjustable bench can be combined with dumbbells for countless other exercise variations.

POWER BAR

Although we began this chapter with the rack, we could have easily placed the barbell first in terms of importance. Although most commercial gyms will blow tens of thousands of dollars on the best cardio and weight machines, I've seen very few that are willing to drop a grand on a few good power bars. In fact, most gym bars are terrible, and seem to be an afterthought for most gym owners.

To lift heavy weights comfortably and safely, you'll need at least one good all-purpose barbell. That barbell, in my opinion, is the Texas power bar. This bar is just plain good at everything. The knurling is solid, the sleeves rotate well, and it can handle plenty of weight without wobbling or bowing.

If you are building a home gym, this should be the first bar you purchase. If you take care of it, it could very well be the last. Even if you are training in a commercial fitness facility, a Texas bar might still be a worthwhile purchase. I've been a member of several gyms that allowed me to bring my own bar, and keep it in a closet somewhere, out of reach of the other members. This is where it pays to be on great terms with your gym's owner and/or manager.

As a side note, I highly recommend picking up a cheap bar for rack pulls and pin presses. A used one from eBay or a cheap sporting goods store bar is fine. These exercises are really hard on bars, and the last thing you want to do is bend a $350 Texas bar.

PLATES

If your goal is to lift *weights*, then you'll need weights. While there are plenty of expensive brands out there, with seemingly cool options like rubber casing, interlocking grooves, handles, and noncircular shapes, I recommend getting just some basic old-fashioned plates. While the other plates may seem cool, the extra features can limit their usefulness in some situations. For example, noncircular plates don't work all that well for the deadlift where you want the bar to be able to roll a bit.

Rubber or plastic-encased weights take up more room on the bar and may actually max out a standard power bar on some movements.

I do recommend getting weights frm a reputable brand like York Barbell so that the weights are reasonably accurate. Some noncalibrated brands can be quite a bit off from their listed weight.

Don't waste space or money on plates that you will not need. Assuming that you will only be doing one exercise at a time, all you'll need will be:

- 2.5 pounds: 2
- 5 pounds: 2
- 10 pounds: 4
- 25 pounds: 2
- 35 pounds: none (instead, just use a 25 and a 10)
- 45 pounds: as many as you need

While most iron plates look alike, there can actually be quite a big difference in how accurate their weights are. Aside from actually weighing them, a simple way to tell the quality of a plate is to look at the back of it. If the back of the plate has a rough, almost textured look to it, it means that the plate was cast. If the plate is smooth with grooves on it, then the plate was machined.

Machined plates are generally more accurate than cast, because they are usually calibrated more carefully during the machining process.

FLOORING

When you're converting a basement or garage into a training space, you're going to need some kind of protection for your floor. You do not need to go so far as to renovate the entire floor, just some protection for the areas where you know that weights will be hitting the floor. The best protection you can get will come from compressed rubber mats, available from either sports supply or industrial flooring companies. Put them wherever you plan to deadlift. For protection against slipping, cover any area where you will need traction with thin carpeting, like you would use on a deck. Most serious lifters will chalk their hands to help their grip on the bar. A thin, rough carpet will help resist slipping from chalk getting on the floor.

If you're joining a gym, pay careful attention to the floor while you're shopping around. A lot of gyms are located in former warehouses or industrial spaces. Since the buildings were often never intended to be gyms in the first place, the floors are not always level. This can be very annoying in lifts like the deadlift, where the bar has the potential to roll.

A great sign is if the gym has separate Olympic lifting-style platforms, because it shows the gym owners are anticipating members handling serious iron and they are trying to accommodate them.

DUMBBELLS

Dumbbells are indispensable for all kinds of assistance work. If you will be training in a commercial gym, you will no doubt have access to them, but you'll want to make sure the place has enough. A good gym will have multiple pairs of dumbbells in the more used weights, (usually the 15- to 65-pound range) so that there are enough for everyone during peak hours.

If you're going to be training at home, the biggest issue with dumbbells is that most lifters don't have the money and/or space for a full rack of commercial quality dumbbells. Fortunately, you can just buy two Olympic sleeve, adjustable dumbbells and you're set. Make sure you have good collars if you use these. There is typically lots more movement with dumbbell work than with barbells.

SQUAT BOX

If you want to use box squats in your training (explained in Chapter 8: The Exercises) you'll need a good squat box. This can really be anything sturdy, including a homemade wooden box, stacked mats, or an adjustable squat box, made specifically for the exercise.

Finding a decent squat box in a commercial gym can be something of a challenge, because box squats are rarely performed (correctly, at least) outside of serious weight rooms. If you're tall, you can probably use a bench. While I can't actually recommend this because they are not made for this purpose, I have on occasion used aerobics steps as a makeshift squat box when in a pinch.

BOARDS

Boards are an inexpensive, yet very effective tool to boost your bench press. A serious gym should at least have board press boards ranging from 1 to 3 boards thick. You can worry about high boards and half boards as your training gets more specialized.

While several strength supply companies make bench boards, you can save money by purchasing them at a hardware store or lumber store.

BENCH PRESS BENCH

The combination of a rack and bench will do the job, but there's nothing like the feeling of benching on a competition quality bench. Not only will it feel more solid, but you'll also be training on the same equipment that you intend to compete on. As with the power rack, there are some things that you want to look for in a good bench:

Adjustable Uprights

Most gym benches have fixed uprights, which means that short guys will have trouble reaching them, and tall guys need to do a half rep to even get the bar out of the rack. I've even seen racks so low that an average height guy could literally throw the bar over the uprights while trying to rack the bar.

Shallow Rack Lip

The higher you need to lift the bar to get it out of the uprights, the harder it is to keep your shoulders set up on the bench. The best benches have a very shallow lip on their racks; just deep enough so that the bar doesn't roll out when racked.

Handoff Platform

The two biggest issues I see with handoff platforms are that they are either too low or too short. If they are too low, your spotter does not have enough leverage to give you a strong handoff. If they are too short, the spotter has to hand the bar way past their center of gravity, throwing them off balance. (Yeah, that's exactly what I want, my spotter struggling to keep his balance while handing me 600 pounds!)

A good handoff platform will be at least about 6 inches high and long enough so that the spotter can stand over the lifter's head while they're lying on the bench normally. A quality bench will also be high enough so that your legs have enough leverage to stabilize you during the lift. Typical gym benches are usually too low.

GLUTE HAM RAISE

Your posterior chain (lower back, hamstrings, and glutes) can never be too strong. A glute ham raise is an apparatus designed to hit these muscles hard. The glute ham raise works a lot like a reverse hamstring curl, the difference being that instead of pulling on a weight in an open chain fashion, your feet are anchored and you pull your body weight as you flex your knees.

While most lifters and coaches prefer the stationary pad, many glute ham raises have a roller that assists you in the movement. While it's not optimal, the majority of fitness centers don't even have a glute ham raise, so beggars can't be choosers. If you are putting together your own training space and are considering either the glute ham raise or the back extension bench, I recommend getting a glute ham raise, because you have more versatility with it. In addition to its intended exercise, you can also perform back extensions and sit-ups on it.

CABLE PULLDOWN

One of the few traditional machines that serious lifters regularly make use of is the cable pull-down. Fortunately, this is one of the most common machines in existence, and you'd be hard-pressed to find a commercial gym without one. If you are going to purchase one, you can either get one with a built-in weight stack, or a plate-loaded model. In addition to pulldowns, you can also use it for triceps pushdowns and face pulls. For even more options, get one with a low cable, which will allow you to perform exercises like pull-throughs, low rows, and biceps curls.

REVERSE HYPER

With the amount of abuse we lifters subject our backs to, restorative exercise is an important piece of the puzzle. The reverse hyper is an odd looking, but extremely effective tool for strengthening and rehabilitating your back. Personally, I like the roller model that has a solid pendulum because I can't cheat as much on it.

PROWLER AND SLED

I grouped the prowler in with the sled because they both accomplish similar goals. The sled is simply a small metal sled with a sleeve for weights and a strap that you attach to a belt or harness. The prowler is a three-runner sled with handles made for pushing.

Both implements can either be used with heavy weights to improve endurance/conditioning or with light weights to speed recovery. The main difference is that the sled can be performed without fatiguing the upper body.

PERSONAL GEAR

While most of us would love the opportunity to pick and choose our own gym equipment, a home or garage gym isn't always an option, and most of us are at the mercy of whatever commercial gyms are in our area.

While we can't always lift in the power rack or on the bench of our choice, we can certainly make the best of things by purchasing the best personal equipment we can. Below are some essential items that every serious lifter should have in their gym bag.

For most gym goers, specialized training gear really isn't necessary. Any workout clothes should be fine. But when you're trying to get as strong as possible, it makes sense to start using gear that will give you the best chance possible to make the lift.

For example, if your lower body training is limited to a few sets on a leg press machine, the type of sneakers you wear won't make much of a difference. But if you are attempting a max squat, wearing the wrong shoes can throw you out of position and increase your chance of serious injury.

A few small investments in some proper training gear can make a big difference in the productivity of your training.

Belt

Next to lifting gloves (more on those later), the belt is the single most ubiquitous piece of gear you will need. You would be hard-pressed to walk into a gym or weight room without seeing at least a few of the more serious lifters wearing a lifting belt. Yet despite their popularity, the vast majority of lifting belts are designed incorrectly.

Contrary to popular belief, the lifting belt doesn't directly support your back, but rather your abdominals. By taking a deep breath into your belly prior to exertion, and pushing your abdominal muscles against the belt, you create more intra-abdominal pressure, which stabilizes the spine.

For an optimal effect, you want a belt that's wide in the front so that you have a lot of surface area to push against. The typical lifting belt by contrast is wide in the back, and skinny in the front. While these belts will certainly offer some additional support, they will not offer *optimal* support.

The best belt for serious strength training is the same width (usually 4 inches wide) all the way around. This is what you will typically see pro powerlifters use to squat weights in the half-ton range. If it will support these monsters, it will be all the support you'll ever need.

Sizing is also important. While most belts have enough holes to accommodate a size range of about 6 to 8 inches, a new belt should be somewhere in the middle hole range when worn snug. This way, you can gain or lose some weight without immediately having to buy a new one.

In addition, look for a belt with tough construction, which will last for decades, not just years. If you are ordering it online (the higher quality belts are usually not sold in stores), look for a belt priced in the $60 to $110 range. Quality costs, and a cheaply priced belt will be cheaply made.

While vinyl belts have become popular in the last few years, nothing comes close to a quality leather belt in terms of performance and longevity. There's no reason a quality leather belt shouldn't last for 20 years.

Shoes

While most casual gym goers will wear just any sneaker to the gym, your shoes can make a big difference in both your technique and your maximal weights. A traditional sneaker has a cushioned sole to protect the foot from ground impact when running and jumping.

While this type of sole is fine for traditional sports, it doesn't work for strength training, where there is no impact and you want as little force to be displaced into your shoes as possible.

The ideal shoe will vary from lift to lift, and from lifter to lifter.

SQUAT SHOES: While most strength coaches agree that a squat shoe should allow maximal energy transfer to the floor, there remains an ongoing debate as to what type of shoe is ideal. Some coaches recommend an Olympic weight lifting shoe which has a thick, dense sole and a raised heel. (It's kind of like wearing ice skates with the blades removed.) Others prefer a minimal shoe, with a very thin sole. Your choice will depend on your style of squat.

Stocky, quad-dominant lifters tend to do well in the Olympic-style shoe, because the raised heel allows them to recruit more quadriceps and hit depth easier. Squatters who prefer Olympic-style shoes also tend to favor lifters with a relatively narrow (shoulder-width) stance.

Olympic shoes can be on the expensive side, with high-end models selling for up to $200, although a decent pair may start at around $80. The upside of the higher cost is that these shoes tend to be durable, and will last a very long time with normal use.

On the other end of the spectrum are so-called "minimalist" shoes. These shoes are generally lightweight, with a thin sole, with the object being to let your foot act as naturally as possible. These shoes favor wider stance squatters who rely more on their hamstrings, glutes, and lower back. The lower heel profile makes it easier to sit back into the squat, and the minimal sole allows you to drive your knees out without risking your foot rolling over.

Minimalist shoes have become extremely popular in the last few years, with tons of models available. Some companies have gone so far as to make shoes with individual toes, which look every bit as goofy as they sound.

The price is often anything but minimal, with some models costing well over of $100.

Fortunately, the perfect minimalist squat shoe might already be in your closet. More world records in the squat have been set in Converse Chuck Taylors than any other single shoe on the market. Their flat, thin sole keeps your feet grounded, and the canvas high-top provides additional ankle support.

Best of all, they remain modest in price, although they show their wear relatively quickly with regular use. Most serious lifters will wear them out within 2 or 3 years.

BENCH PRESS SHOES: At first glance, shoes might seem somewhat unimportant for the bench press, since you are lying on your back. But as you'll learn in the techniques section, the lower body plays a vital role in the bench press, and the right shoes can make a noticeable difference with maximal weights.

Some lifters will bench in the same shoes they squat in, which might be okay, depending on how you're built. Traditional squat shoes with a raised heel might be fine for shorter lifters because the raised heel can improve your leverage and help you get more leg drive which will stabilize your upper body.

Taller lifters might prefer a minimalist shoe, which lets you drive hard into the floor with less chance of butt-lift. A minimalist shoe will also make it easier to drive your knees out for additional support, without worrying about your ankles rolling.

Some lifters are fine benching in traditional sneakers, but if you do, make sure you use a pair with a fairly firm sole, which will give you a nice, reliable transfer of force from your feet to the floor. Running shoes would generally *not* be optimal here.

DEADLIFT SHOES: Almost all serious deadlifters prefer a minimal shoe because the closer your feet are to the ground, the less distance you will need to pull. Additionally, the lack of a heel helps you to lean back during the pull, which will improve your mechanics. Some lifters will even go so far as to pull barefoot, or in specially made slippers.

Chalk

While a block of chalk may not seem like a piece of "gear" per se, it certainly counts as one of the more indispensable items in your gym bag.

While the average gym goer might

rely on gloves to maintain a secure grip, serious lifters know that nothing beats a naked, chalked-up hand. Chalk provides friction because it reduces moisture on your hands, and allows the knurling of the bar (the rough, file-like surface where you grasp the bar) to dig into the skin of your hands (it sounds painful, but it's not).

Despite the increased comfort, gloves can actually hinder grip strength because they interfere with tactile feedback; your nervous system's ability to sense the pressure of the weight in your hands. With the extra layer of material between you and the weight, gloves can also cause you to lose your grip on heavy weights.

Plus, the more serious lifters in your gm will know you're just a pretender.

The one drawback to chalk is that commercial gyms often don't allow it. There are, however, some lotions on the market that will dry on your hand to form a chalky-like surface. Liquid Chalk and Dry Hands are two of them. While not as ideal as chalk, both are better than gloves.

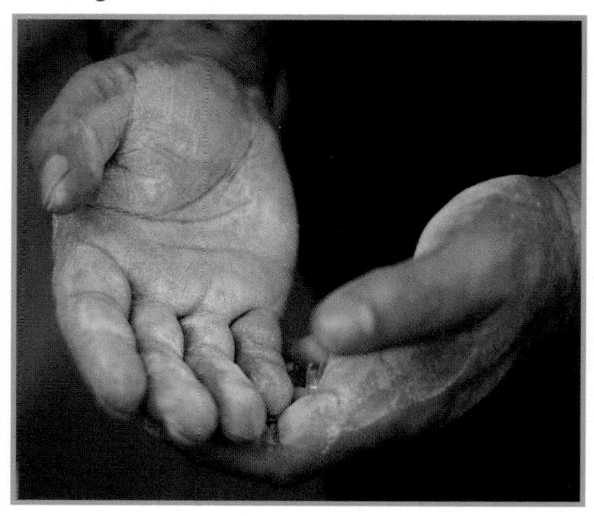

Wrist/Knee Wraps

Resembling thick bandages, wrist and knee wraps are designed to stabilize and assist the wrist and knee joints during squatting and pressing movements.

While wraps are often sold and used as a means to protect the wrist, knee, and sometimes elbow joints, their true function is to allow the user to handle more weight. A tight wrap acts as a spring, stretching as the joint is flexed, and releasing elastic energy as it extends. High quality knee wraps are so effective at this that most powerlifting organizations recognize separate records for lifters who choose to wear them. Elbow wraps are generally not allowed in powerlifting competitions.

While knee and elbow wraps rely on joint flexion/extension to work, wrist wraps work by immobilizing and stabilizing the wrists, minimizing force displacement and making the weight feel lighter in your hands.

For non-competitive lifters, I find wraps to be unnecessary in most instances. If functional strength and muscle gain is what you're after, you'll be better off allowing your joints to function naturally. Occasionally wrapping to try and break a long standing pr is fine, but limit your training gear to your belt for the majority of the time.

And please, if you do choose to use knee wraps, don't be one of those weight room showoffs that uses knee wraps on a loaded up 45-degree leg press. Either use them on squats, or don't bother.

Elbow/Knee Sleeves

If you don't want the additional support of a wrap, but you do want some measure of protection around the elbow and knee joints, knee and elbow sleeves are a great alternative. Essentially neoprene tubes, sleeves keep your knee and elbow joints warm, which can help reduce the risk of injury while offering minimal support. Rehbands are the most popular brand, but other companies such as Tommy Kono and Metal Sport also have high quality offerings.

Wrist Straps

Not to be confused with wrist *wraps,* wrist straps are small canvas straps, about a foot long and an inch wide, with a small loop on one end. Straps are used to assist you in holding onto a barbell, when the weight is either too heavy, or the reps are too high with a given weight to hold onto it for the entire set.

Straps are often looked at as kind of a "cheat," but they do have their applications. While you should hold on to the weight yourself for your main lifts, straps can be a valuable tool on assistance work (mostly back exercises to push past the point where your grip would normally fail).

To put them on, make a slip knot by snaking the unlooped end through the loop, then put your wrist through the hole. The free end of the strap should cross the space between your thumb and forefinger. Next, wrap the strap around the barbell, and grasp the bar over the strap. The pressure of the weight of the bar against your hand will keep the bar secure in your hands.

Gloves

No. While popular with the general fitness and bodybuilding crowds, gloves are rarely used by serious strength athletes. Gloves put a cushion between you and the bar, which can negatively affect your body's ability to sense the weight in your hands (known as proprioception). Having a barrier between your hands and the bar on the deadlift can cause the bar to slip. Whatever gear you choose to use when lifting, make sure that you are using, and not *relying* on it. The majority of your training, with the exception of your heaviest work, should be performed with no gear at all. The only gear that should be used throughout the entire workout would be your lifting shoes and chalk.

"A few small investments in some proper training gear can make a big difference in the productivity of your training."

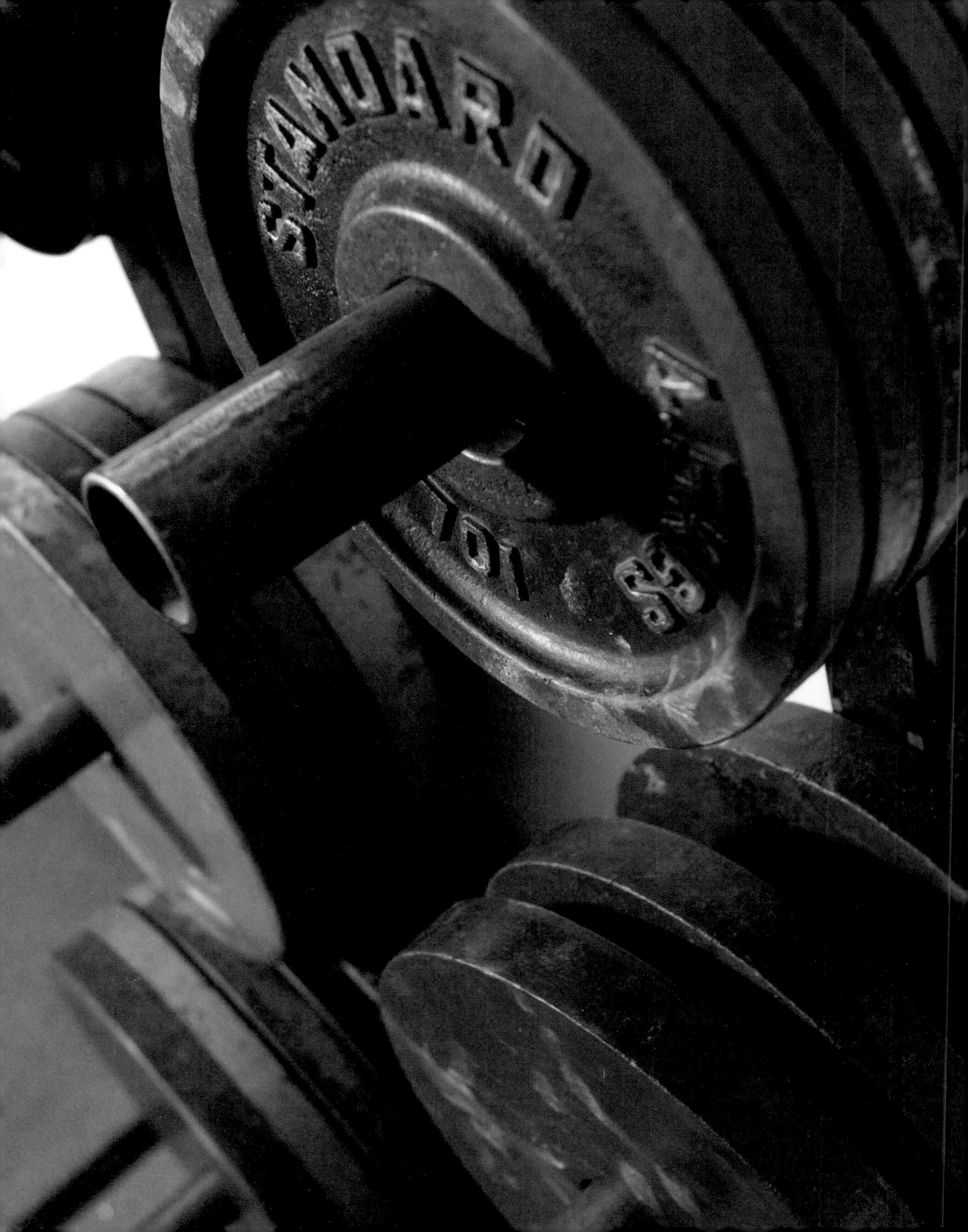
STANDARD

WARMING UP

A proper warm-up is critical to hoisting heavy weights, but warming up incorrectly could be just as detrimental as skipping it completely. Preparing to lift heavy weights means warming up like a lifter, not like a runner.

OVER-STRETCHING

Stretching before training is so ingrained in most exercisers minds, it's practically gospel. However, for strength training, a long, thorough stretch actually sends your nervous system the wrong message.

Your body relies on a mechanism called a stretch-reflex in order to help the muscles produce force. Initiated by a structure called the muscle spindle, which detects changes in muscle length, the stretch reflex is a protective mechanism that causes a muscle to contract in opposition to a stretch. The stretch reflex is critical to injury prevention because it prevents muscle tears due to over-stretching.

You've likely seen this process firsthand at your doctor's office. When a doctor taps a patient's knee with that little rubber hammer, what he's really doing is testing the patient's stretch reflex. Tapping the knee causes an abrupt stretch in the patellar tendon. In a healthy patient, the body's normal response is to contract the quadriceps, resulting in the reflexive kicking motion that should follow.

Your body uses this same reflex to assist in the lifting of heavy weights. For example, as you descend into the bottom position of a squat, your hamstrings and glutes are stretching and building elastic tension. When you reach the "the hole" (the bottom position) your muscles, aided by the stretch reflex, use this elastic energy to initiate the contraction which lifts the weight.

The better you are at maximizing the stretch reflex, the stronger and more explosive you will be.

While pre-workout stretching is usually prescribed for injury prevention, the result is often the opposite. Muscles protect the various structures (such as tendons, ligaments, bones, and discs) by remaining tight and creating stability. If injury prevention is your goal, why would you ever want to handicap this process with stretching?

While stretching is great for relaxation and recovery after a hard workout, thorough stretching before lifting will generally make you loose and weak, as opposed to explosive and strong.

Now just to be clear, stretching isn't *always* bad. Stretching *after* training is an effective way to speed recovery and improve range of motion. Even some pre-workout stretching is fine if it is to address a specific muscle group that tends to be too tight.

When I'm preparing for a lifting session, I will get through my first few light warm-up sets to see if there is any tightness I need to deal with before progressing. If I notice any pain or restricted range of motion, I will address the problem. If I feel fine, I just proceed without any stretching.

For a more appropriate pre-lifting warm-up, try the following upper and lower body circuits.

"A proper warm-up is critical to hoisting heavy weights, but warming up incorrectly could be just as detrimental as skipping it completely."

WARM-UP CIRCUITS

To provide you with some further clarity on the importance of warming up, below are two warm-up circuits that can be completed in less than 10 minutes. Please note that these are not merely stretching circuits; they are meant to warm up your body for your full workout. These circuits are recommended because they:

- "Excite" the nervous and muscular systems response
- Increase blood flow
- Improve mental preparedness

UPPER BODY CIRCUIT

Sets: 1
Reps: 15
Tempo: Continuous, smooth tempo. Expect slight perspiration and elevation in heart rate.

Arm Circles

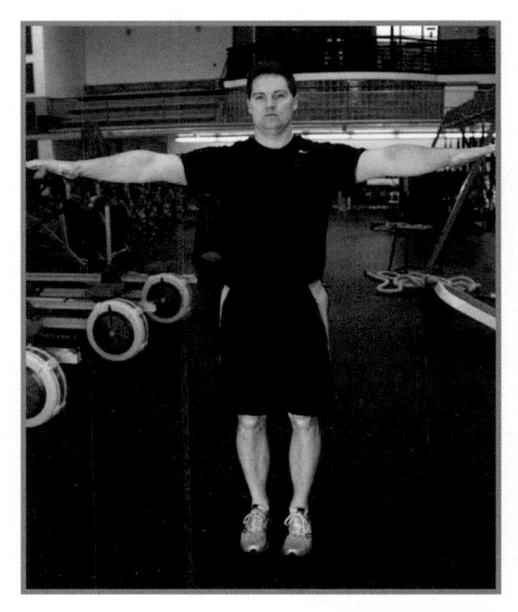

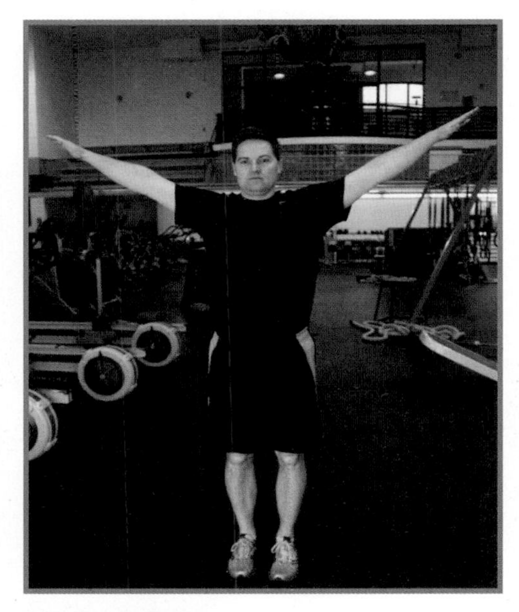

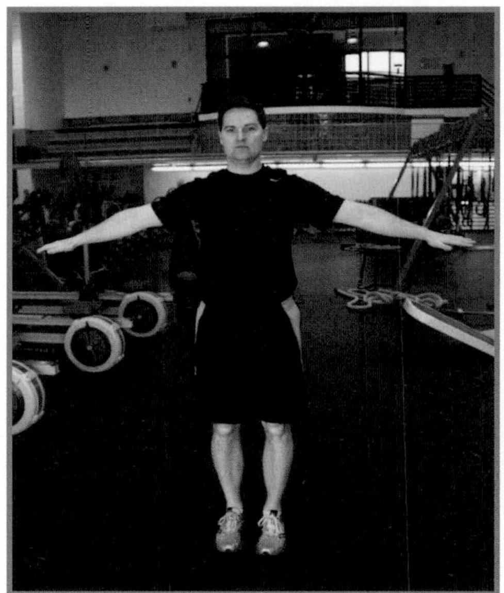

DESCRIPTION: Begin in a sitting or standing position. Position your arms straight out to the sides. Start the movement with small circles forward and progress to large circles. Reverse the movement backward.

MUSCLES USED: Focus on using the chest, shoulders, and arm muscles during this movement.

Spinal Whips

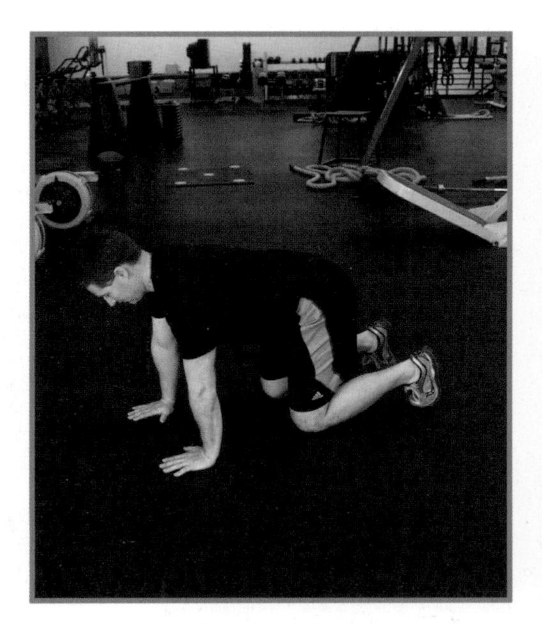

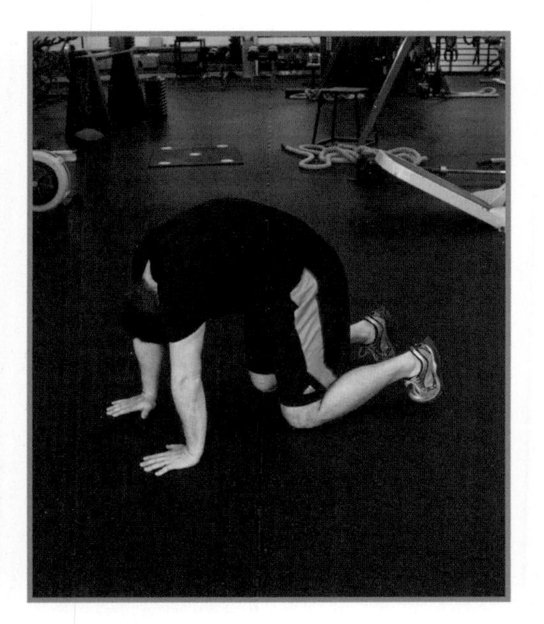

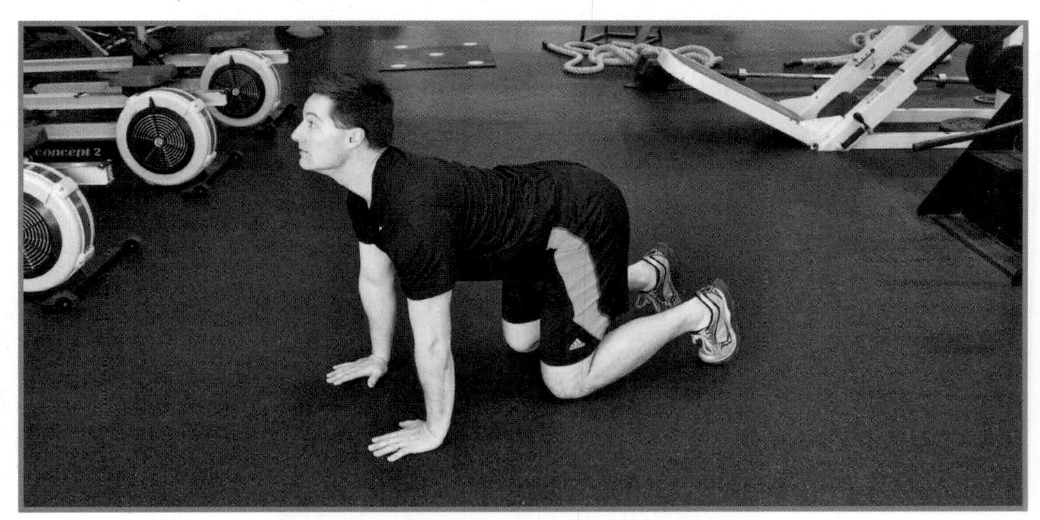

DESCRIPTION: Begin in an all-fours position. Your hands should be positioned under the shoulders and your knees should be under the hips. Arch the spine up using the stomach muscles, return to neutral starting position, and drop the hips back over the feet. Return to neutral, repeat sequence.

MUSCLES USED: Focus on using the abs, lats, and lower back.

Bird Dog

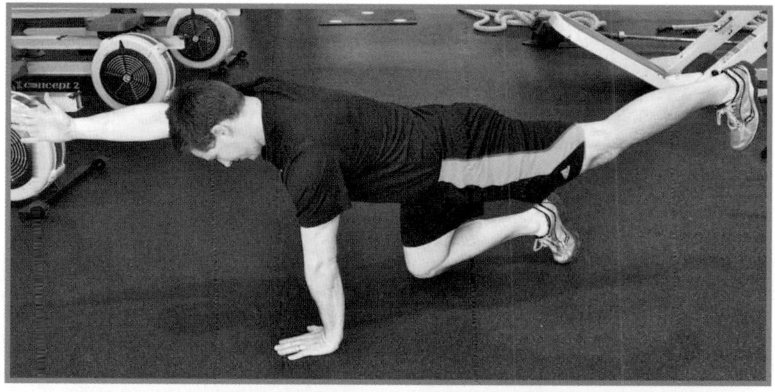

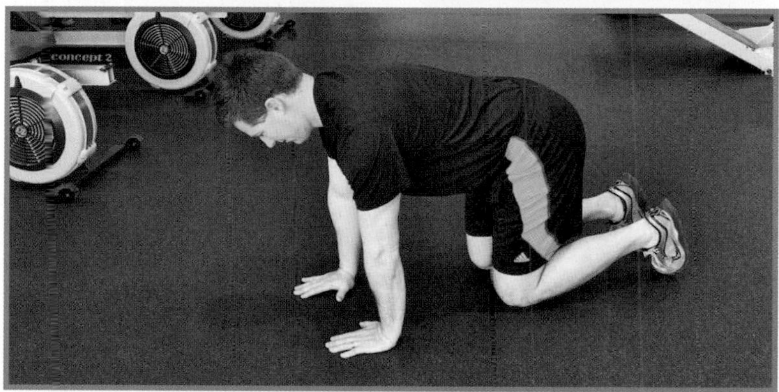

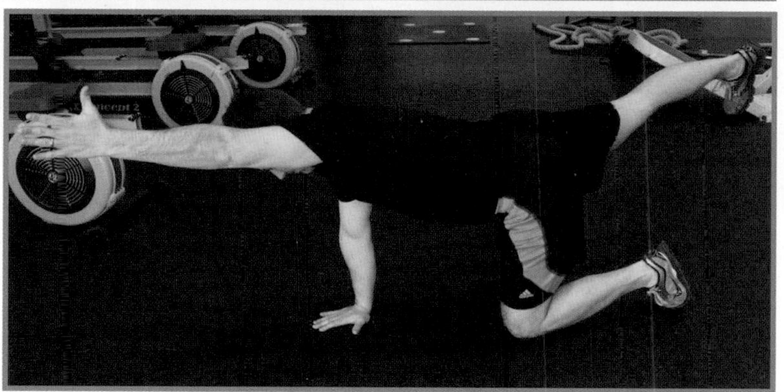

DESCRIPTION: Begin in an all-fours position. Extend the opposite arm and leg, hold, and return to starting position. Repeat sequence on same side.

MUSCLES USED: Focus on using the shoulders, core, and hips.

Jumping Jacks

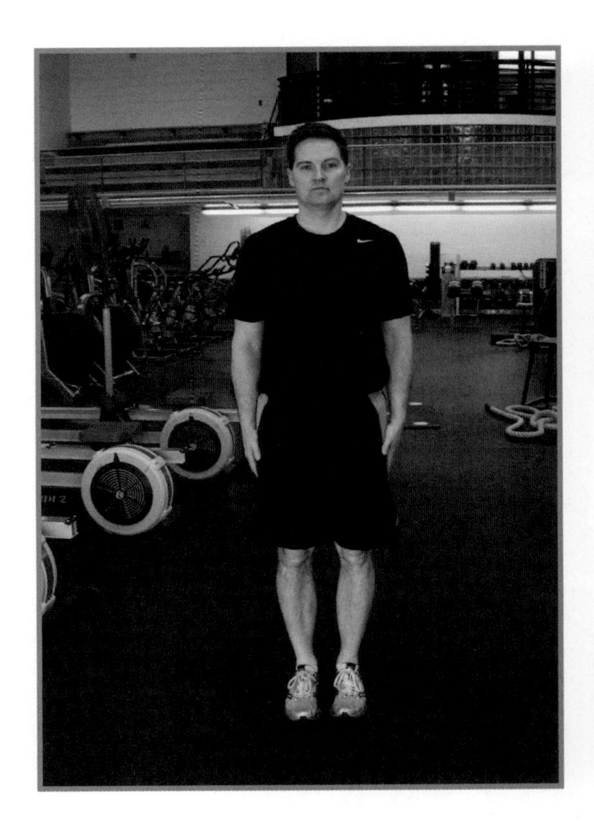

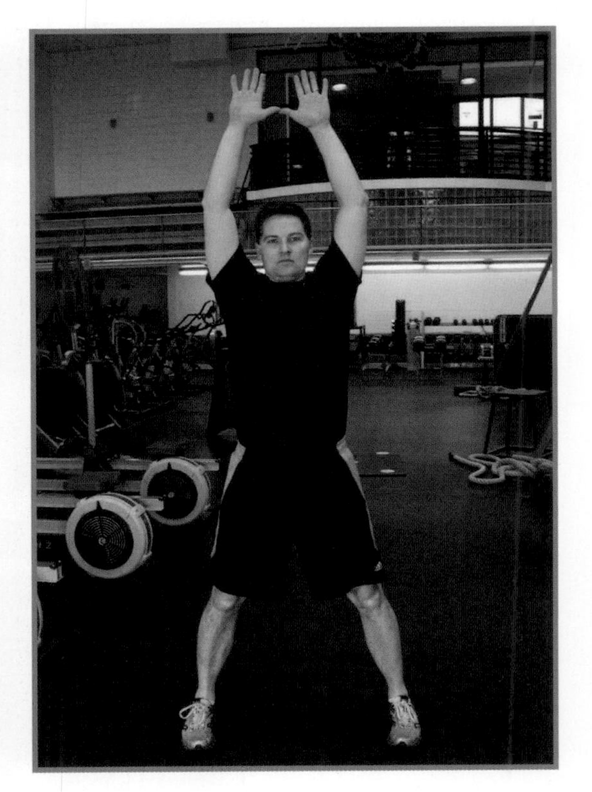

DESCRIPTION: Begin in a standing position with your hands relaxed on either side. Simultaneously raise the arms out to the sides and above the head, and "kick" both legs out to the sides. Return and repeat sequence.

MUSCLES USED: Focus on using the arms, shoulders, and legs.

T-Jacks

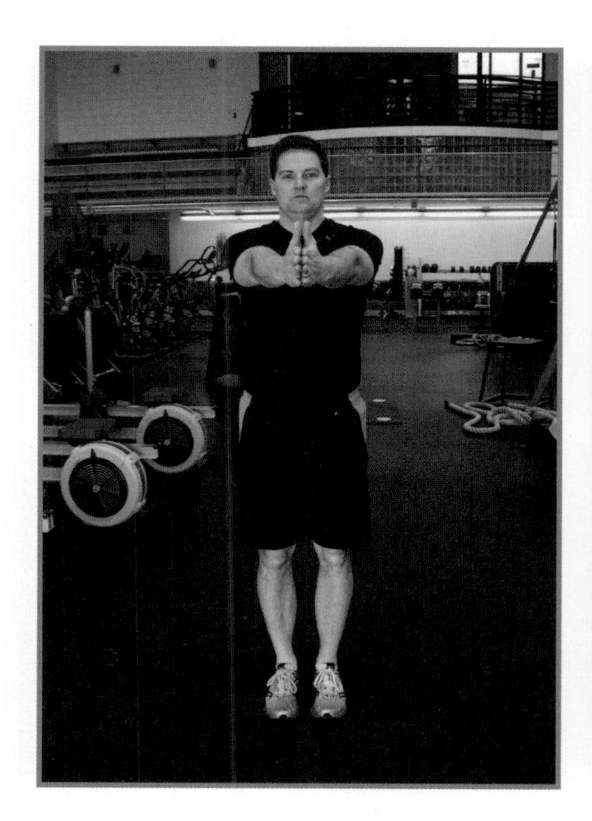

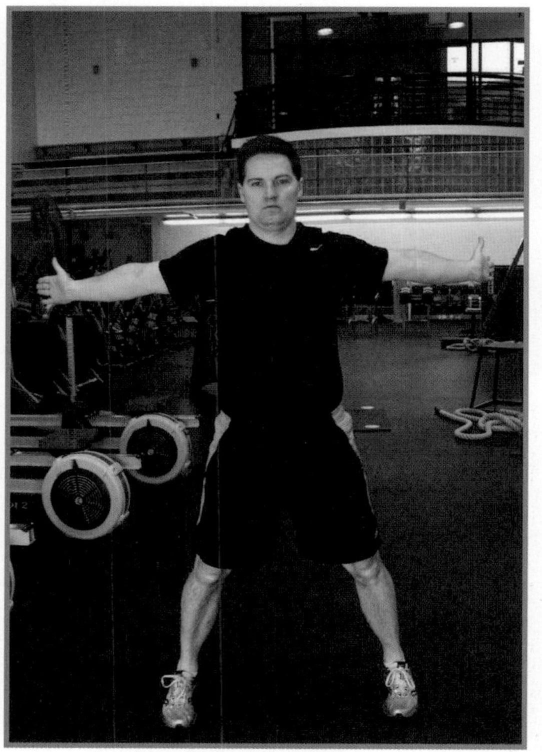

DESCRIPTION: Perform the same execution as Jumping Jack, while keeping your hands out in front of you.

MUSCLES USED: Focus on using the chest, back, and legs.

Inch Worm

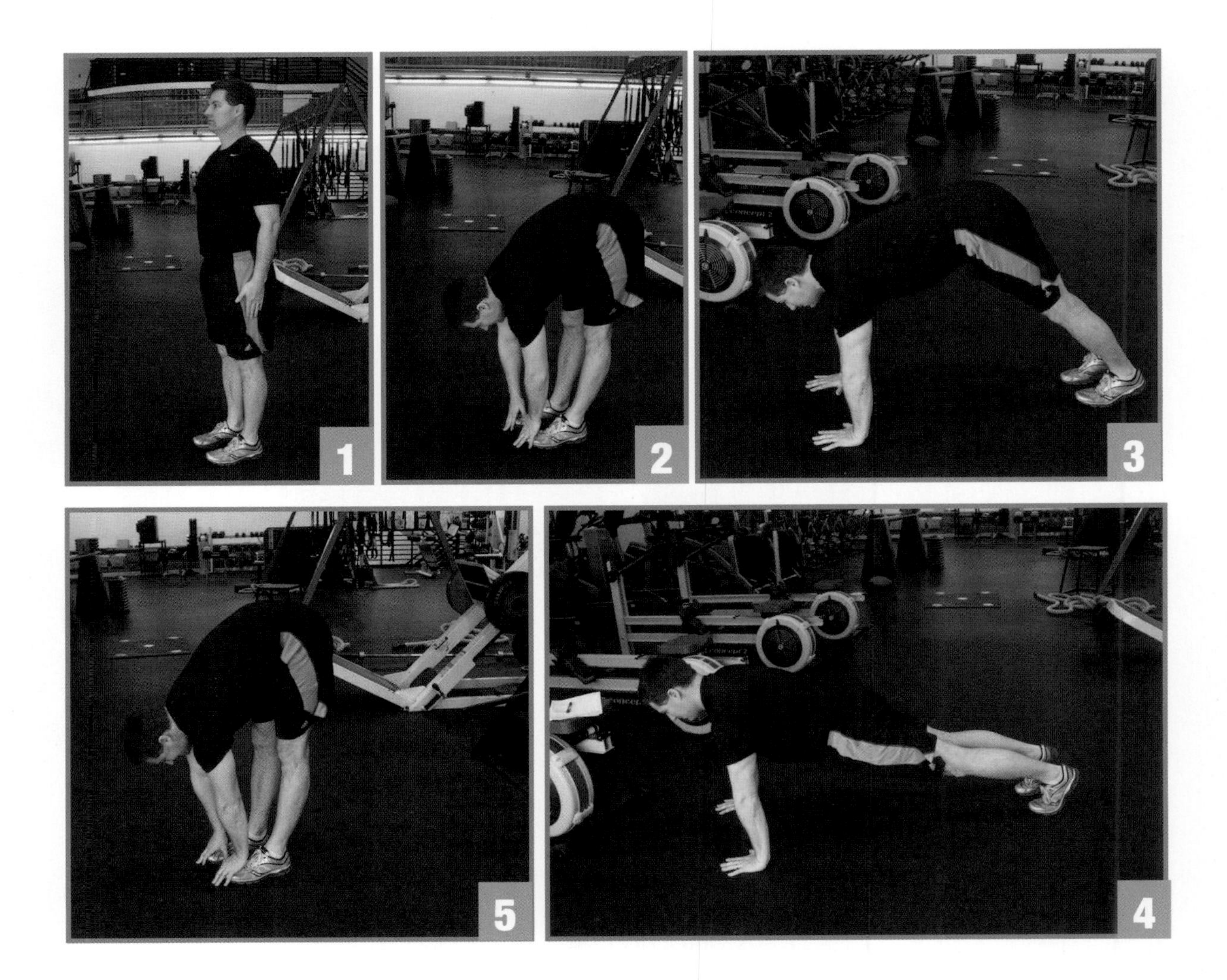

DESCRIPTION: Begin in a standard push-up position. Walk your hands back towards the feet until the body is in a vertical tuck position. Walk the hands out to the starting position.

MUSCLES USED: Full body movement.

LOWER BODY CIRCUIT

Sets: 2
Reps: 10
Tempo: Pause between the first and second sets.

Hip Hinging

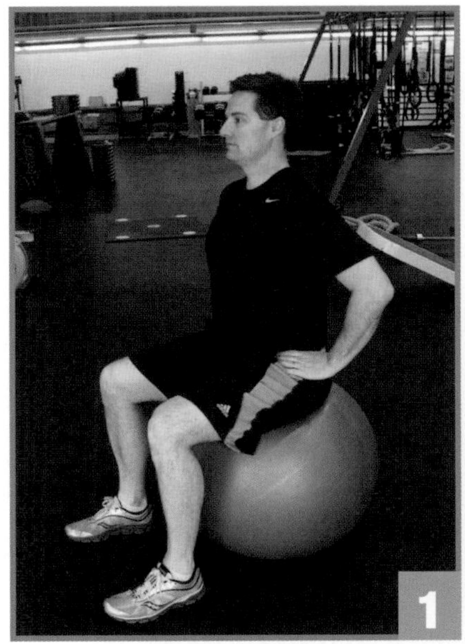

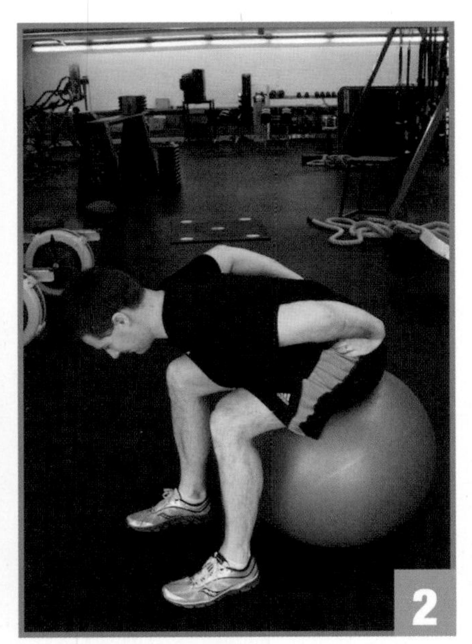

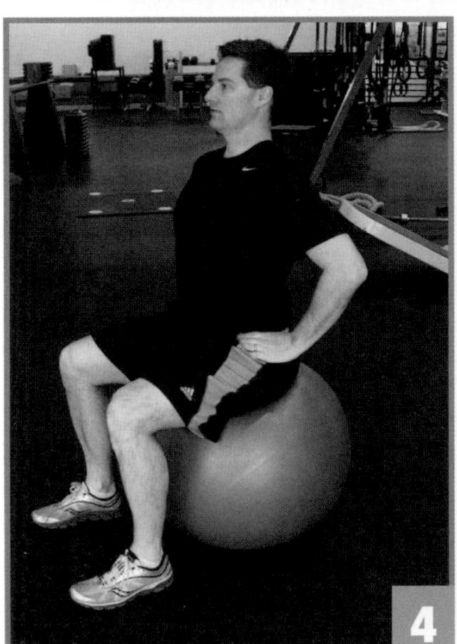

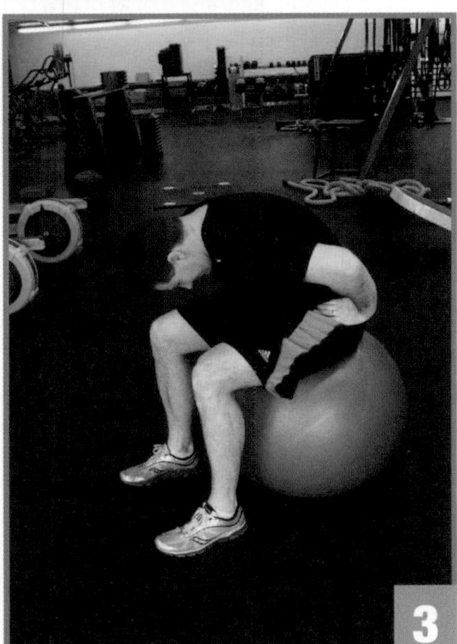

DESCRIPTION: While standing, begin by placing your hands on your hips. Keeping your back straight, hinge at your waist sticking your hips out. A good teaching cue is to imagine a broomstick is lying vertical on your spine. Keep it straight. Hinging the hips is one of the most important basic movements. *(Note: The last photos demonstrates what* not *to do.)*

MUSCLES USED: Focus on the hips and hamstrings.

Kneeling Hip Flexor Rock

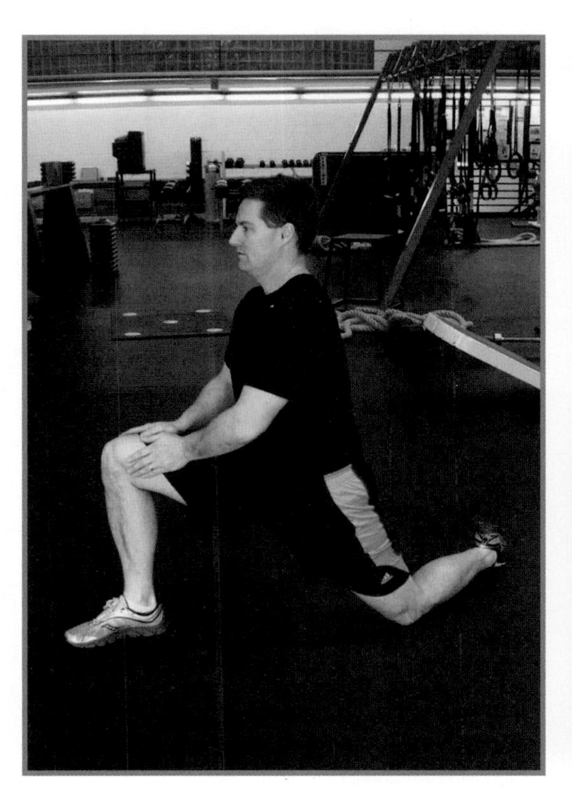

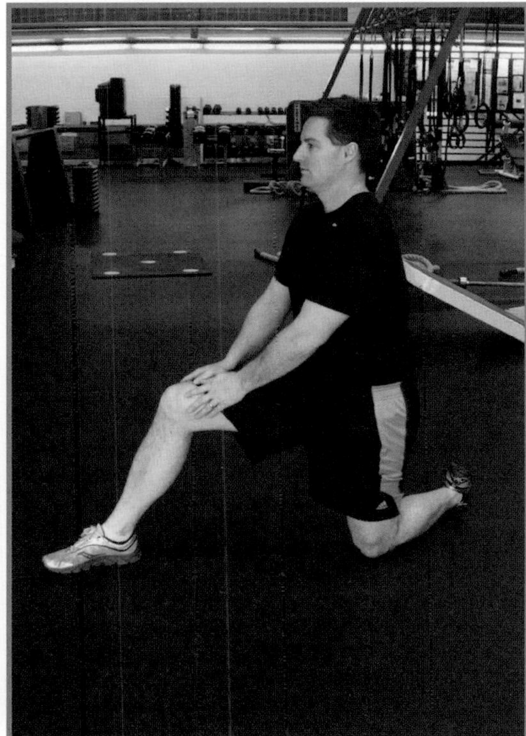

DESCRIPTION: Begin in a lunge or split stance position with one knee on the ground. Gently push the hips forward feeling a stretch in the front of the hip. Reach a maximum end point without arching your lower back; pause, and return to starting position.

MUSCLES USED: Focus on the hips and legs.

Drop Squat

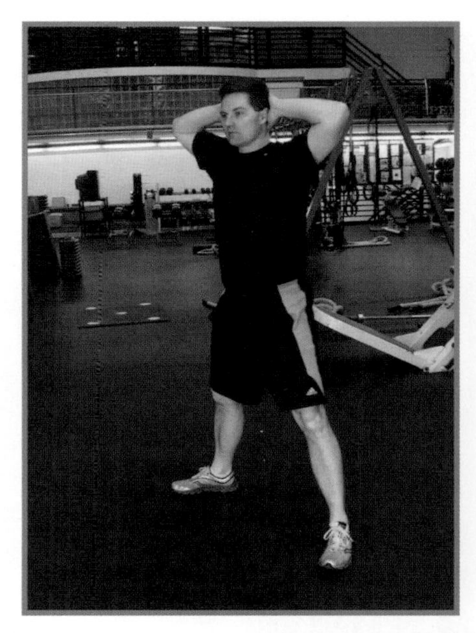

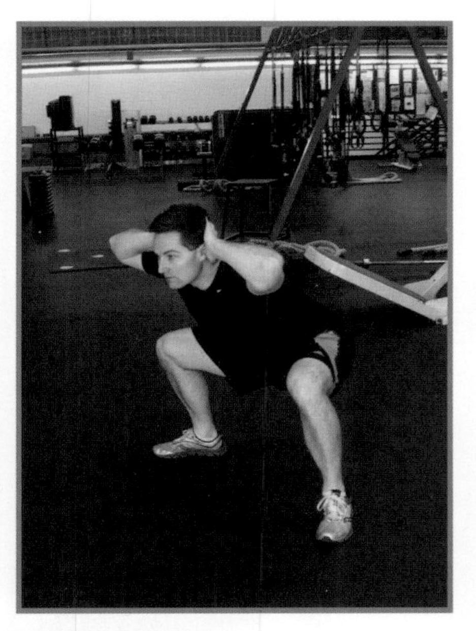

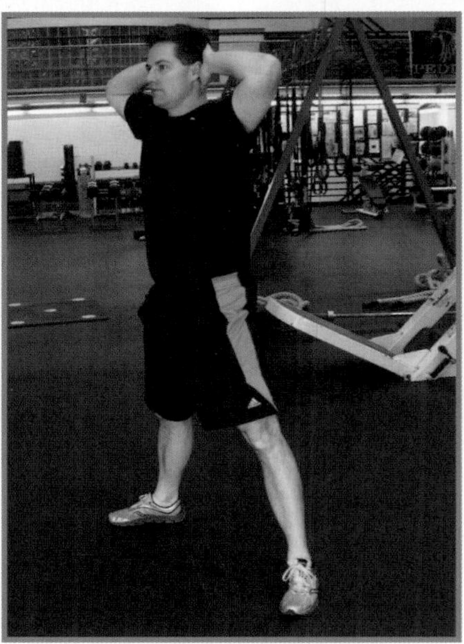

DESCRIPTION: Position your feet slightly outside your hips. Drop your hips down as if performing a squat. Gently use the elbows to push the knees out, feeling the stretch in the groin and hips. Keep the chest up during the movement.

MUSCLES USED: Focus on the hips, groin, and legs.

Forward Lunge into Lateral Lunge

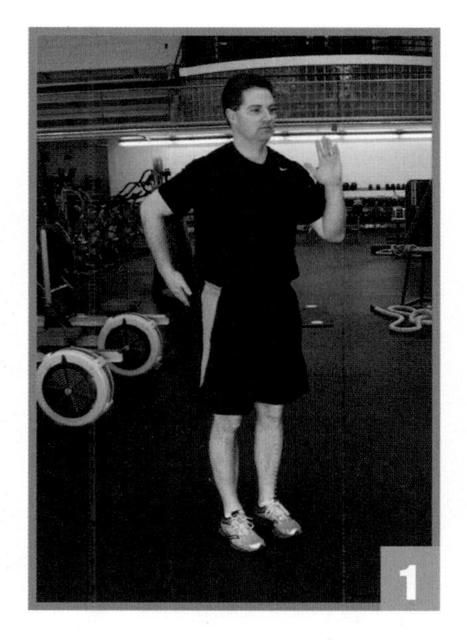

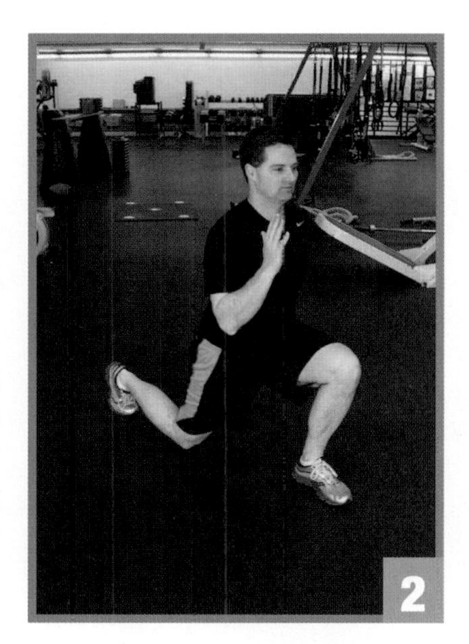

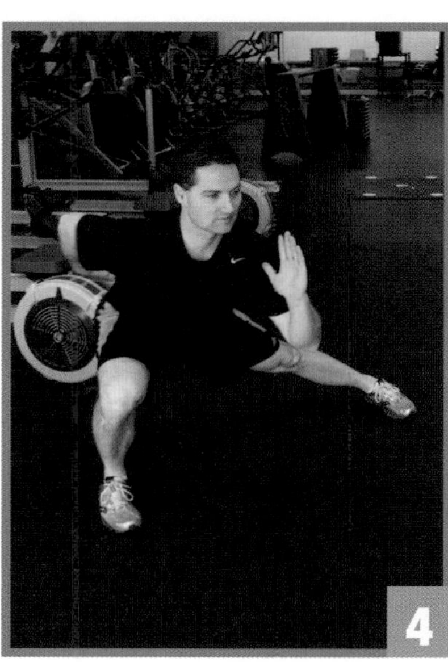

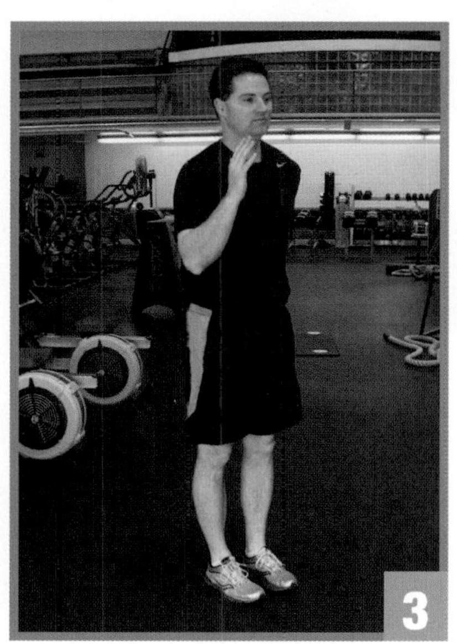

DESCRIPTION: Begin in a neutral, standing position. Perform a standard forward lunge. Return to starting position. Perform a lateral lunge to the side.

MUSCLES USED: Focus on hips and legs.

Jumping Jacks

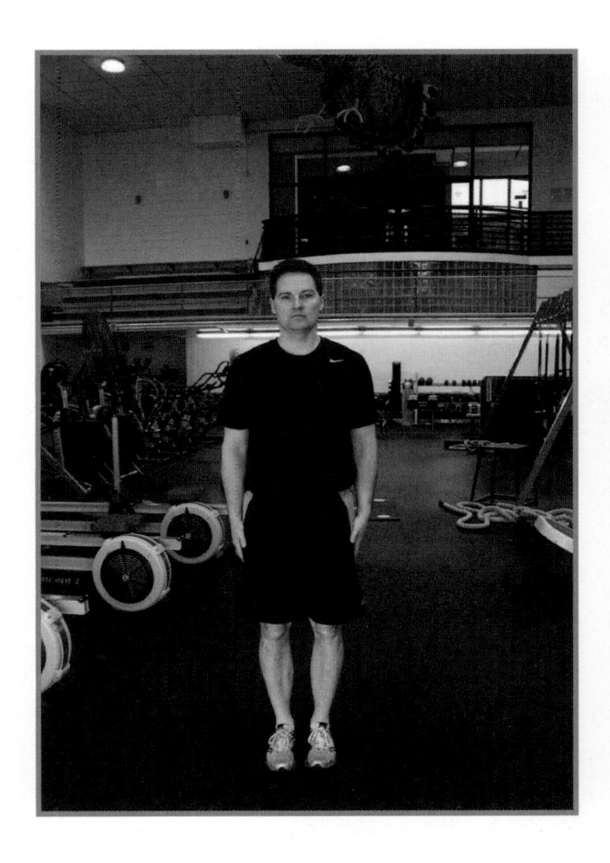

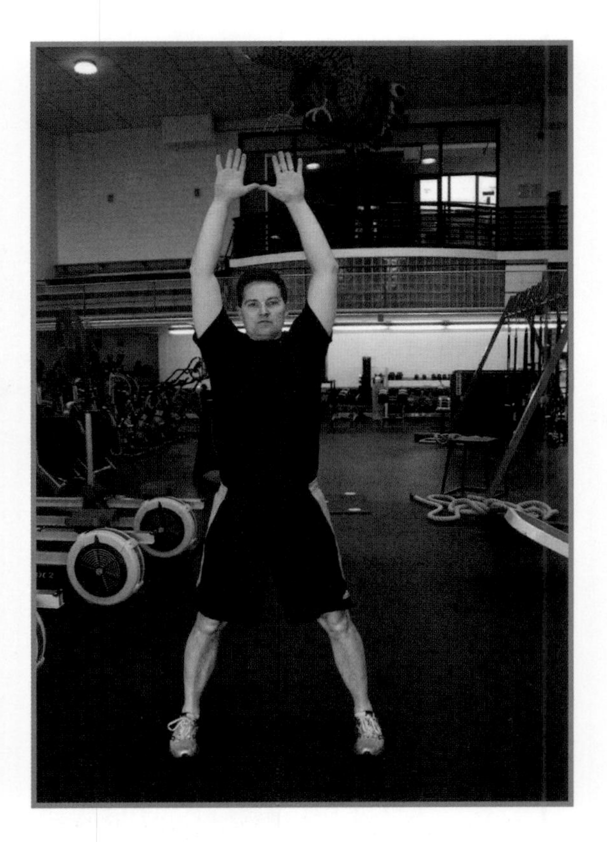

DESCRIPTION: Begin in a standing position with your hands relaxed on either side. Simultaneously raise the arms out to the sides and above the head, and "kick" both legs out to the sides. Return and repeat sequence.

MUSCLES USED: Focus on using the arms, shoulders, and legs.

THE EXERCISES

When I explain strength programming, either to athletes or coaches, I often describe your program as a roadmap to your goals. Using the same analogy, think of your exercises as the car. If you were to take a cross-country road trip, it wouldn't matter how detailed your map is if you're driving a shoddy car. At some point, you'll break down and never make it to your destination. In our case, that breakdown would be either a plateau in your progress, or a literal breakdown in the form of an injury.

When I'm working my athletes, either in a training or seminar format, I tend to spend far more time on exercise technique than anything else because without the ability to perform the core lifts correctly, even an intelligently written program will end in either a plateau or an injury.

I've done my best to go into detail with each exercise I've included in the programming for this book, but remember that no matter how experienced you become, your technique will never be perfect, and even world champion lifters constantly strive to identify and correct mistakes. If you do not have access to an experienced coach or training partners, I highly recommend you periodically take video of yourself on the main lifts, to make sure that you aren't developing any bad habits.

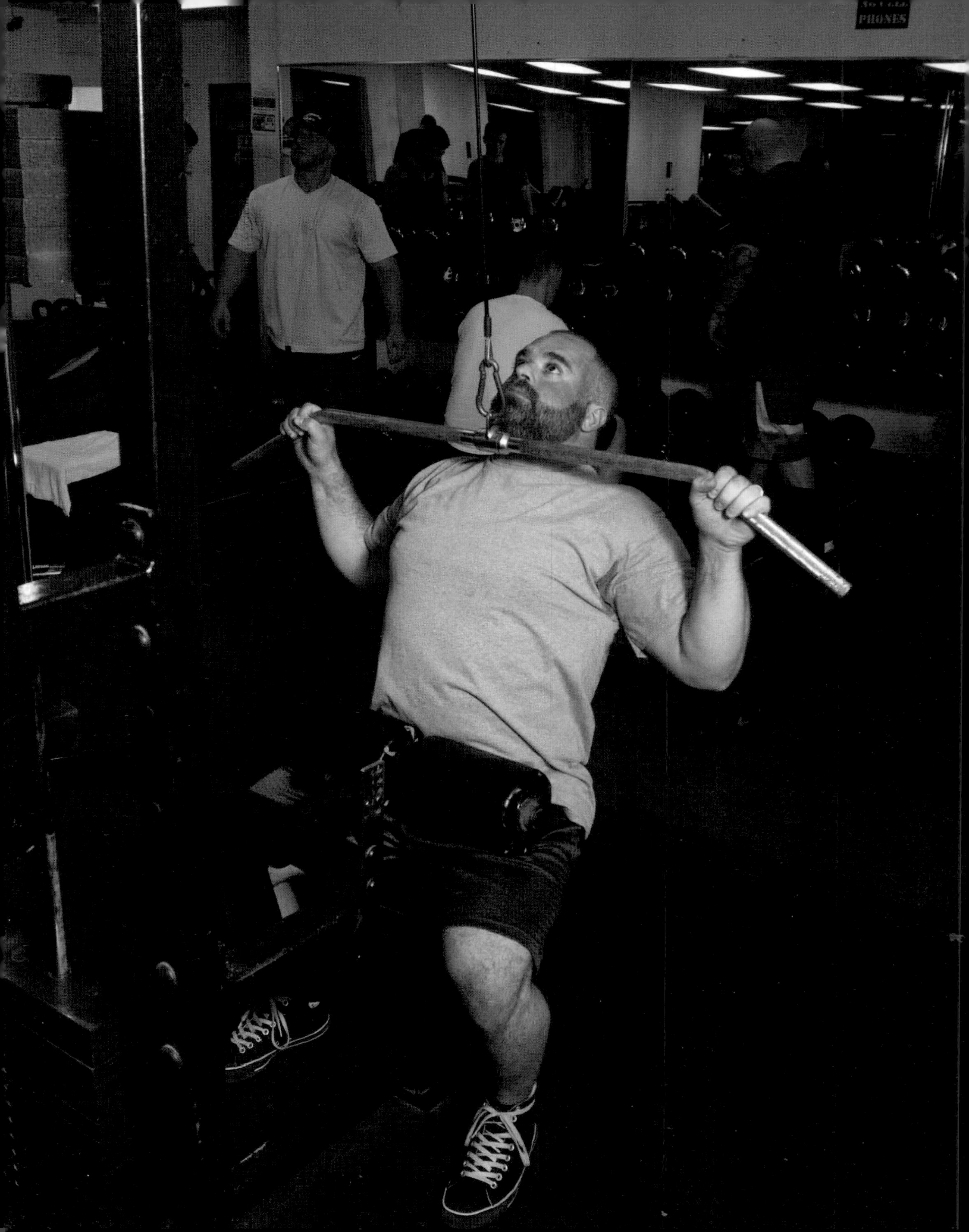
PHONES

MACHINE EXERCISES

While of limited use to most serious strength athletes, resistance machines can serve a valuable purpose for beginners. The fixed range of motion of the typical resistance machine, while not enough of a stimulus for serious athletes, does offer beginners the ability to safely get into the routine of training, even if they lack the technique necessary for free weight training.

Machines are not going to be something you'll want to rely on beyond the first month or so, but if you've never weight trained before, they will be a user-friendly way to get your feet wet.

> Please note that there are numerous variations of each machine on the market, so the equipment pictured in this book may not at first glance resemble the machines available to you. For this reason, we have kept our advice as to their operation fairly general. Specific operation instructions unique to each machine (such as mechanisms for changing seat or pad settings) are usually explained on instruction panels on the machine.

The two most common types of resistance machines are plate loaded and selectorized.

PLATE-LOADED MACHINES are mechanically the simpler of the two. As the name implies, plate-loaded machines require the user to place the weights directly onto the cam, just like with a barbell. The main advantage to plate-loaded machines is that due to their simpler mechanics, they have a smoother, more natural feel than selectorized machines. The major disadvantage is that the user must pick up and load the plates themselves, which can be a little more of a hassle, especially on exercises like the leg press, where you might need to load six or more 45-pound plates to get the resistance high enough.

SELECTORIZED MACHINES use a weight stack attached to an intricate pulley and cam system to supply the resistance. The biggest advantage of selectorized machines are their ease of use. Typically, all the user needs to do is stick a pin into the stack at the desired weight. This ease of use makes selectorized equipment significantly more popular in most fitness centers than plate loaded. The biggest disadvantage to selectorized machines is that their complex mechanisms create more friction, and can add more resistance than intended if the machines are not well cared for. Another possible drawback to selectorized machines is that the cam and pulley system utilized by most machines feels less like free weights than the simpler plate-loaded machines.

In either case, the drawbacks of machines are largely mitigated by the fact that you won't be using them for very long. However, an important point to remember is that regardless of the type of machine you use, the weights you use on machines will generally not translate to free weights. So if you can handle 200 pounds on a chest press, it is not an indication that 200 pounds will be an appropriate weight for the bench press. When it's time to transition from machines to free weights, you will need to reestablish your training weights.

ONLY YOU CAN PREVENT LEG PRESS ABUSE

When used properly, the 45-degree leg press is a great piece of equipment. However, the leg press is misused all the time, especially by young men (although we have seen some female culprits as well).

The scenario typically goes something like this: The lifter starts his leg workout with the leg press. He'll start at around two or three 45-pound plates per side and work up to eight or nine. He'll mostly use half reps and may even wrap his knees for the top set. Between sets he'll stand around looking intense. Before the last set he will make sure to get a big psych by grunting, yelling to himself or a training partner, and basically making a scene. (We're not even going to get started on the guys who, when finished, walk away from the leg press leaving nine plates on each side.)

For all their theatrics, these guys never seem to have the legs to match the effort. The main reason for this is that leg presses (along with leg extensions and leg curls) do not train the legs in a manner that they are designed to function.

Our lower bodies are designed to propel our bodies from a solid base of support, not to lift separate implements themselves. Leg pressing removes a very important element from lower body training: the back.

The lower back, hamstrings, glutes, and quads are designed to work together during squatting, jumping, or running movements. When training for strength and functionality, the body needs to learn how to properly transfer force from the lower body to the upper body. If properly used, the 45-degree leg press is a great piece. It's fantastic as a secondary movement or when you need to give the back a break from spinal loading. In either of those scenarios, modest weights and full reps would be in order.

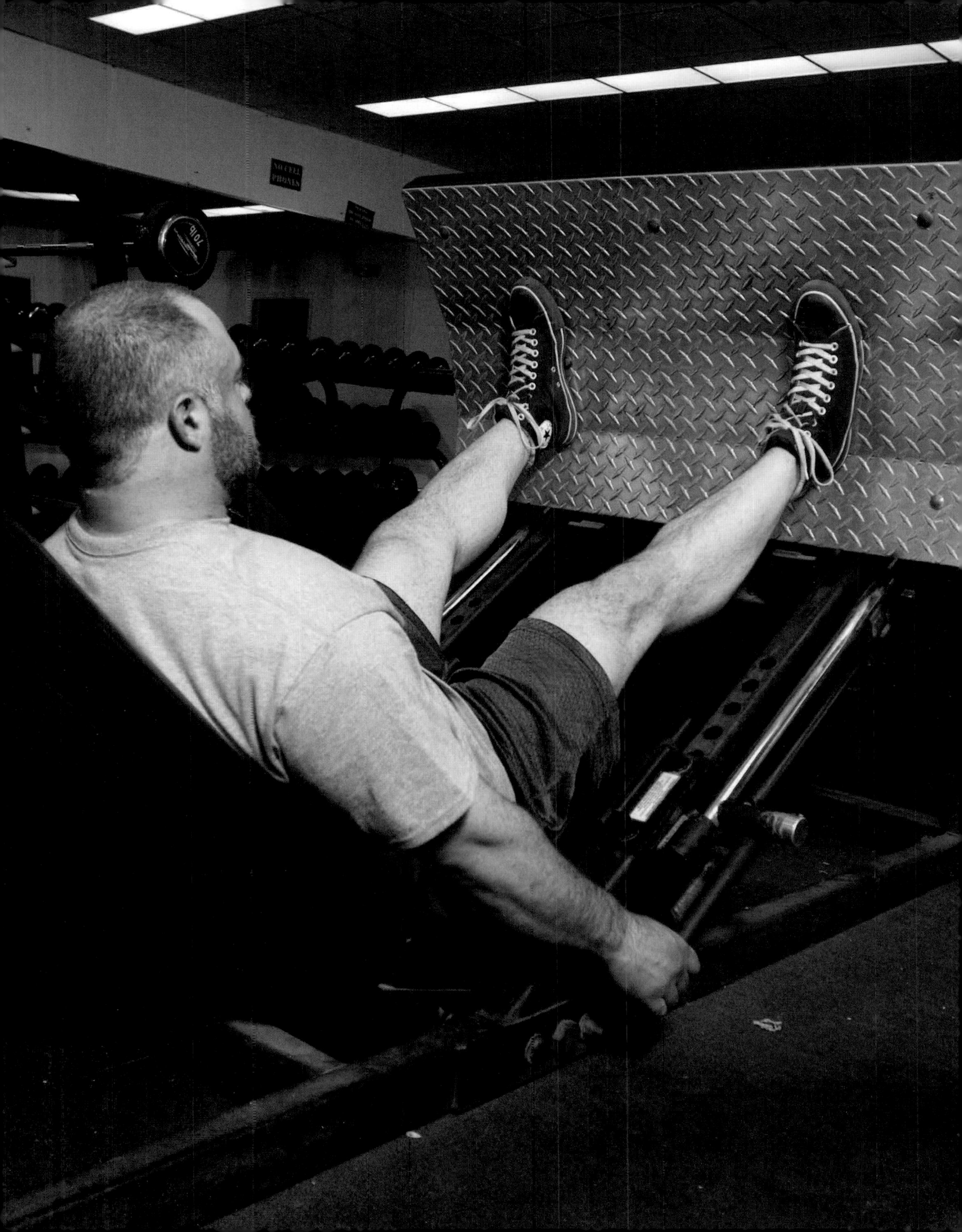

MACHINE LEG PRESS

Muscles targeted: Glutes, quadriceps, and hamstrings

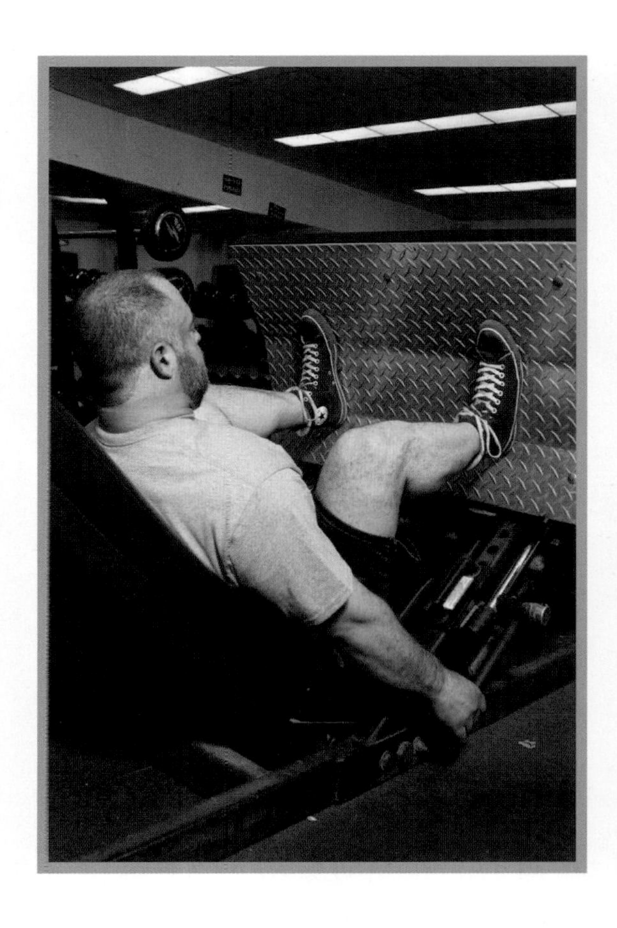

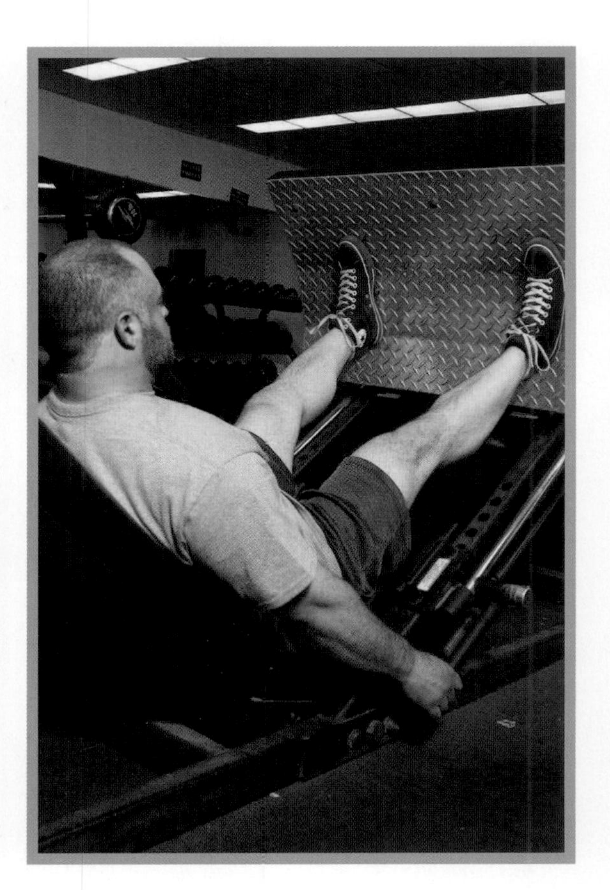

Set-Up

Leg press technique will vary based on your use of either the selectorized or plate-loaded 45-degree machine. If you have a choice, use the plate-loaded variety because it will allow you to start the movement with your legs extended, and start the loft with the descent, just like you would in a squat.

Most leg presses allow you to adjust for leg length, either with multiple height rack positions or an adjustable seat. The starting height on the 45-degree leg press should be with your legs just short of completely straight, requiring you to only push the weight a couple of inches to clear the racks. If you must use a selectorized model, set the plate so that both your hip and knee joints are at about a 45-degree angle. If you must round your lower back to get into position, set the foot platform a bit further from the seat until you can maintain a neutral lower back.

Your feet should be set on the center of the foot platform, slightly wider than shoulder width, with your toes pointed slightly out.

If using the 45-degree leg press, get into the start position by pushing against the foot platform until your legs are completely extended, then releasing the safety racks (the handles are usually on the sides of the machine, just below your hips).

The Exercise

For the 45-degree plate-loaded variety, lower the platform until your hip and knee joints are at about 45 degrees. Keep your back in a neutral (straight) position throughout the entire lift. If you find your lower back rounding at the bottom of the descent, you've gone too far. If you are on a selectorized model, you will be starting the exercise from the bottom position.

Using only your legs, press against the foot platform until your legs are fully extended. Keep your knees tracking over your toes throughout the entire lift, and do not try to buck your hips off of the seat.

If using the 45-degree model, re-rack the weight by holding the foot platform at full extension while returning the safety racks to the original position.

If using the selectorized model, just return the foot platform to the start position in a controlled manner.

Variations

You can change the difficulty of the leg press, as well as the targeted muscles by changing your foot position on the platform. A wider, foot forward stance will be easier, and will focus more on your hamstrings and glutes while removing stress from the knee joint. A narrower stance, with your feet further under you will place more stress on the quadriceps, but will also place more stress on the knees.

HACK SQUAT

Muscles Targeted: Glutes, quadriceps, and hamstrings

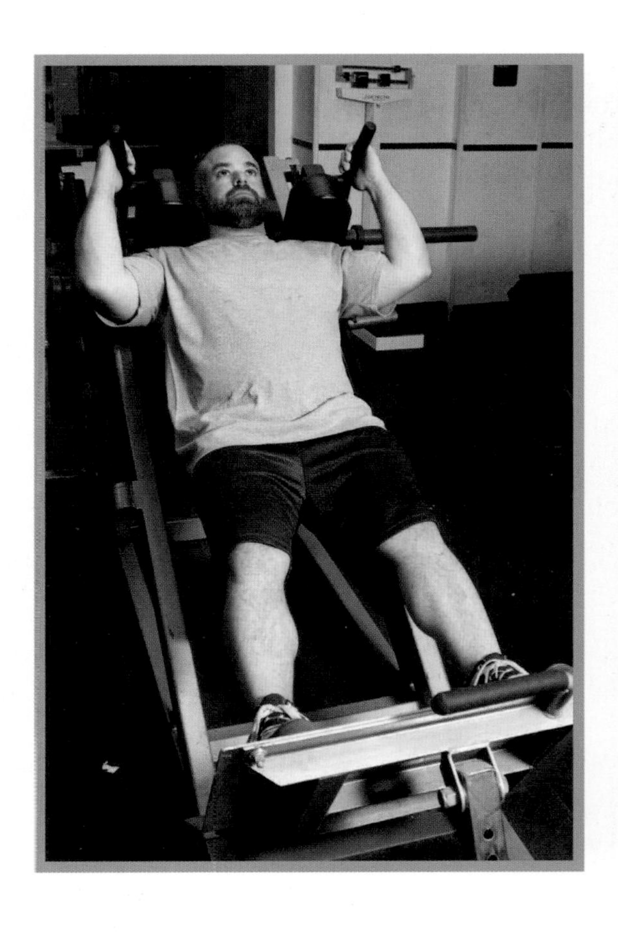

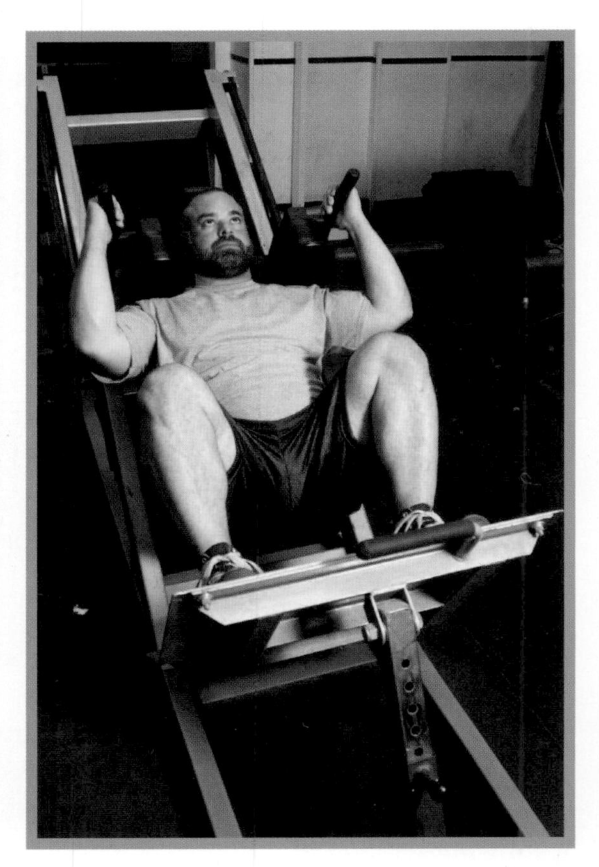

The hack squat machine looks a little like an upside-down 45-degree leg press. Instead of pushing a weighted sled up and away from you with your legs, your feet remain stationary on a solid platform while pressing your body along with the sled up along the tracks. The hack squat is a bit closer to the barbell squat not only because your feet are grounded, but because your hips reach full extension, while they do not get much past 90 degrees on the leg press.

Set-Up

Lean back onto the back pad of the sled with your shoulders against the two shoulder pads. Place your feet in the middle of the platform, slightly wider than shoulder width apart, with your toes pointing slightly out. You should only need to lift the sled a couple of inches to clear the safety racks. Most hack squats will have multiple heights on the safety racks, so if the height is not correct, just press up on the sled, release the safety racks, and reset them at your desired height. On most hack squats the handles for the safety racks will be on the sides of the machine, at about waist height, although they can also be up by the shoulder pads.

The Exercise

Once the safety racks are released, you will be able to begin the descent. Lower the sled by flexing your knees and hip joints. As you descend, your knees should remain in line with your toes and track out slightly. Your lower back should remain neutral, with no rounding as you approach the bottom position. Assuming you are able to maintain a neutral spine, descend until your knees and hips are at about a 45-degree angle.

Once you've reached the bottom position, reverse direction and press the sled back up to the start position. Reset the safety racks to complete the set.

Variations

You can change the difficulty of the hack squat, as well as the muscles being targeted, by changing your foot position on the platform. A wider, foot forward stance will be easier, and will focus more on your hamstrings and glutes while removing stress from the knee joints. A narrower stance, with your feet further under you will place more stress on the quadriceps, but will also place more stress on the knees.

CHEST PRESS MACHINE

Muscles Targeted: Pectorals, deltoids, and triceps

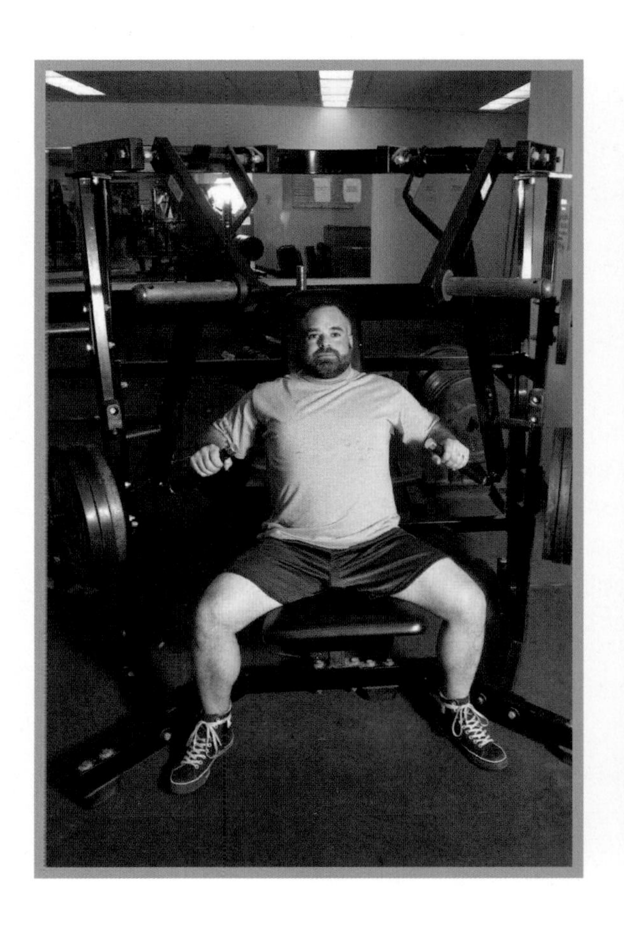

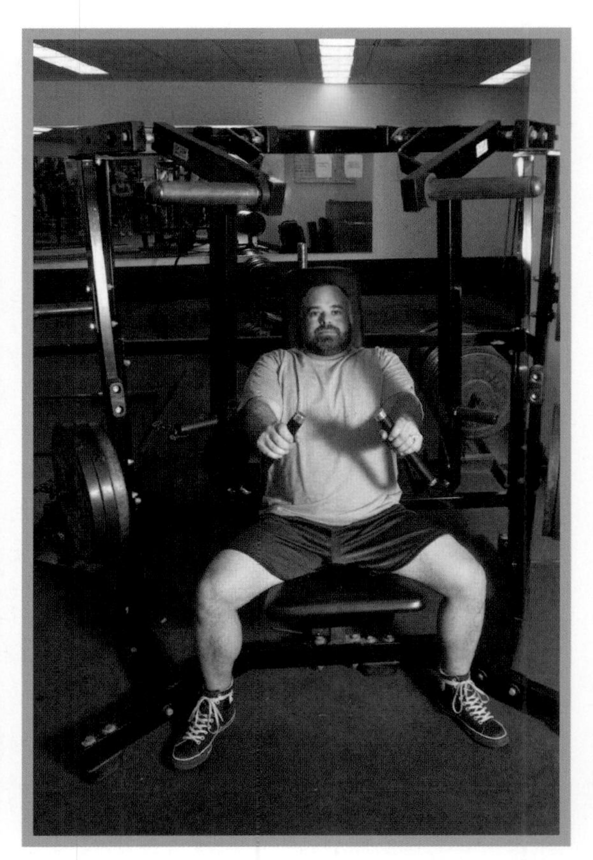

Aside from the weight loading mechanism, most chest press machines, either selectorized or plate loaded, have almost identical operation. The main difference will be that the plate-loaded version's handles will usually move independently of each other, while the selectorized version will usually have both handles attached to the same cam so that they move together.

Set-Up

Most chest press machines will allow you to select the seat height. Some will also allow you to change the starting point of the handles.

Adjust the seat height so that the handles are in line with your mid-chest, about 2 inches below your armpits. If the handles themselves are adjustable, set them at a starting point where you feel a slight stretch at the chest/shoulder, but not enough so that you feel like you are straining to get the weight moving.

Some chest presses will have a pedal that allows you to assist the initial press with your feet. Use this option if you have it because it will reduce the risk of a shoulder/pec strain, but only use it on the first rep to get the weight moving from the dead stop at the start.

Just before starting the exercise, tighten your upper back muscles by pulling your shoulder blades together and holding them there for the entire set. This will stabilize the shoulder joint during the exercise.

Keep your feet firmly planted on the floor during the exercise. A wide stance works well to keep you stable during the exercise.

The Exercise

Most chest presses start the movement from the bottom position (or what would be the bottom of a bench press), so you will start with the ascent.

Press the handles until your arms are fully extended. Throughout the movement, keep your upper back muscles tight, with your shoulder blades pinned together. Keeping your upper back tight will keep the shoulders stable during the lift, minimizing the chance of injury and increasing power.

Your upper arms should remain at about a 45-degree angle from your torso.

Return the handles to the starting position in a controlled manner.

Variations

Most chest press machines will allow you to take multiple grips. An overhanded grip with your hands slightly wider than shoulder width will place more stress on your pecs and shoulders. A parallel grip, with your palms facing each other will shift the resistance to your triceps.

LAT PULLDOWN

Muscles Targeted: Latissimus dorsi and biceps

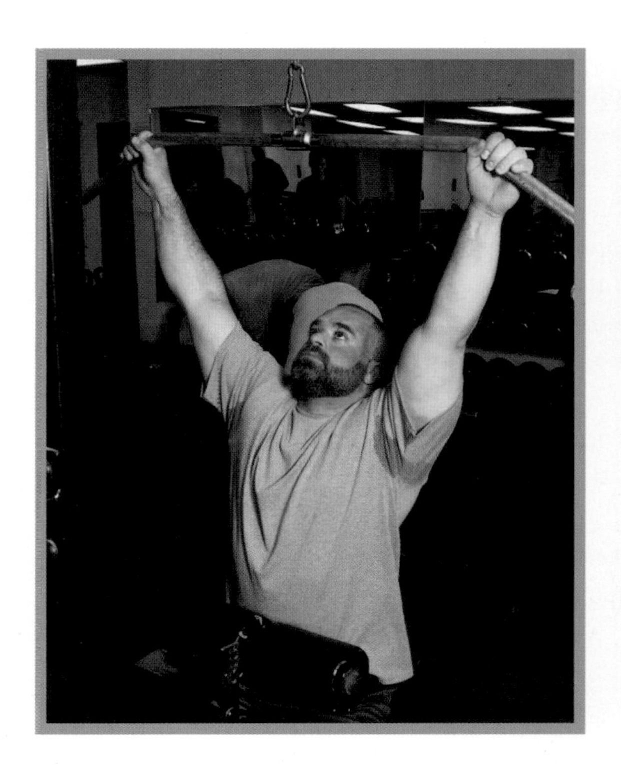

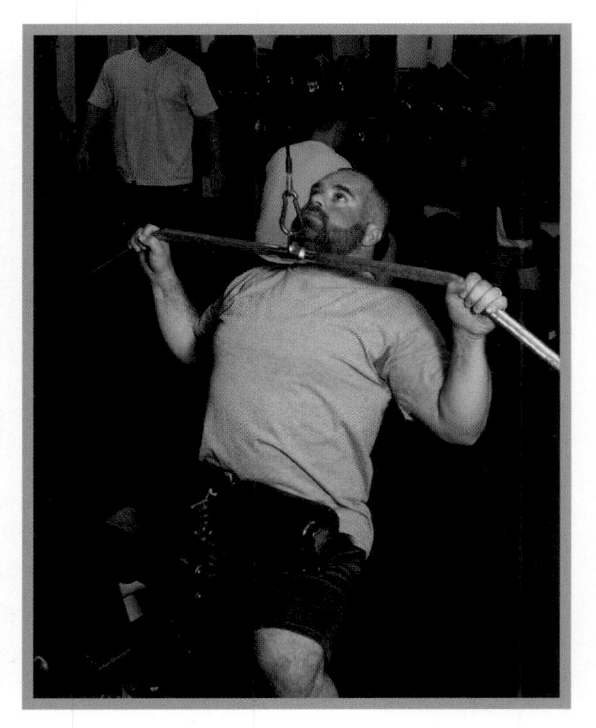

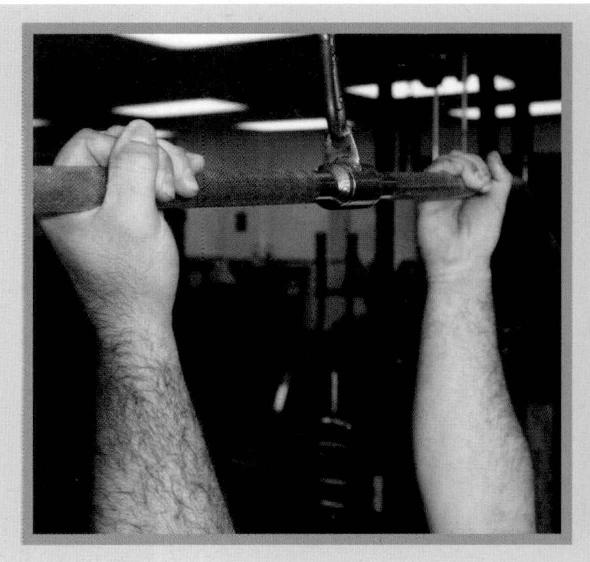

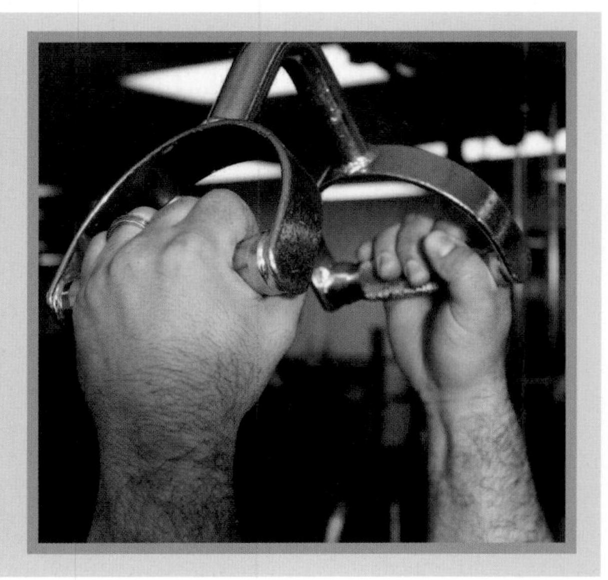

The lat pulldown is a standard machine with little variation from model to model. The basic pulldown machine is essentially a cable machine with a high pulley, a seat, and a pad to hold you in place during the exercise.

Set-Up

Lean back onto the back pad of the sled with your shoulders against the two shoul-Most pulldown machines have a pad over the seat that locks your legs into place during the exercise and prevents the weights from actually lifting you off of the seat. If it is adjustable you'll want to start by setting it to the correct height. Just sit on the seat facing the machine and pull the pad down so that it covers your thighs. It should be snug, but not tight.

Once you've set the pad to the correct height, stand up and grab the bar overhead. Still holding the cable handle, Sit back down (the weight will slow your descent) and place your thighs back under the pad. With the cable attachment still at arm's length, pull your shoulder blades down and back and lift your chest up. This is your start position.

The Exercise

Unlike most machines and all free weight exercises, you are actually lifting the weight as the bar/handle descends. Pull the bar down, keeping your shoulder blades together and lifting your chest as you pull. You can lean back slightly, but don't lean excessively to try to use momentum to pull the weight. A few degrees is okay. When the weight touches your upper chest, just below the collarbone begin the ascent.

Return the handle to the start position in a smooth and controlled movement. At the end of the set, stand up before letting go of the handle in order to avoid slamming the weight stack.

Variations

You can vary the lat pulldown either by changing your grip on the pulldown bar, or swapping the bar for another attachment entirely. By taking a shoulder-width underhand grip, the bar will recruit more of your biceps, and usually allow you to handle a bit more weight.

You can also switch the long bar out for a v-grip, which will let you take a close, parallel grip. This grip also recruits more biceps than the overhand wide grip, and will also give you more of a stretch in your latissimus.

MACHINE OVERHEAD PRESS

Muscles Targeted: Deltoid, triceps, and pectorals

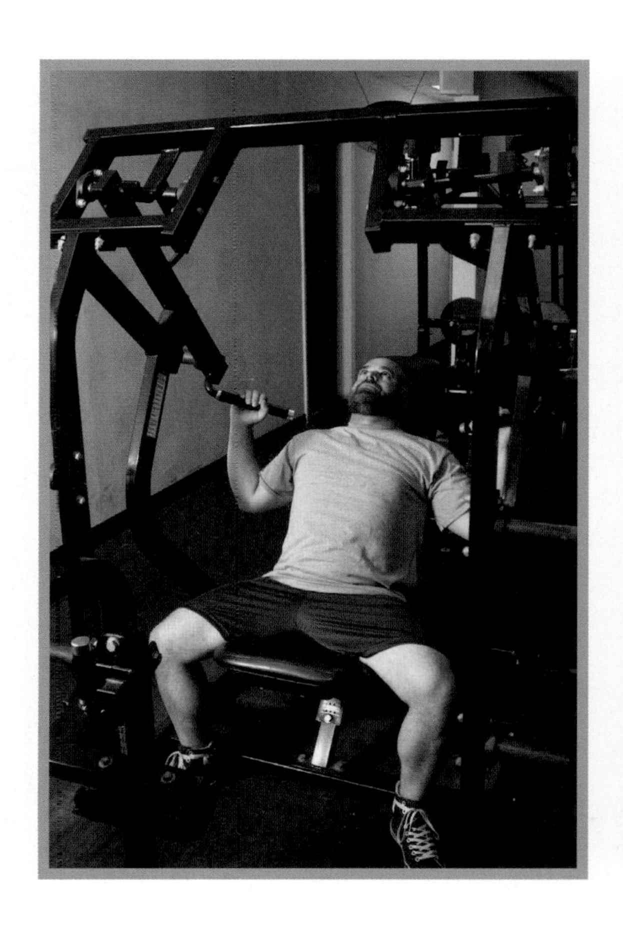

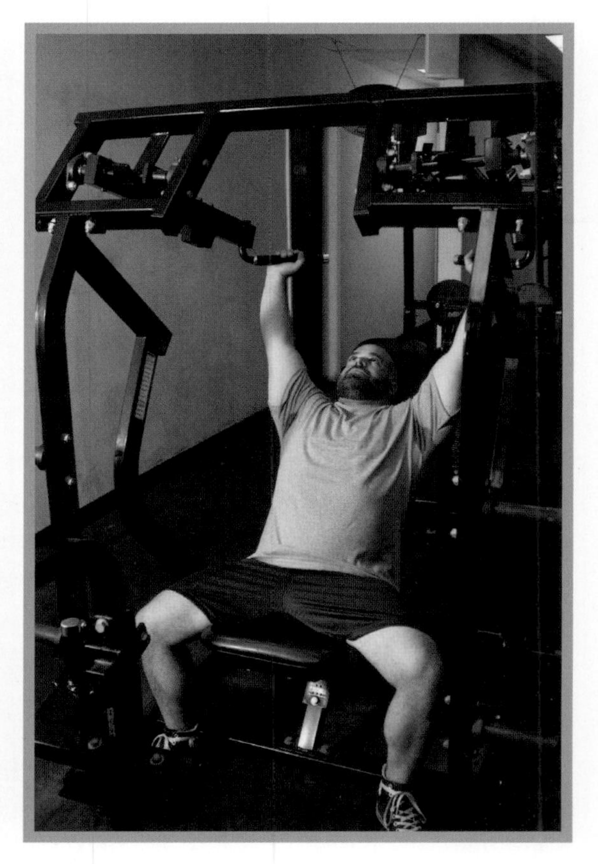

Aside from the weight loading mechanism, most overhead press machines, either selectorized or plate loaded, have an almost identical operation. The main difference will be that the plate-loaded version's handles will usually move independently of each other, while the selectorized version will usually have both handles attached to the same cam so that they move together.

Set-Up

Most overhead press machines will have an adjustable seat. Before starting the exercise, adjust the seat so that the handles are level with the top of your shoulders. Before pressing the handles overhead, pull your shoulder blades down and lift your chest.

Place your feet flat on the floor in a wide stance so that you can use them to brace yourself during the exercise.

The Exercise

Press the handles overhead to arm's length and pause for a second before lowering the handles down to the start position.

Variations

Most overhead press machines will have handles for either wide, overhand grip or a palms-in parallel grip.

MACHINE ROW

Muscles Targeted: Latissimus dorsi, biceps, rhomboids, and rear deltoids

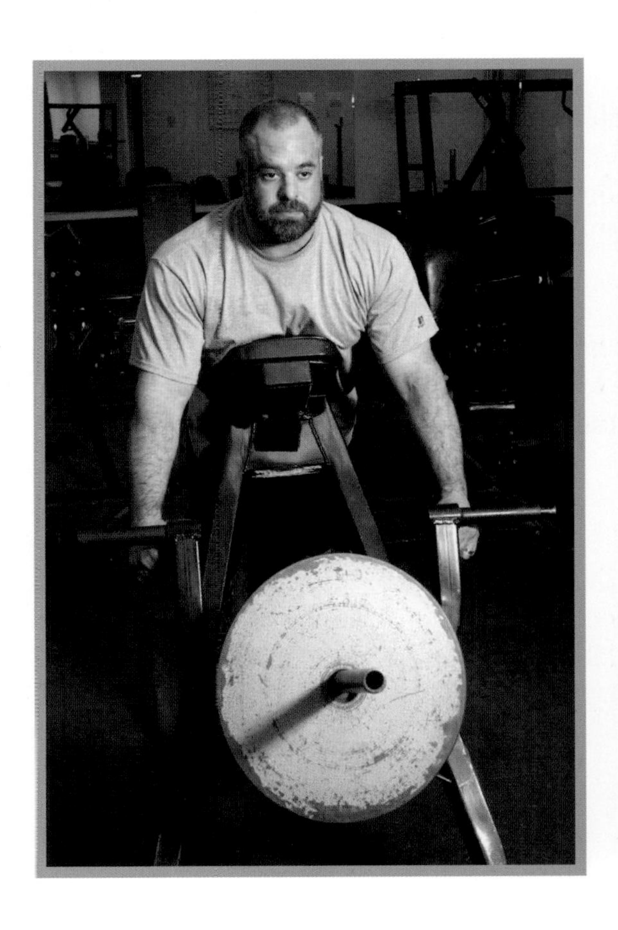

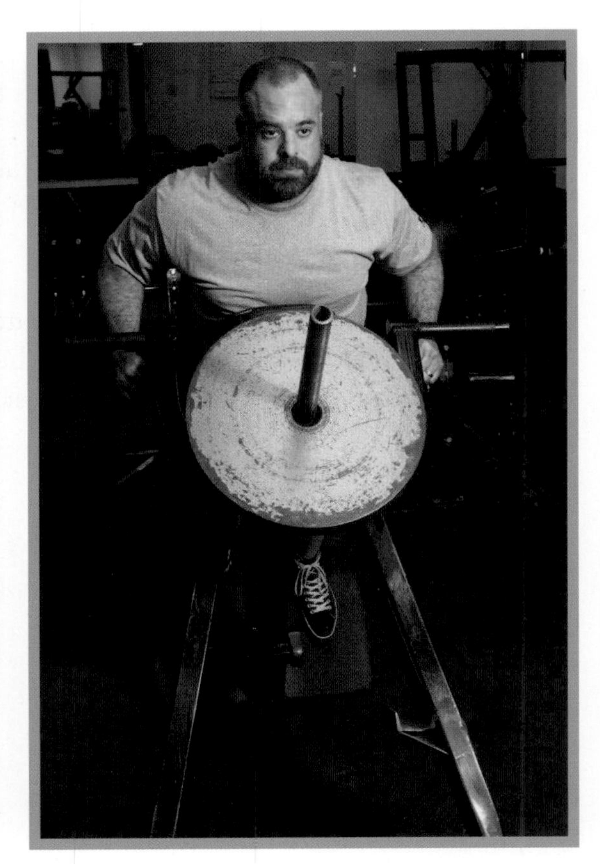

Aside from the weight loading mechanism, most row machines, either selectorized or plate loaded, have almost identical operation. The main difference will be that the plate-loaded version's handles will usually move independently of each other, while the selectorized version will usually have both handles attached to the same cam so that they move together.

Set-Up

Sit on the machine with your chest against the support pad and your arms outstretched toward the handles. The handles should be just far enough away that you can touch them with your fingers, but not quite the palm of your hands. Keep your chest flush against the pad. If the handles are not the correct distance, you should be able to adjust either the handles or pad until they are. Your hands should also be about even with your mid-chest. If not, you should be able to adjust the seat height.

To get into the start position, reach forward and grasp the handles, one hand at a time. Lift your chest up and pull your shoulder blades back. This is the start position.

The Exercise

As with most machines, there is no descent before the start of the exercise. Keeping your upper back and your chest up, pull the handles toward your chest until your hands are at about chest level. After a brief pause, return the handles to arm's length.

Variations

Most row machines will have handles for either wide, overhand grip, or a palms-in parallel grip. The wider overhand grip will focus more on your upper back, including rear deltoid/rhomboid area, while the parallel grip will recruit more biceps.

SMITH MACHINE PUSH-UP

Muscles Targeted: Pectorals, triceps, and deltoids

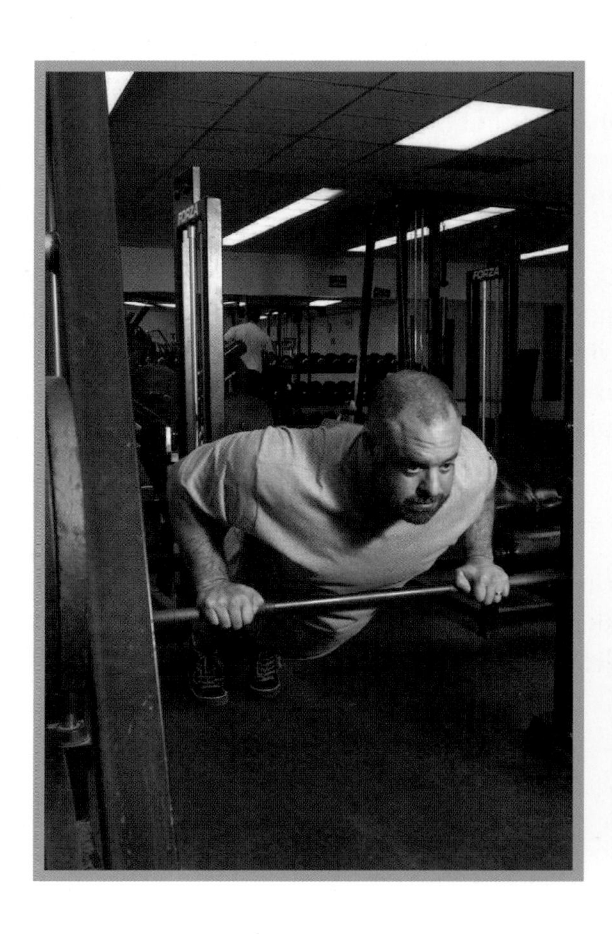

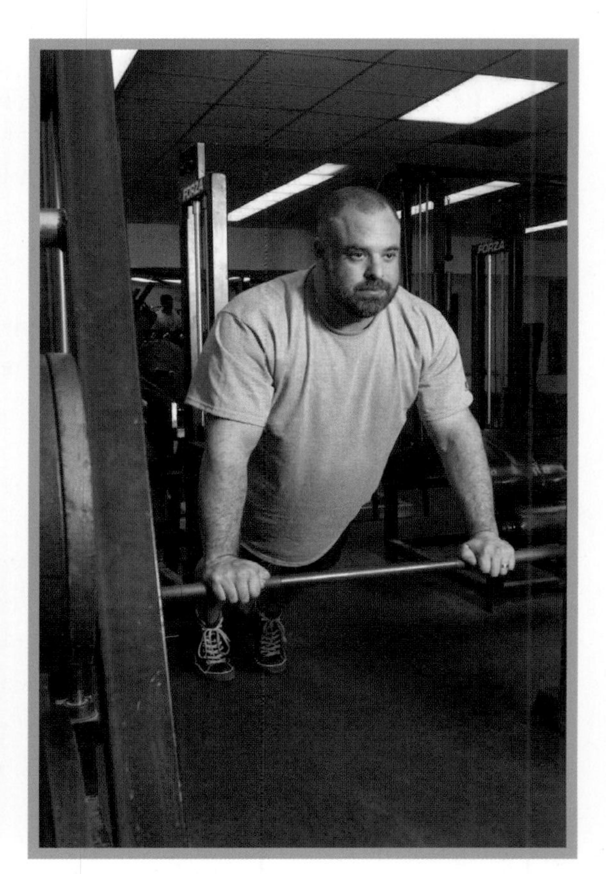

The Smith machine push-up utilizes the barbell in a fixed position to provide variable resistance in the push-up. Since many beginners are unable to perform 10 to 15 push-ups, the Smith machine allows you to change the angle on the exercise, subtracting body weight until you develop the strength necessary to perform them from the floor.

Grasping the bar is also more comfortable for most people than placing the hands on the floor because it allows you to maintain a neutral wrist.

Set-Up

Set the bar anywhere from 1 to 3 feet from the floor. To change the height of the bar, lift it up an inch or so, then twist it so that the hooks disengage from the frame. Move the bar up or down to your desired height, then twist the bar back to re-engage the hooks. Most Smith machines have pegs every four inches or so to allow you to rack the bar at any height you wish.

The higher you rack the bar, the lower the percentage of your body weight you'll be lifting and the easier the push-up will be.

To get into the start position, grasp the bar with an overhand grip and your hands slightly wider than shoulder width. Walk your feet back so that you are supporting your body weight evenly between your feet on the floor and your hands on the bar. When your arms are about perpendicular to your body and your body is straight, you are ready to go.

The Exercise

Keeping your chest up and your head neutral, lower yourself to the bar by bending your arms. When you reach the bottom position, the bar should touch your chest at about the mid-chest level. If you touch too low, you will need to walk your feet a step or two backward. If you touch too high, walk your feet a step or two forward.

Keeping your chest up and your head neutral, press yourself back up to arm's length.

Variations

You can perform the Smith machine push-up with a wider grip to focus more on your chest, or with a narrower grip which will put more emphasis on your triceps. If you do not have access to a Smith machine, you can just place a standard barbell in a standard rack at your desired height and use that. Since only gravity will be holding the bar in the rack, it would be a good idea to put at least one 45-pound plate on each side to make the bar a bit more stable in the rack.

ASSISTED PULL-UP

Muscles Targeted: Latissimus dorsi and biceps

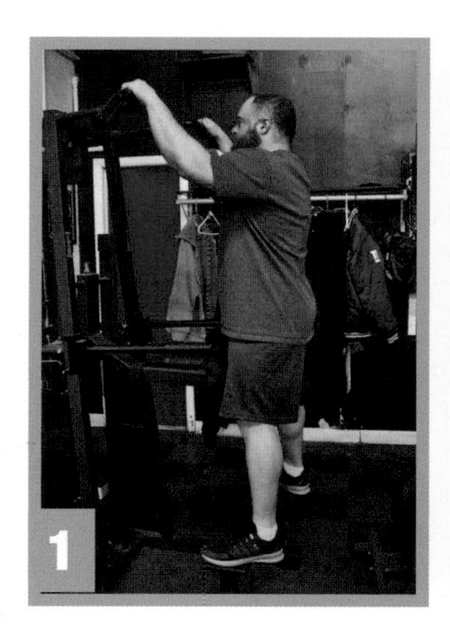

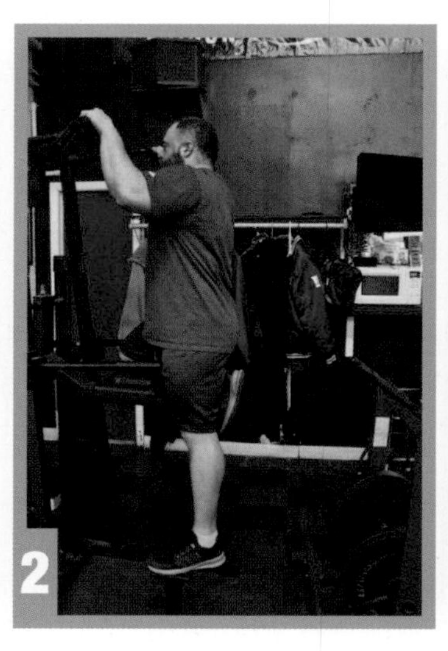

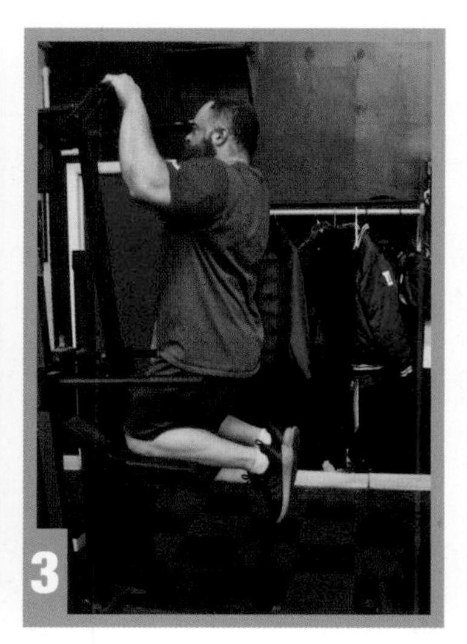

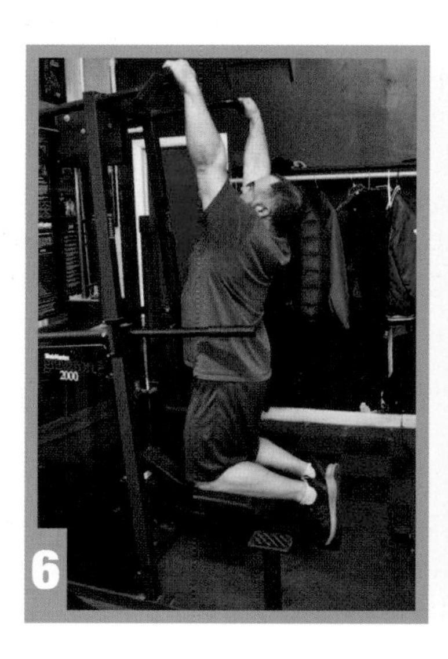

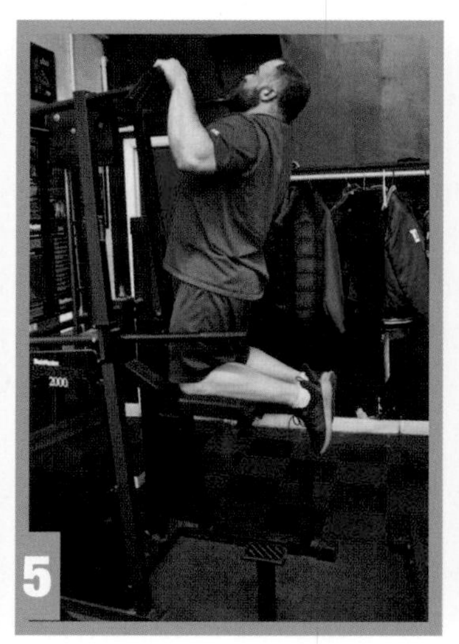

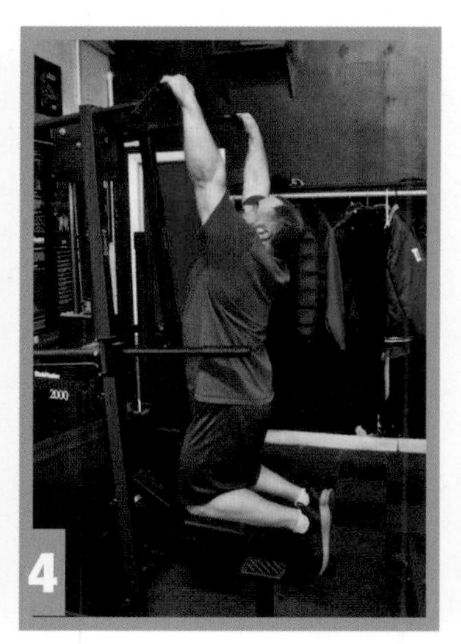

The assisted pull-up machine is unique in that the weight stack does not provide resistance against you as it does in other machines. Instead, the resistance is used to assist you in performing body weight exercises that you would otherwise be unable to perform, either at all or in the necessary rep range.

Usually combined with parallel bars for dips, assisted pull-up machines usually consist of a platform that you either stand or kneel on, a bar or handles to pull yourself up to, and the weight stack which gives you the resistance. A few years ago, assisted pull-up machines using an air compressor/hydraulic system were popular, and they can still be found in some older gyms, but these have largely been phased out by the more compact, less expensive plate-loaded version.

Set-Up

The assisted pull-up is easily the most difficult machine to set up on the first time you try; however, once you get the hang of it, it won't be a big deal.

The most important factor to remember about the assisted pull-up is that since the weight assists you, the higher the weight you select on the stack, the *easier* the exercise will be. In order to get a feel for the machine the first time you use it, start with a lot of weight assistance, gradually lowering the weight until you are at a comfortable (but sufficiently challenging) training weight.

Most assisted dip machines have a couple of steps leading up to the platform. Step to the highest step and grasp the pull-up handles.

Make sure you are holding the handles tightly before trying to step onto the platform! Remember that the platform will move once you step on it, so you must be prepared to hold yourself up with the handles.

Once the handles are firmly in hand, carefully step onto the platform, allowing it to descend under your weight. As the platform drops, you should notice the weight stack rising, which means the weight will assist you on the way back up. When you are supporting all of your body weight between the handles and the platform, you will be ready to begin the exercise.

The Exercise

With your head and chest up, pull yourself up toward the handles until your chin is about level with your hands. Pause briefly and lower yourself back down to the bottom position, still keeping a firm grip on the handles.

In order to get off, it's usually easier to step back onto the step at the top of your last repetition.

Variations

Most row machines will have handles for a wide grip, overhand grip, or a palms-in parallel grip. The wider overhand grip will focus more on your upper back, including rear deltoid/rhomboid area, while the parallel grip will recruit more biceps.

SMITH MACHINE OVERHEAD PRESS

Muscles Targeted: Deltoids and triceps

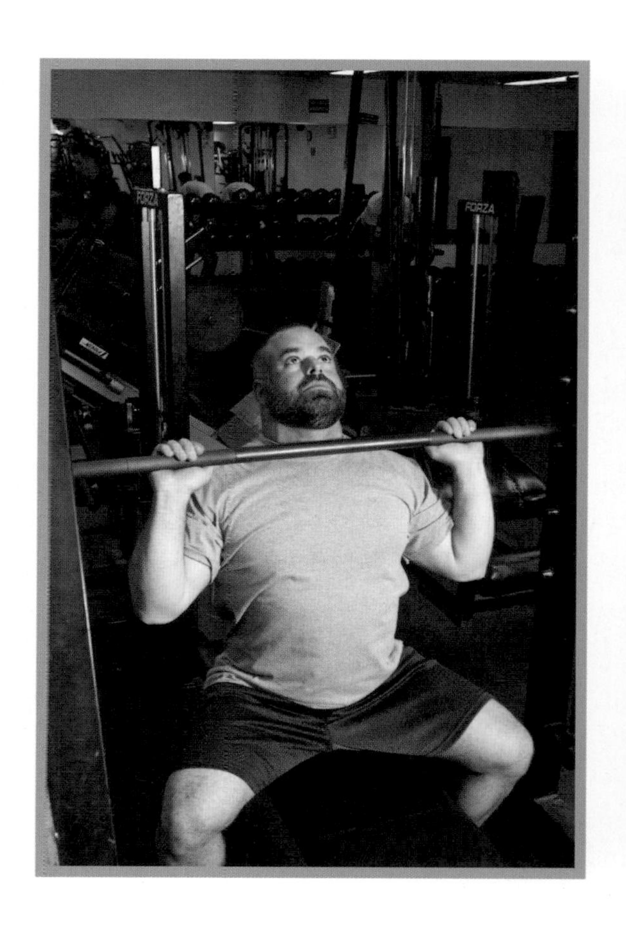

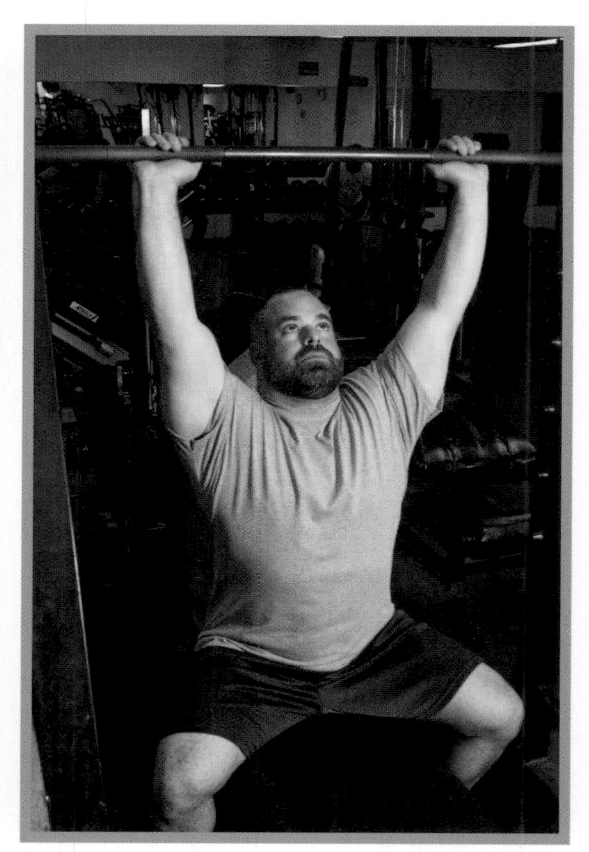

The Smith machine is a multipurpose machine that can be found in most weight rooms and fitness centers. Relatively simple in design, the Smith machine is essentially a fixed barbell that moves up and down on a track, usually counter-weighted so that the empty bar weighs less than a standard 45-pound barbell. To add resistance, you will slide standard plates on and off the outer sleeve of the bar, just like you would a regular barbell.

The Smith machine is a common machine in most fitness facilities because of its versatility. You can do almost any exercise on it that requires a straight up and down bar path. While still inferior to free weights for serious strength training (due to the decrease in neuromuscular stimulus common to most machines) it can be a useful tool for beginners and certain assistance exercises for more advanced lifters.

Set-Up

The overhead press can be performed either sitting or standing, however most Smith machines are not tall enough for a standing overhead press. I recommend using an adjustable bench set at the highest incline, however if you do not have access to one, you can also sit up straight on a flat bench.

To ease the stress on your shoulders I recommend starting with the bar at arm's length, rather than shoulder height. It's much easier on your musculature to start the lift with the descent, as opposed to grinding out of a dead stop at the bottom position. For the sake of ease, make sure you adjust the bar height *before* loading it with weights.

To change the height of the bar, as well as rack and unrack it, lift it up an inch or so, then twist it so that the hooks disengage from the frame. Move the bar up or down to your desired height, then twist the bar back to re-engage the hooks. Most Smith machines have pegs every four inches or so to allow you to rack the bar at any height you wish.

Once you have your bench and bar height set up, load the desired weight onto the bar and sit on the bench, under the bar. The bar should not be directly overhead, but slightly to the front so that when you lower it, it will just clear your face.

Before unracking the weight, get set by grasping the bar with your hands just wider than shoulder width. Lift your head and chin up, and pull your shoulder blades down and back to stabilize your shoulder girdle. If using an incline bench, keep your upper back in contact with the bench throughout the entire set.

Unrack the weight by pressing up and twisting the bar just enough to release the hooks.

The Exercise

Lower the weight to just below the chin. Throughout the descent, keep your elbows directly under the bar.

Once the bar dips below your chin, press it back up to arm's length. Upon completion of the set, twist the bar to engage the hooks and re-rack it.

SMITH MACHINE INVERTED ROW

Muscles Targeted: Latissimus, rear deltoids, and biceps

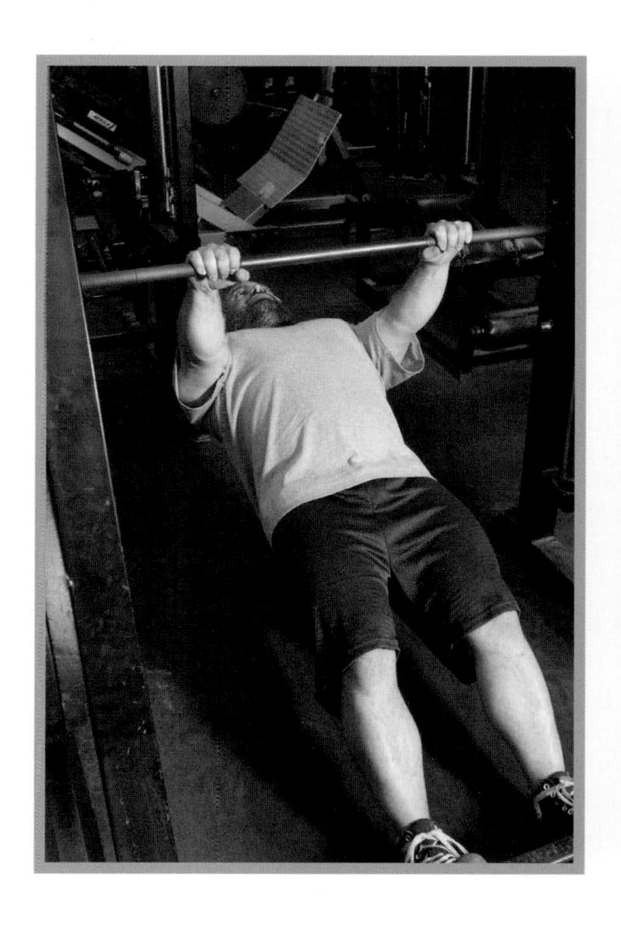

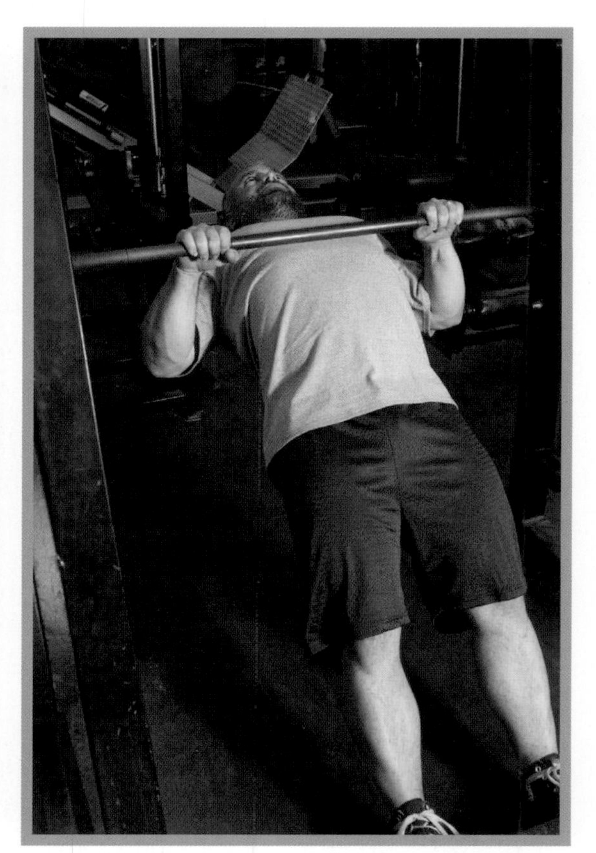

Similar to the Smith machine push-up, the inverted row uses the fixed barbell as means to support your body weight at various heights.

The inverted row is somewhat of a cross between the pull-up and the barbell row. Like the pull-up, you are using your own body weight for resistance. However, the actual plane of motion is closer to the barbell row, because you are pulling the bar toward your chest. The inverted row can be used as its own exercise, or as a way to transition into full pull-ups.

Set-Up

Most people will set the bar a notch or two higher for inverted rows than they will for Smith machine push-ups. Grasp the bar with your hands a little wider than shoulder width apart. Holding onto the bar tightly enough to support your weight, walk your feet forward until your arms are straight and the bar is over your mid chest.

Before starting the lift, pull your shoulder blades together and lift your chin and chest.

The Exercise

Keeping your shoulder blades pulled together and your chin up, pull yourself up toward the bar. The bar should touch your torso at the middle of your chest (an inch or two below your armpits). If the bar touches much higher than this, walk your feet back a few steps. If it touches too low, walk forward a few steps.

BACK EXTENSION MACHINE

Muscles Targeted: Glutes, lower back, and hamstrings

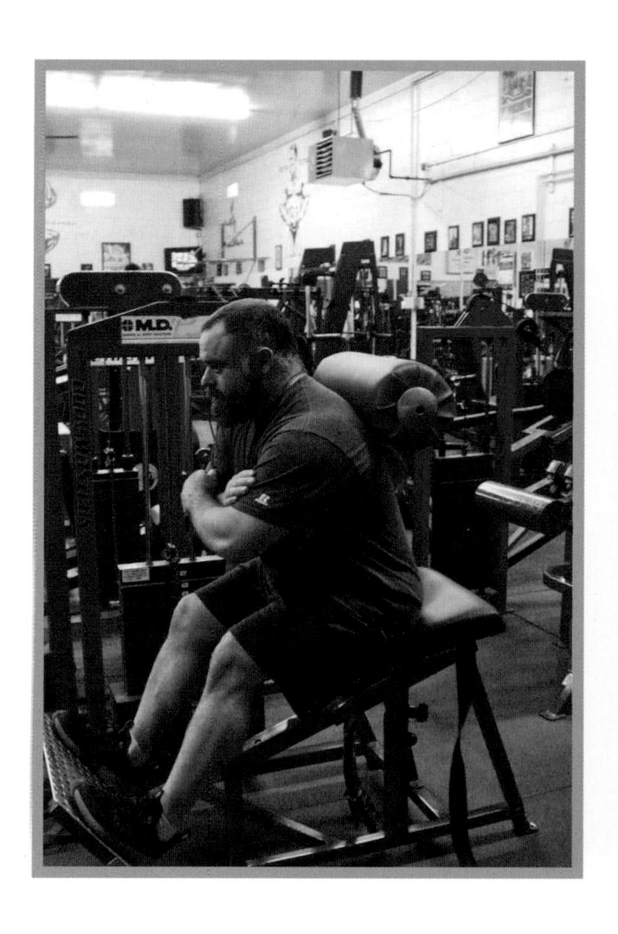

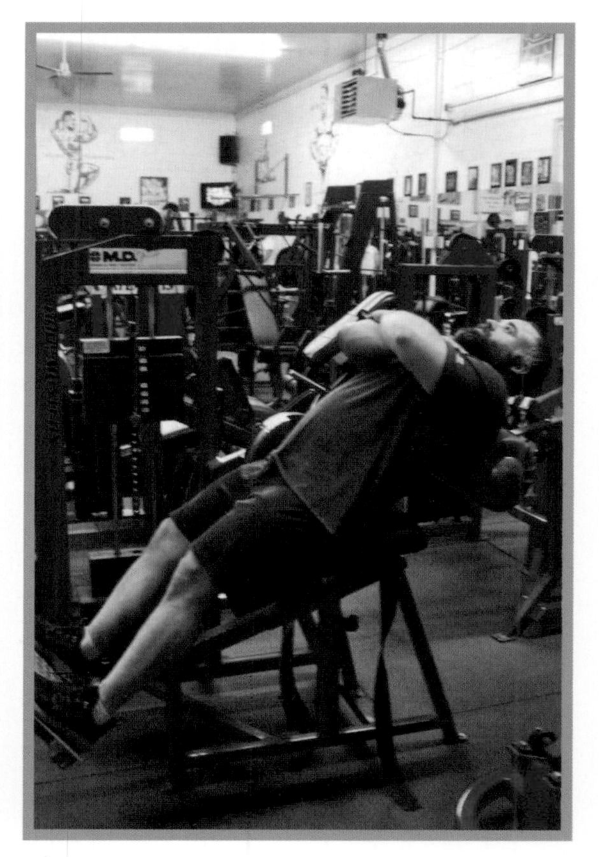

Unlike most of the machines on this list, the lower-back machine is usually selectorized, and rarely has a plate-loaded counterpart.

Set-Up

Sit on the machine with your back against the pad. On most machines, the pad should be across your upper back. There may also be a seatbelt to keep your hips from bucking up during the exercise. At the start position, your hips should be at about a 45-degree angle and your spine should be neutral (straight). Cross your arms in front of you and lift your elbows to cue yourself to keep your chest up. There will usually be a small platform to put your feet on.

The Exercise

Keeping your chest up, push back on the pad until your hips are fully extended. Do not try to extend past 180 degrees. Pause briefly and return to the start position

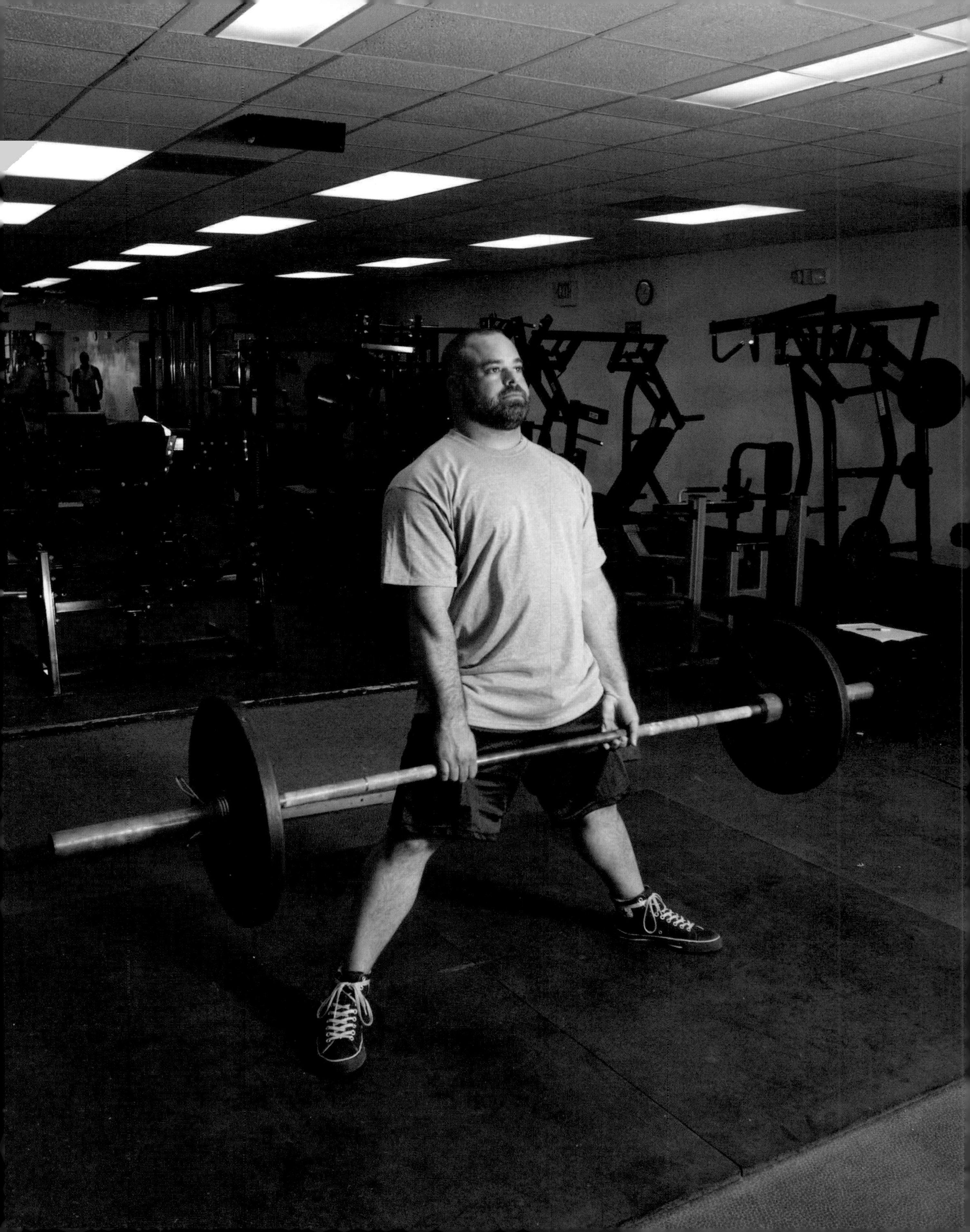

MAIN LIFTS

Once you are through with the Introductory Cycle, which primarily focuses on machines, you will begin the transition to a free-weight based program. While machine exercises can serve a purpose throughout your lifting career, most experts on strength training agree that a free-weight based program will ultimately produce better results, in less time.

However, the trade-off for this increased efficacy is that free weights require more attention to technique than machines do. Pay attention to the exercise descriptions, and if you have any doubt you are performing an exercise correctly, either plug in a similar exercise as a substitute, or find someone qualified to take a look at your form.

In today's age of smart-phones and tablets, take advantage of your device's camera, and record yourself performing a main lift periodically to make sure you are doing it correctly.

Beginning with the Intermediate Cycle, these main lifts will serve as the foundation of your programming.

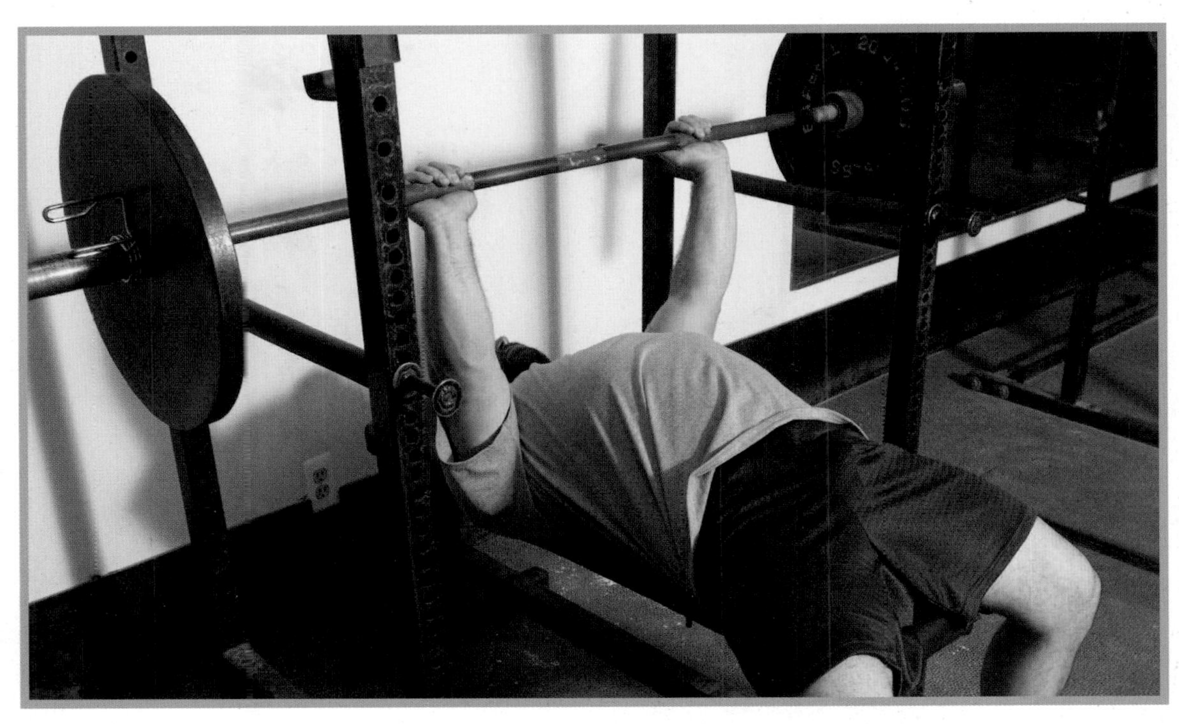

SQUAT

The Foundation of Strength Training

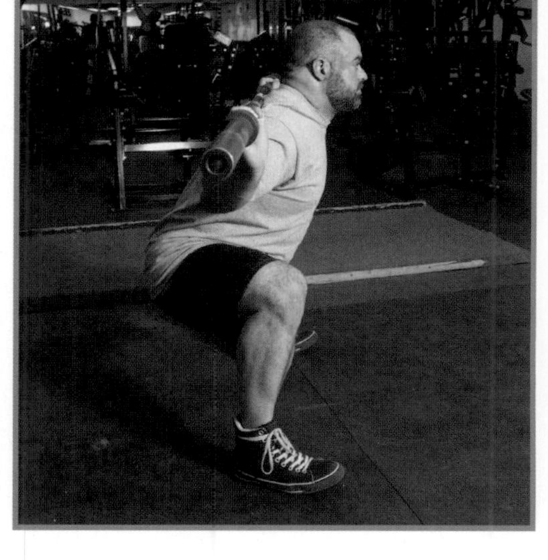

It all starts with the squat—quite simply, the king of the lower body lifts. While it is true that some people have gotten strong without squatting, many more have gotten strong by relying on the squat and its variations. Unfortunately, the squat is a lift that is commonly performed incorrectly. Even many experienced trainers do not teach the squat properly. By performing the squat correctly you will not only improve the strength of your legs, but also your back, hips, glutes, and abdominals.

One of the most common mistakes made while squatting is allowing the knees to move forward over the toes. This action not only increases stress on the knee joints, but also prevents activation of the hips and back muscles.

A correct squat is similar to sitting down in a chair but without actually settling on it. Many people find it hard to squat without lifting their heels off the floor. This can frequently be corrected by slightly lifting your big toes. Other mistakes include looking down and allowing the knees to track inward. Keep the eyes looking straight ahead by giving them a focus point and keep the knees in line with (but not drifting in front of) the toes.

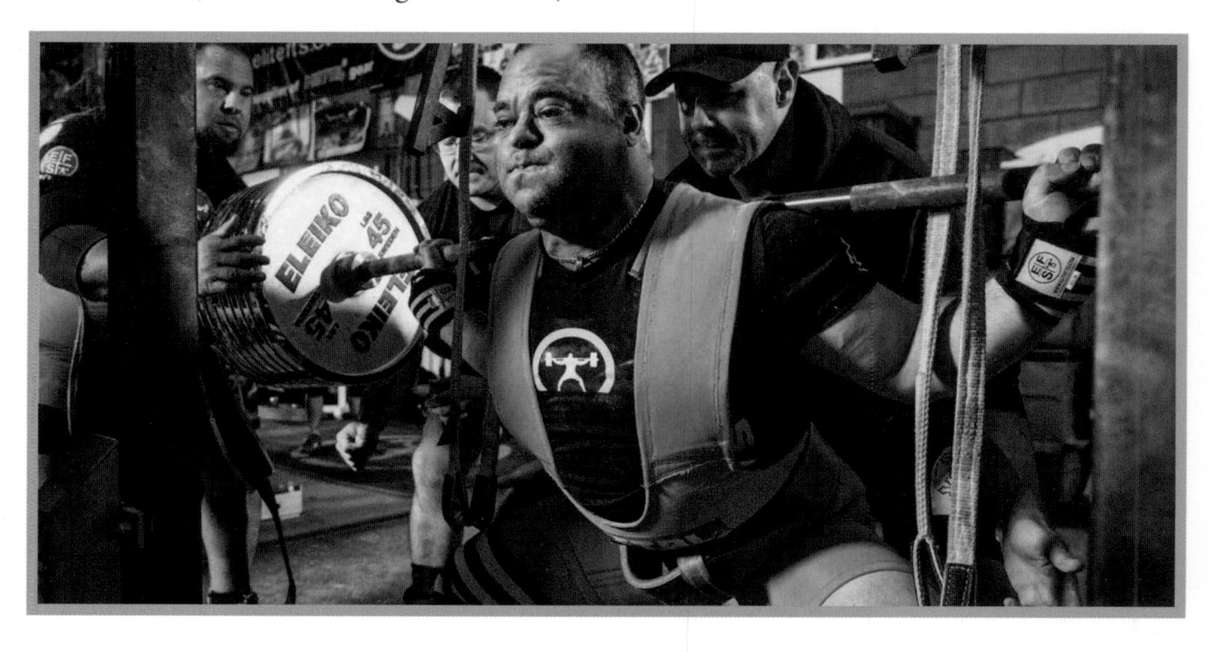

Finding Parallel

Of all the mistakes made during the many variations of the squat, the most common is squatting "high." By this, I mean stopping before you have reached parallel. Breaking parallel is defined as the crease of the hip dipping below the top of the knee. Many trainers avoid teaching the full squat for fear of knee injury, but with some simple corrections the full squat is perfectly safe. The full squat is a natural position for the human knee.

The problem is that due to sedentary lifestyle, many adults lack the hip flexibility necessary to reach a full squat position. By improving flexibility, most people should be capable of squatting correctly. In our opinion high squatting is more dangerous because it allows you to use heavier weights than you should be using, and it does not recruit the muscles and joints through their full range of motion.

TO PAD OR NOT TO PAD?

Many gyms have foam tubes that fit over the bar to make squatting more comfortable. Since power racks in most gyms are used by the general population for curling rather than squatting, you can typically find these pads on Smith machine bars. While many lifters feel the pad makes the exercise more comfortable, there is a cost to this comfort. Putting anything between you and the bar limits tactile feedback from the bar and increases the likelihood that the bar will roll off, especially in an unsecured foam tube. By relying on your upper back muscles to carry the bar, you will learn to find the "sweet spot," where the bar feels most comfortable and secure. This is much safer than the false sense of comfort the pad provides. Also, keep in mind that the pad forces you to carry the bar higher, making your torso a longer lever arm and making it more difficult to maintain a neutral spine throughout the squat.

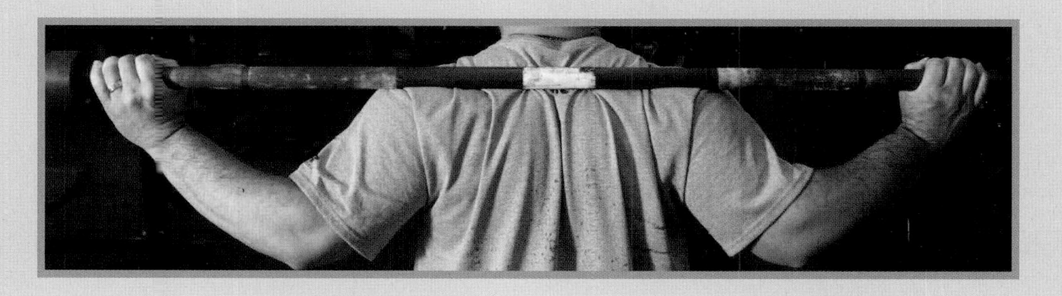

BARBELL SQUAT

Muscles Targeted: Glutes, Lower back, Hamstrings, and Quadriceps

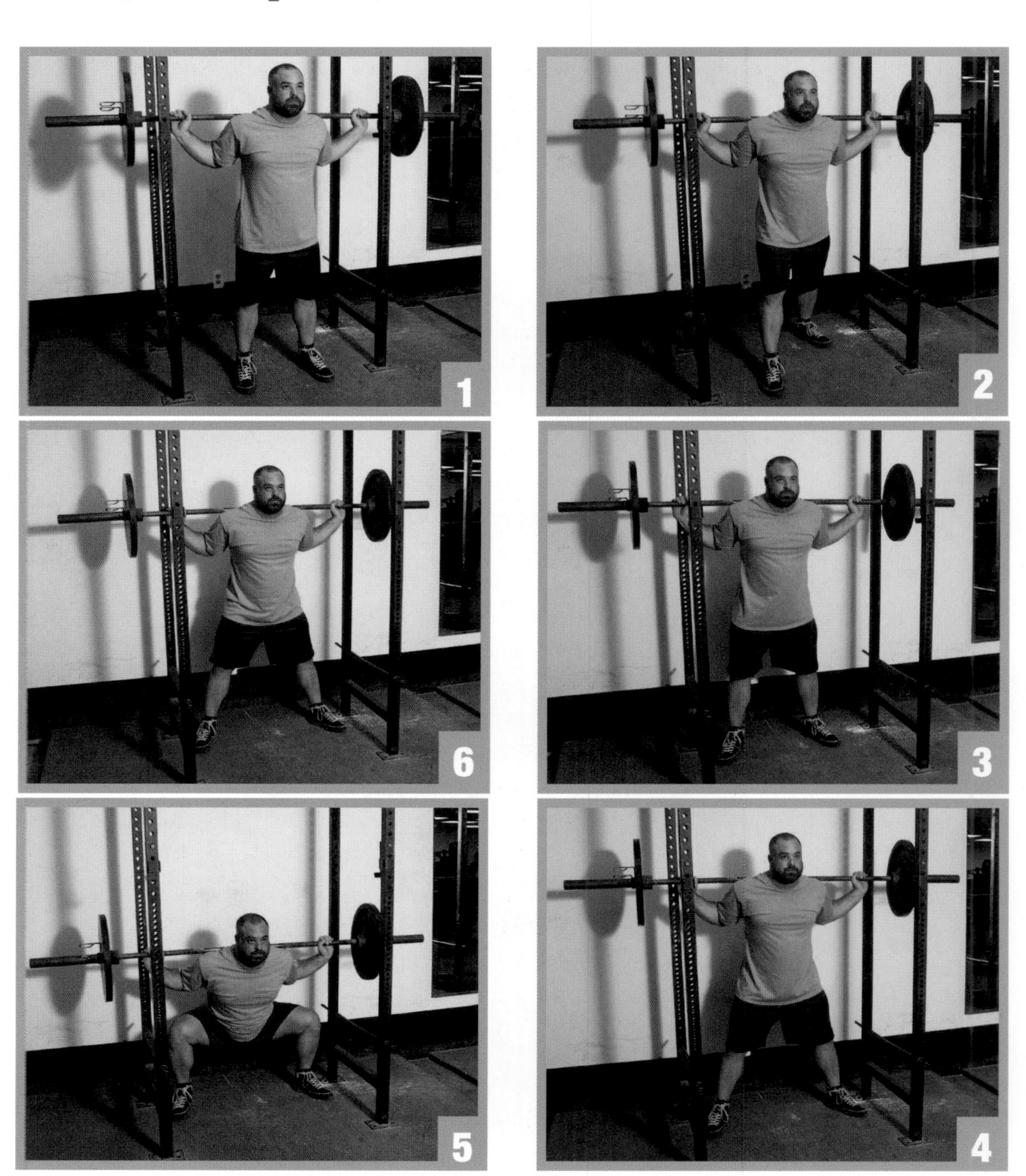

There's a reason that the standard barbell squat is the foundation of just about every serious strength program. It's because it just may be the single most effective exercise for gaining muscular size and strength. While I normally shy away from referring to an exercise as the "best" at anything, the squat just might be the exception. If you polled most strength coaches and asked them which exercise they would choose if they could only use one, the barbell squat would probably come out on top.

Despite the affinity most training experts hold for the squat, the exercise remains both underused and/or corrupted by the general fitness crowd. On the rare occasion you see someone squatting in the average fitness center, it's usually with terrible technique, eliminating most (if not all) of the benefits from this exercise. In fact, for every 100 commercial gym members I've seen perform the squat, fewer than 10 got it even close to correct.

Common mistakes include (but are certainly not limited to):

- Failing to squat to the correct depth
- Upper or lower back rounding out
- Knees collapsing inward or excessively forward
- Heels lifting off the floor

Set-Up

One of the most common errors I see in the squat occurs before the lift even starts. Setting up is a critical skill that, due to either over-psyching or carelessness, most beginners rush through. A strong, steady set-up sets up the rest of the lift because it cues you to start the lift properly.

Hand Position

The first step in unracking the bar is to set your hands. The closer to center you can keep your hands on the barbell, the more stable the shelf you can create with your upper back. Lots of lifters, however, opt to keep their hands wider to lessen the stress to their shoulders. Most will do best with their hands somewhere between having the pinkie and the pointer finger on the line on a standard power bar, although very large people may need to go wider. You'll need to experiment to find what is most comfortable for youth.

Foot Position

Before even placing the bar across your shoulders, I recommend setting your feet where you'll want them for the unrack. An easy way to do this is to place your chest against the center of the bar with your feet slightly forward, so that the bar is over the center of your feet. Your stance will be closer for the unrack than it will be for the squat itself, so set them at about 12 inches apart.

Setting your feet too wide can result in a side-to-side motion during walkout which will cause the plates to bump against the rack. Setting your feet before you place the bar on your back helps you to be sure that the bar will be centered on your back, because you can see where your feet are in relation to the middle of the bar.

Bar Position

Next, keeping your feet where they are, set the bar across your upper back. *Do not rest the bar across your neck!* Instead, pull your shoulder blades together, creating a "shelf" for the bar to rest on. If you set the bar too high, you will place too much pressure on the cervical vertebrae which will make you more likely to round out your upper back. If you set the bar too low, you'll likely wind up flopping over at the bottom of the squat to keep it from slipping off of your back.

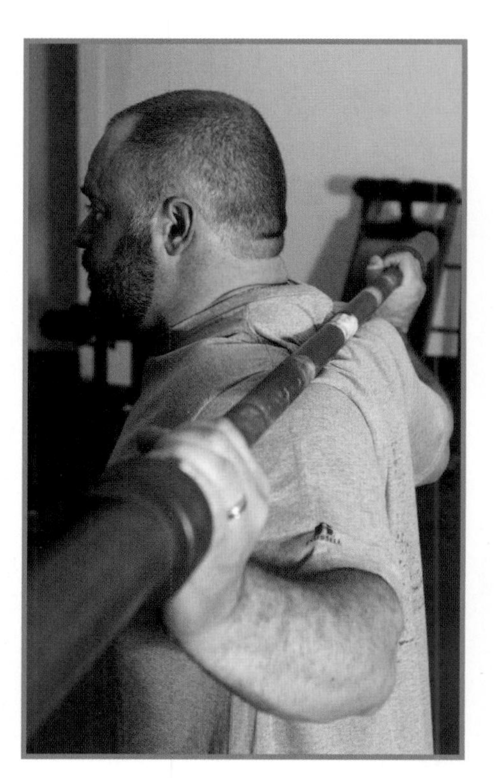

Your elbows should be pointed at a downward angle and remain there for the duration of the lift.

A very common novice mistake is to point the elbows backward during the squat. Not only is this bad for the shoulders, but it also creates a poor foundation for the bar to rest on and makes it easier for you to round out in the bottom of the squat. Having the elbows pointing straight back usually results from holding the bar too low across your back.

The Unrack

Take a deep breath into your belly, and hold it as you unrack the weight. Lift the bar out by pushing your hips forward and arching it out. You should be performing the unrack primarily with your hips, and using minimal knee flexion/extension to move the weight. Unracking the bar with your knees will cue you to squat into your knees, rather than your bigger, stronger hips. Pause for a moment to allow the weight to settle on your back.

Do not step back until you are totally stable under the weight.

The Walk-Out

Once you've stabilized under the weight, begin your walk-out. When you're walking backward with a heavy barbell on your back, efficiency is the name of the game. Any unnecessary movement is wasted energy that you could have saved for the squat itself.

An efficient walk-out should only require three steps.

1. Keep a straight back
2. Move back and out to the side
3. Move out to the other side, leaving your stance at a few inches wider than shoulder width.

The Descent

Once you've stabilized after the walk-out, take another deep breath into your belly, and begin your descent.

Start the descent by arching your back and pushing your hips back, as if you were about to sit in a chair. I recommend breaking the hips slowly and deliberately at first, in order to be sure you are squatting into your hips. I also prefer a slow initial break because it is extremely difficult to correct any mistakes once the descent has started.

Breaking the hips quickly can easily throw you off balance. After you've descended a few inches, you can pick up a little speed in order to conserve energy and gain some rebound out of the bottom position. While you will need to relax your hips somewhat in order to descend, your torso should remain tight and ridged. Loosening up on the descent can cause you to round over when you try to reverse your direction.

Keep your chest up and drive your gaze slightly above eye level for the entire descent.

The Ascent

When you know you've hit depth (either by feel, or by a training partner's call), reverse the process to stand up. Keep your head and chest up, drive your belly out, and push your hips forward as you stand up. You should be holding your breath for each entire repetition, taking a breath between reps when you are standing up straight.

When you gain control over the weight at the top, take another deep breath and begin your next descent. Upon completion of the set, take another moment to settle, and walk back into

BOX SQUAT

Muscles Targeted: Glutes, lower back, hamstrings, and quadriceps

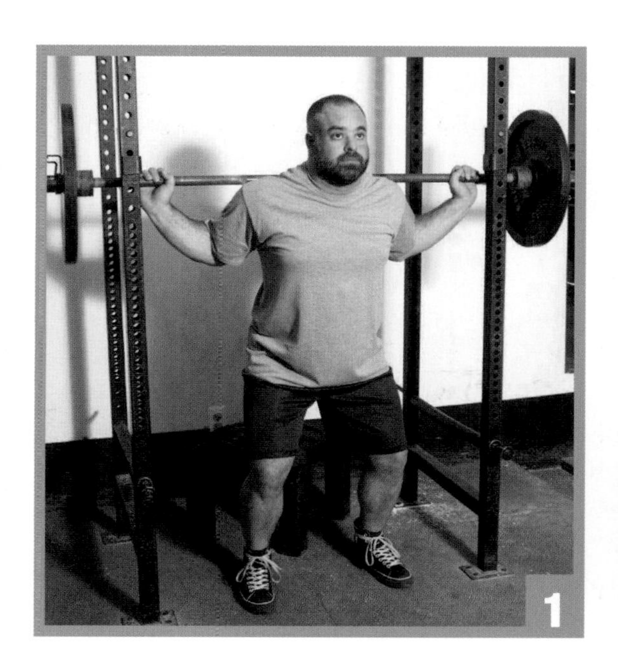

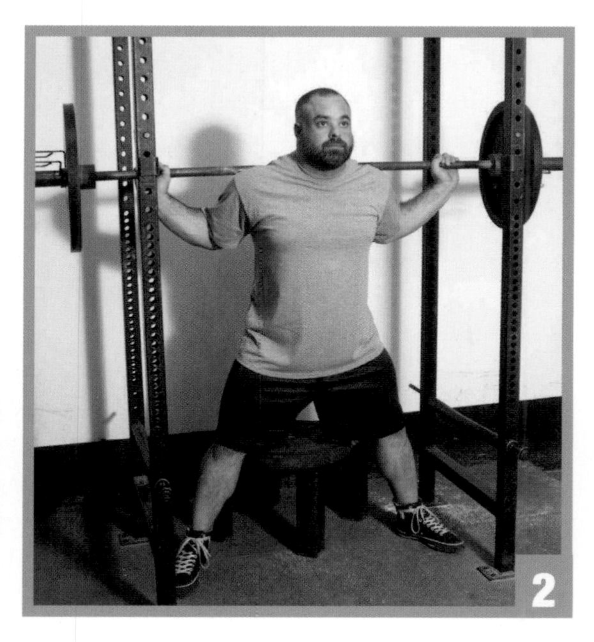

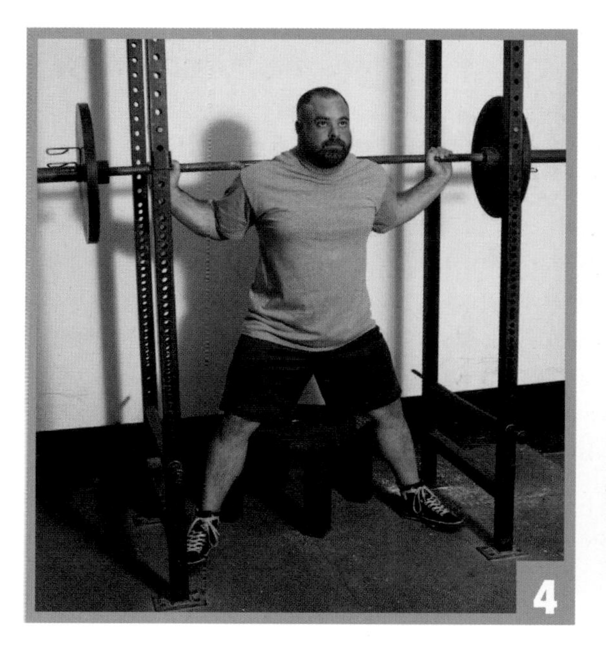

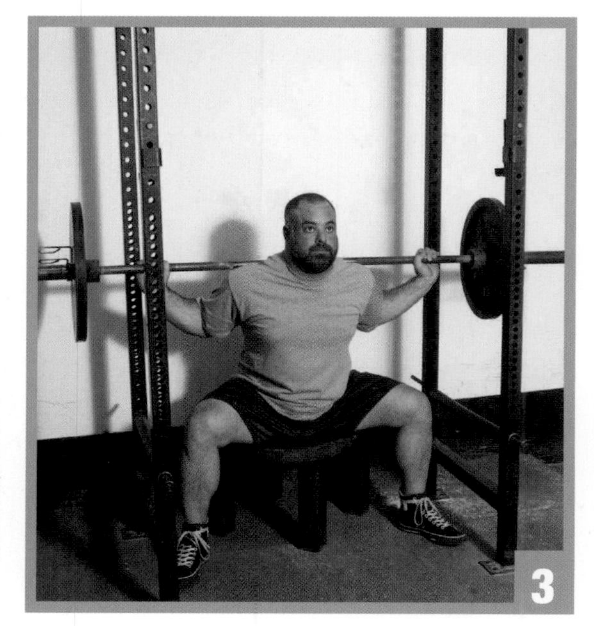

The box squat is an excellent tool for both learning the traditional squat and strengthening the necessary muscles in a similar recruitment pattern. Countless elite powerlifters have used the box squat to perfect their squat technique because when properly executed, the box squat allows you to exaggerate the technical cues used in the traditional squat.

In addition to the barbell and rack, you will need a sturdy platform to sit on. Plyometric boxes, or specially built box squat platforms, are best, but homemade wood boxes topped with mats will also work well. The reason box squats are so effective is that the sitting motion is essentially an exaggerated squat. Another advantage to this exercise is that you will hit the desired depth every time.

Set-Up

Place the box or platform about two feet behind the squat rack and set up exactly as you would for a typical barbell squat. The box should be set at a height that puts you at slightly below parallel when seated on it. The rest of the set-up should mimic the set-up of the traditional barbell squat. The only difference is that you will set your feet about two inches wider. When you finish your walk-out, you should be in your squat stance with your heels in line with the front of the box.

As with the free squat, a belt is not absolutely necessary, but it will enable you to handle heavier weights.

The Descent

When most novice lifters try to execute the box squat for the first time, it looks like little more than a free squat with their butt touching a box at the bottom. However, a true box squat means that you will actually sit back onto the box like a chair.

Start the box squat by pushing your hips back, your knees out, and your head back, just like you would start a free squat. Instead of decelerating at the bottom by yourself however, continue sitting back until you are actually seated on the box. The idea is to sit further back than you would be able to without the box being there.

The sitting motion shifts the load from your quadriceps to your hamstrings and glutes. Once you are on the box, try to relax your hips while still keeping your midsection tight. Following a brief pause (just long enough to stop completely), begin your ascent.

While most lifter's knees will shift forward slightly at the bottom of a traditional squat, you should be able to box squat with no forward motion at all, minimizing stress on the knee joints. Some experienced powerlifters can even box squat with the knees shifting slightly back, really maximizing the hamstring/glute/lower-back recruitment.

The Ascent

To begin the ascent, push your head back hard, drive your knees out, and imagine jumping as high as you can from that stance. A good cue to remember is to try to spread the floor with your feet while you drive your knees out. Imagine standing on a wrinkled rug, and trying to stretch out the wrinkles as you squat. Keep your head and chest up, just like you would in a traditional squat.

Due to the motions of sitting back and spreading the floor, the box squat tends to work best in a minimal Chuck Taylor–type shoe. Even if you free squat in traditional squat shoes, I would recommend squatting in Chucks.

Box squats can be performed with chains, anchored bands, or reverse bands.

Variations

Almost all variations of the squat can also be performed on the box, including the dumbbell squat, front squat, and Zercher squat. In all cases, the idea is to sit further back than you would normally be able to, with the goal being to recruit more posterior chain musculature, and to build strength out of the bottom position.

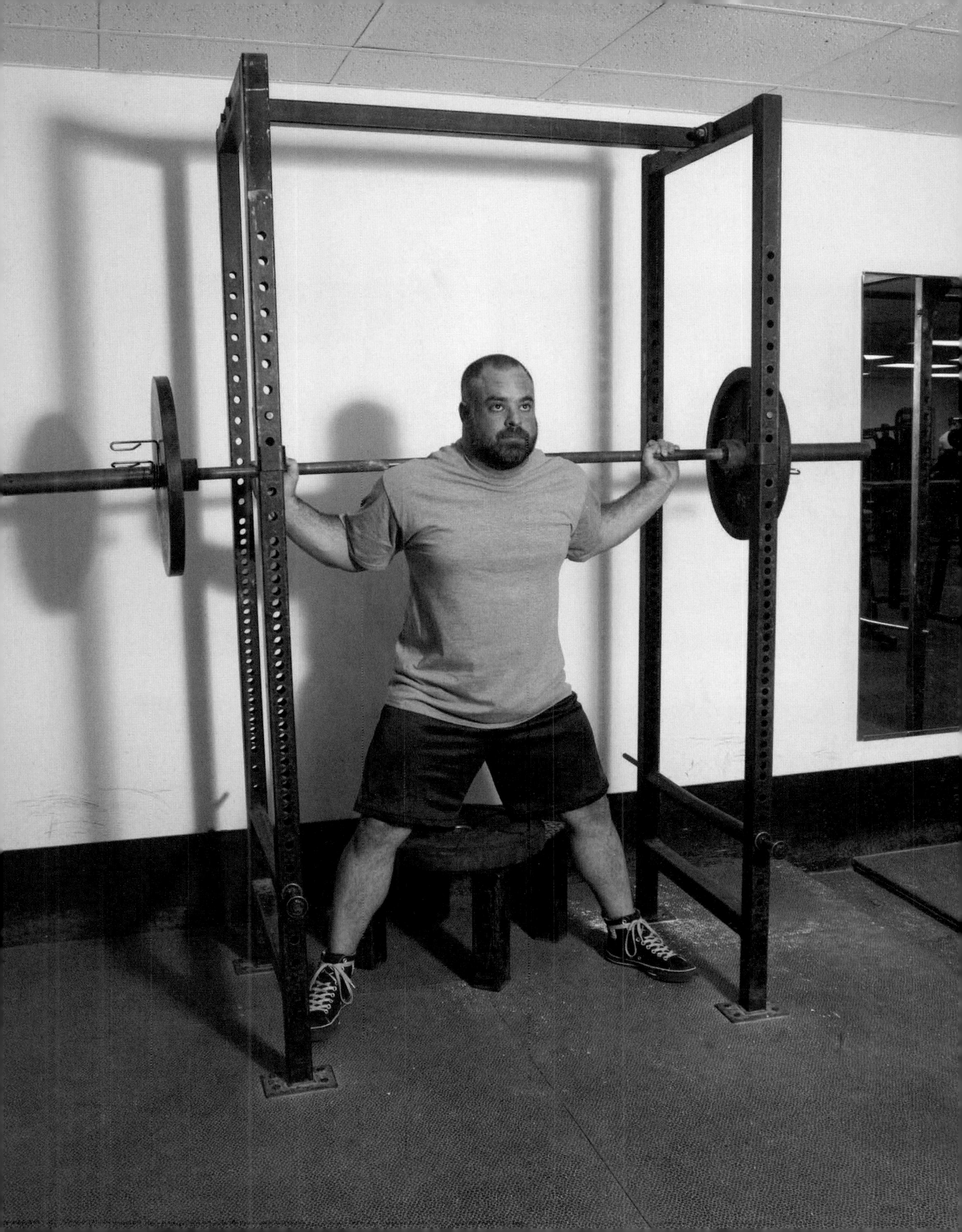

DUMBBELL SQUATS

Muscles Targeted: Glutes, lower back, hamstrings, and quadriceps

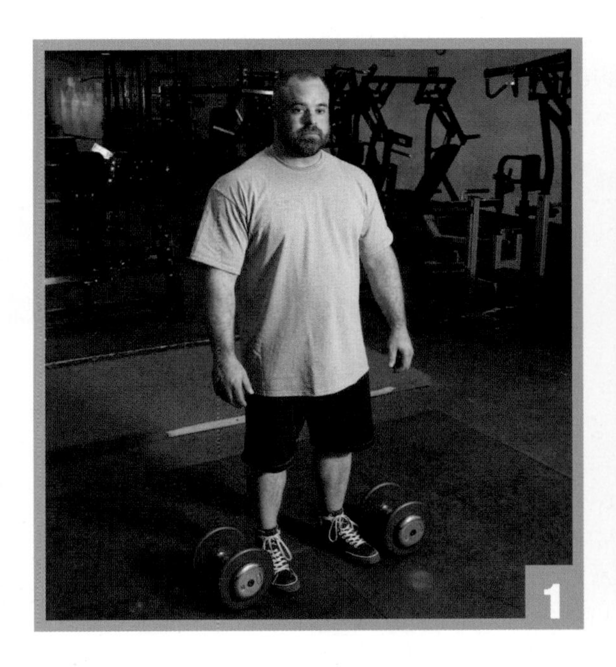

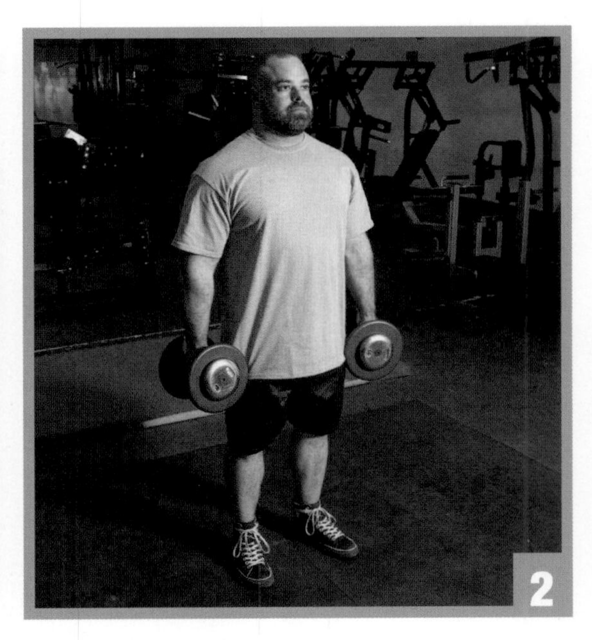

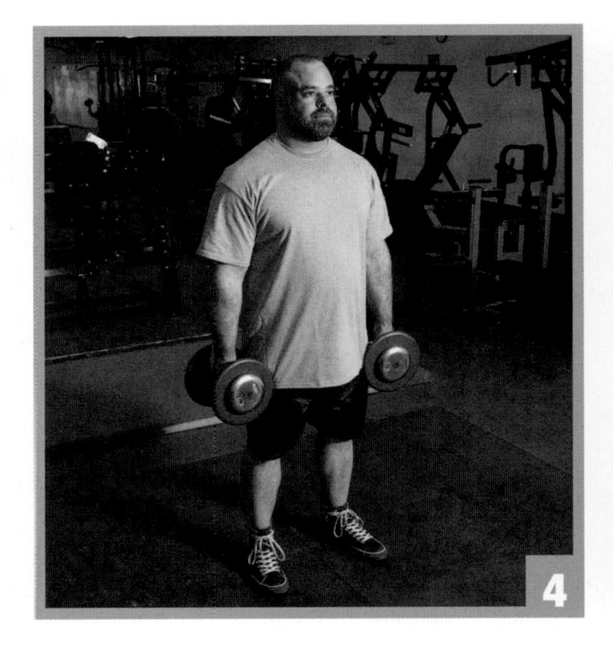

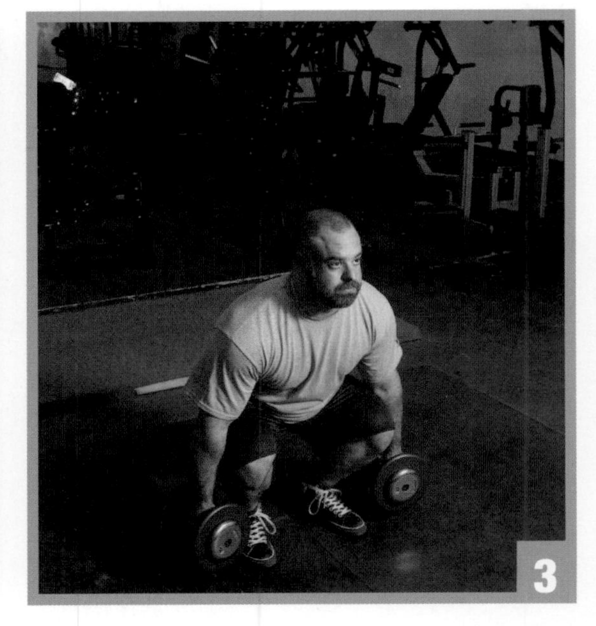

Instead of a barbell, you can also hold dumbbells at your sides like suitcases. The dumbbell squat is an easier lift for most people to perform because the dumbbell position lowers your center of gravity and allows for some arm movement in the event you find yourself off balance.

Set-Up

Select the appropriate dumbbells and place them on a bench in front of you about shoulder width apart. Make sure you have a few feet of space behind the bench. When you're ready to begin, grasp a dumbbell in each hand and hold them at your sides with straight arms. Take a couple of steps back and take a slightly wider than shoulder-width stance. Your arms should not bend at all during the exercise. In fact, the more relaxed you can keep your arms, the better.

The Descent

Start the descent by arching your back and pushing your hips back, as if you were about to sit in a chair. I recommend breaking the hips slowly and deliberately at first, in order to be sure you are squatting into your hips. I also prefer a slow initial break because it is extremely difficult to correct any mistakes once the descent has started.

Breaking the hips quickly can easily throw you off balance. After you've descended a few inches, you can pick up a little speed in order to conserve energy and gain some rebound out of the bottom position. While you will need to relax your hips somewhat in order to descend, your torso should remain tight and ridged. Loosening up on the descent can cause you to round over when you try to reverse your direction.

Keep your chest up and drive your gaze slightly above eye level for the entire descent.

The Ascent

When you know you've hit depth, reverse the process to stand up. Keep your head and chest up, drive your belly out, and push your hips forward as you stand up. You should be holding your breath for each entire repetition, taking a breath between reps when you are standing up straight.

When you complete the set, walk back toward the bench and place the dumbbells back on it.

FRONT SQUAT

Muscles Targeted: Glutes, lower back, hamstrings, and quadriceps

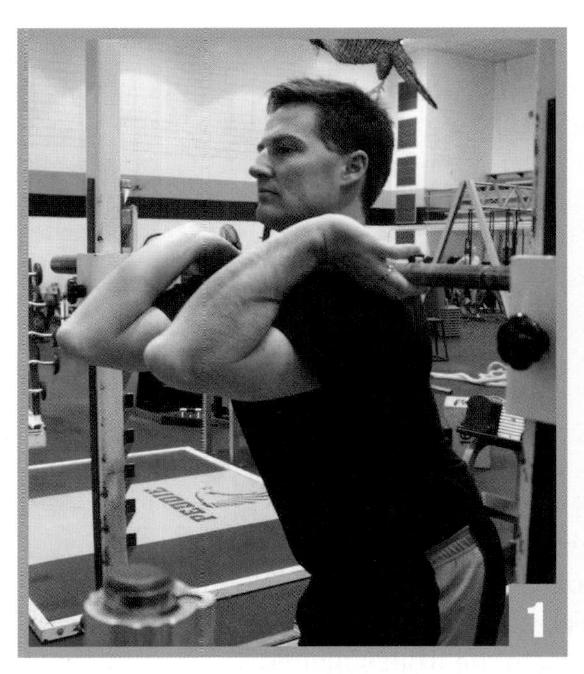

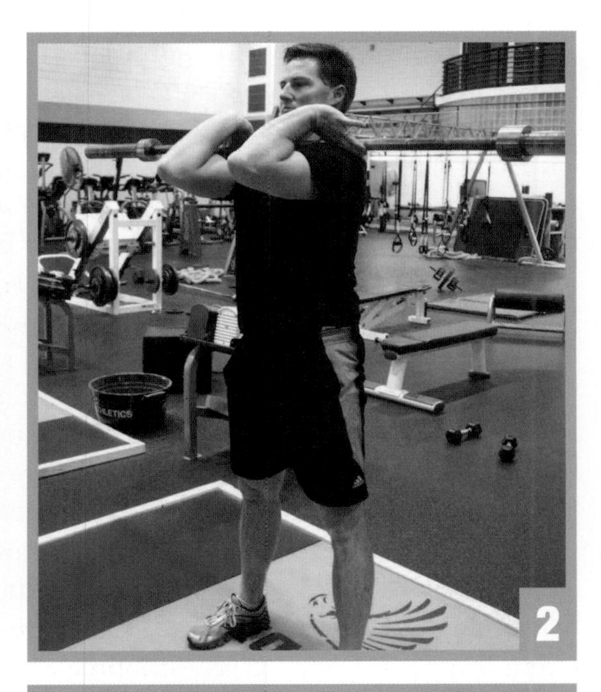

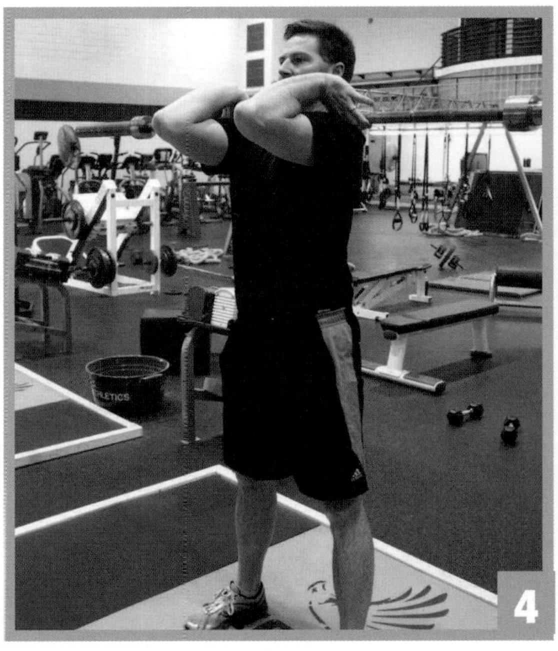

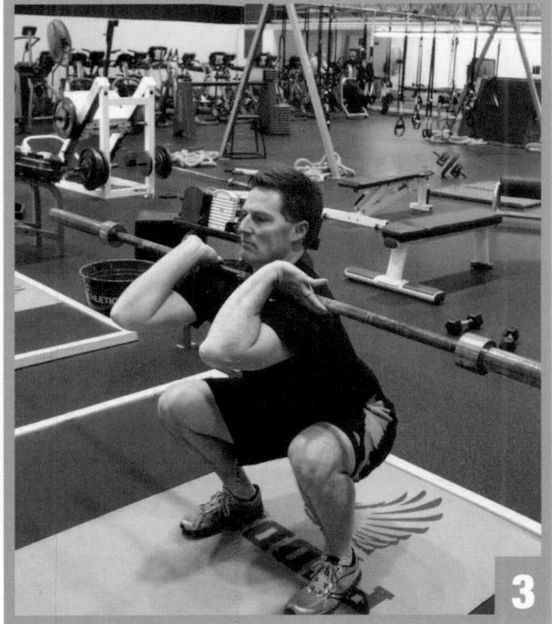

For a more challenging version of the squat, you can perform a front squat, which requires you to hold the barbell across the front of your shoulders and your fingertips (called the rack position). The front squat is challenging because it requires a more upright torso position, and will place more emphasis on the quadriceps.

Set-Up

Place the barbell in the rack at about the same height you would for the traditional barbell squat. Place your hands the bar slightly wider than shoulder width. Instead of grasping the bar tightly as you would with the traditional squat, keep your hands open. Point your elbows forward and keep them as high as you can. The barbell should be resting on the front of your shoulders and in your fingers at the second knuckle.

Press the bar out of the rack using your legs and walk the bar out. Your stance should generally be a little bit more narrow than it would be in the traditional squat because you will need more knee flexion to squat all the way down.

The Descent

Keeping your chest up and your head neutral, lower yourself to the bar by bending Because of the bar position, you will not be able to push your hips back as much as you would be able to in the traditional squat. In order to keep the bar in the rack position you will need to maintain a more upright torso position. However, despite the different torso position, you will still break parallel in the front squat. Take a big breath into your belly immediately before beginning your descent, and hold it for the entire repetition.

The Ascent

When you know you've hit depth, reverse the process to stand up. Keep your head and chest up, drive your belly out, and push your hips forward as you stand up. You should be holding your breath for each entire repetition, taking a breath between reps when you are standing up straight.

ZERCHER SQUAT

Muscles Targeted: : Glutes, lower back, hamstrings, quadriceps, and upper back

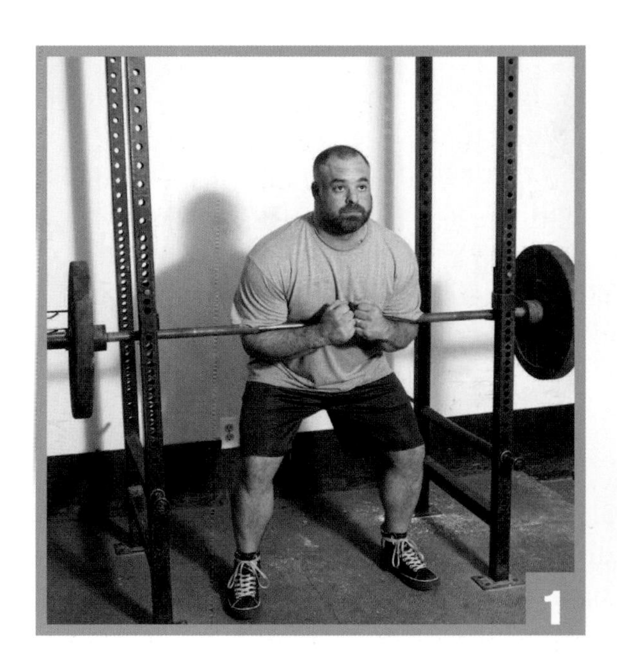

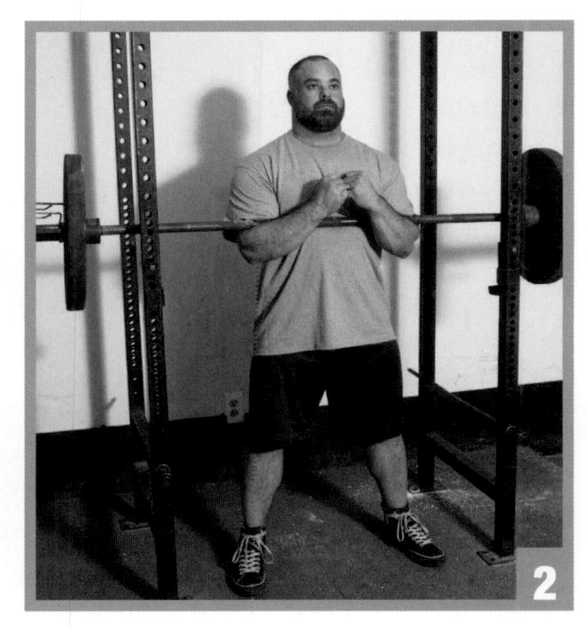

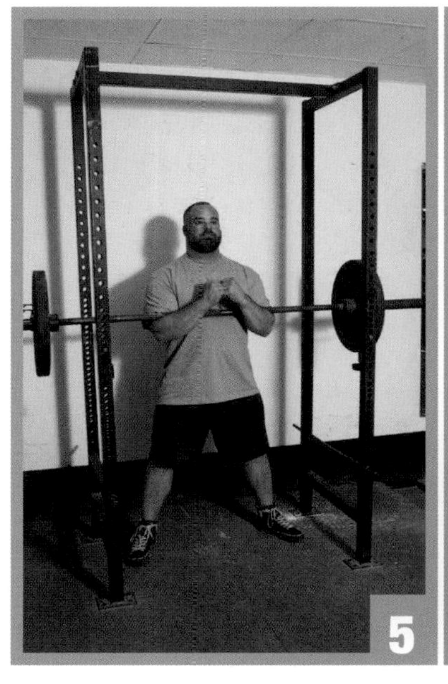

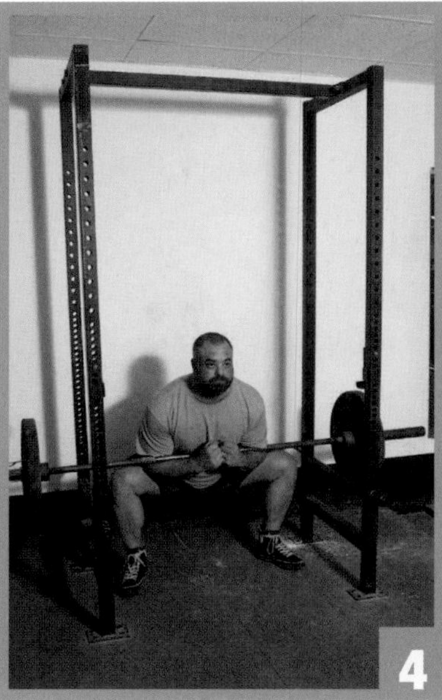

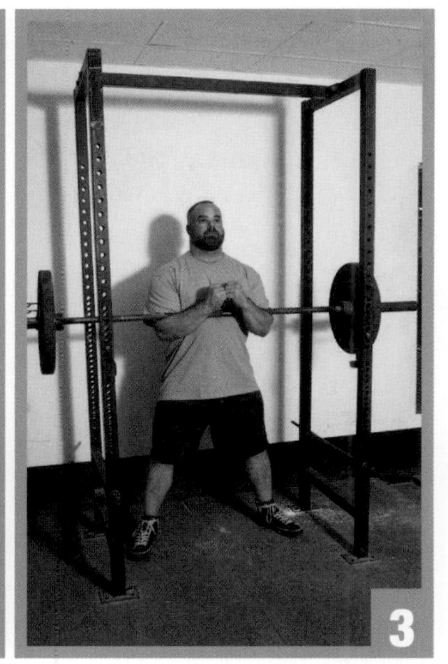

Still another version of the squat is the Zercher squat. This is a rather odd-looking squat variation that you rarely see performed in typical commercial fitness centers, although it's an effective way to build a strong back. While technically a squat, it's been used by powerlifters for years as a way to build the deadlift because of the demand it places on the middle and lower back.

Set-Up

For this technique, you'll set the rack at about belly-height and unrack the bar holding it in the crooks of your arms. To displace the weight on your elbow joints, I recommend wrapping the barbell in a towel, or using one of those squat pads common in many commercial gyms (this incidentally is the only time I recommend the pad).

Once your arms are in place, stand up with the weight and walk it out of the rack, just as you would the traditional barbell squat. The Zercher squat works best with a wide-to-moderate stance. At minimum, place your feet just outside shoulder width.

The Descent

Once you've stabilized after the walk-out, take another deep breath into your belly, and begin your descent. Despite the unconventional bar position, the actual squat technique is almost identical to the traditional squat. Start the descent by arching your back and pushing your hips back, as if you were about to sit in a chair. I recommend breaking the hips slowly and deliberately at first, in order to be sure you are squatting into your hips. I also prefer a slow initial break because it is extremely difficult to correct any mistakes once the descent has started.

Breaking the hips quickly can easily throw you off balance. After you've descended a few inches, you can pick up a little speed in order to conserve energy and gain some rebound out of the bottom position. While you will need to relax your hips somewhat in order to descend, your torso should remain tight and rigid. Loosening up on the descent can cause you to round over when you try to reverse your direction.

Keep your chest up and drive your gaze slightly above eye level for the entire descent.

The Ascent

As far as technique, try to pull exactly as you would for a traditional deadlift. Due to the awkward starting position, it's easy to get bent over at the start. Keep driving your head back and try to lean back against the weight.

CONVENTIONAL DEADLIFT

Muscles Targeted: Glutes, lower back, hamstrings, and upper back

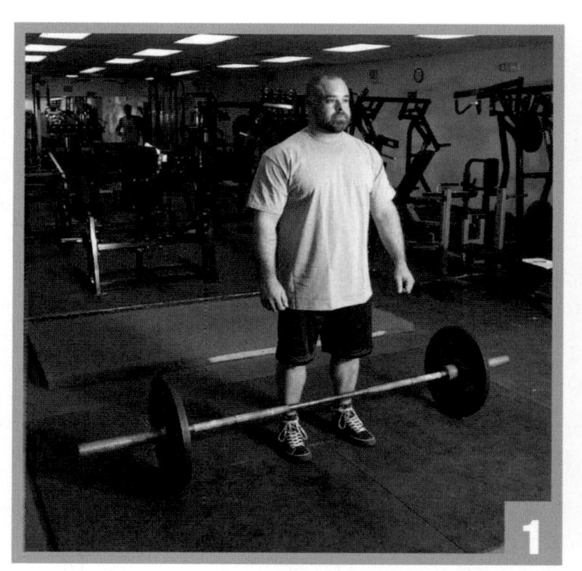

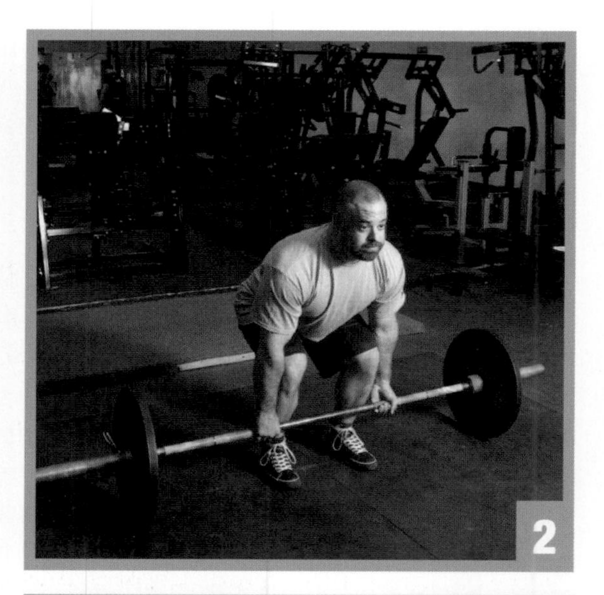

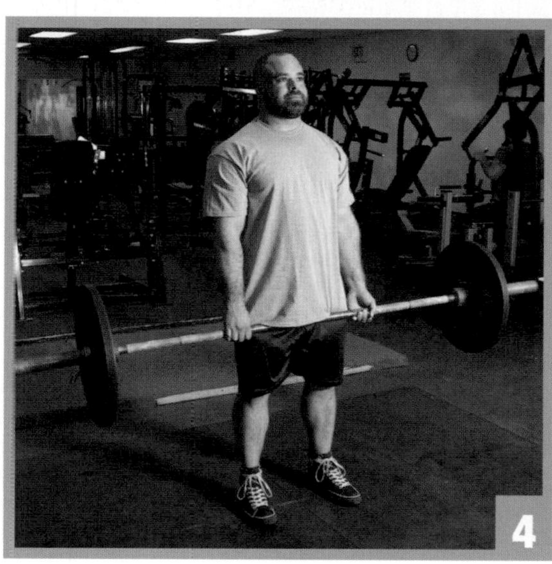

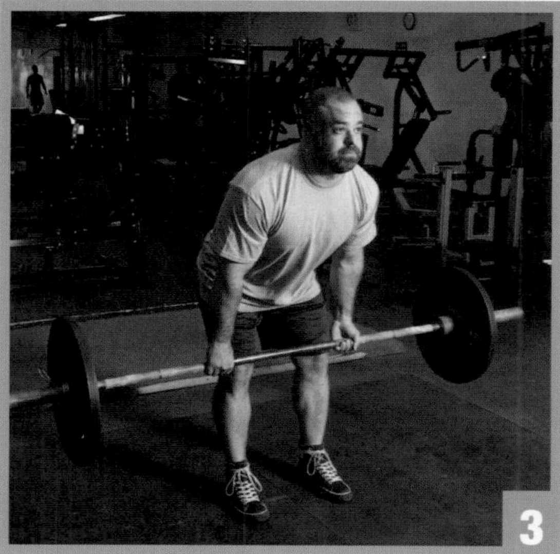

The conventional deadlift is regarded by many lifters as the truest test of strength, and with good reason. The deadlift in general presents a challenge that the other power lifts do not, in that you must start the lift from a dead stop at the bottom. By contrast, the squat and bench press allow you to lower the weight first, building elastic energy as the muscles stretch.

Incidentally, this is where the deadlift gets its name. You must start the lift from a dead stop.

Set-Up

For the conventional deadlift, the set-up seems simple. Just walk up to the bar and take your grip. But there is a bit more to it than that if you want to lift the most possible weight. Your set-up will vary depending on how you are built.

To start, your shins should be about 2 to 4 inches from the bar at the start of the pull, so that your shoulder joint is not in front of the bar at the start of the pull. If you have a large midsection, you'll want to start from about the 4-inch range. Smaller wasted lifters will usually be most efficient closer to 2 inches from the bar. The further the bar tracks from your body, the tougher the lift will generally be.

Larger lifters who might have trouble getting into this position can start with the bar further out and then roll the bar toward them, "catching" it in the proper position as they start the pull. This method takes some practice to learn, but it can be very effective.

The ideal grip width will usually put your hands directly under your shoulders. If they are too wide, you will be at a mechanical disadvantage because you will have to pull a longer distance. If they are too narrow, your hands will drag against your legs during the lift, which can cause them to open. Bigger lifters however, may have no choice but to set their hands wider in order to avoid their hands catching on their big midsections.

The most popular grip by far is the over-under grip. This means that one hand takes an overhand grip while the other takes an underhand grip. This hand position is stronger than a double overhand grip because it allows you to torque the bar into your own hands as you pull. Just make sure that you are placing your hands on the bar correctly. The pinky on your under- hand side should be in the same place (relative to the lines on the bar) as the pointer finger on the overhand side.

Some lifters prefer a hook grip as used by Olympic lifters. The hook grip looks like a double overhand grip except that you are grasping the bar with your thumbs between the bar and your fingers. Although uncomfortable, this grip can be advantageous because your upper body is more aligned and you are reducing the risk of a biceps tear, which the underhand grip leaves you more susceptible to.

As stated on the previous page, unlike the squat and the bench press, which have an eccentric (lowering) phase, followed by a concentric (lifting) phase, the deadlift has only a lifting phase. While this makes for a simpler lift, you do miss out on the elastic energy that the lowering phase provides. With the right set-up however, you can create a similar effect.

Before starting the lift, allow your hips to remain high. When you are ready to pull, start by actually pulling your hips down against the bar. This will create tension as well as a pre-stretch in your posterior chain and will give you a smooth transition from a dead stop into the lift. If you are wearing a belt, take this opportunity to take a deep breath and push your abdominal muscles against the belt.

You will be ready to pull when your hips are down, your lower back is arched, your head is up, and your shoulders are slightly behind the bar.

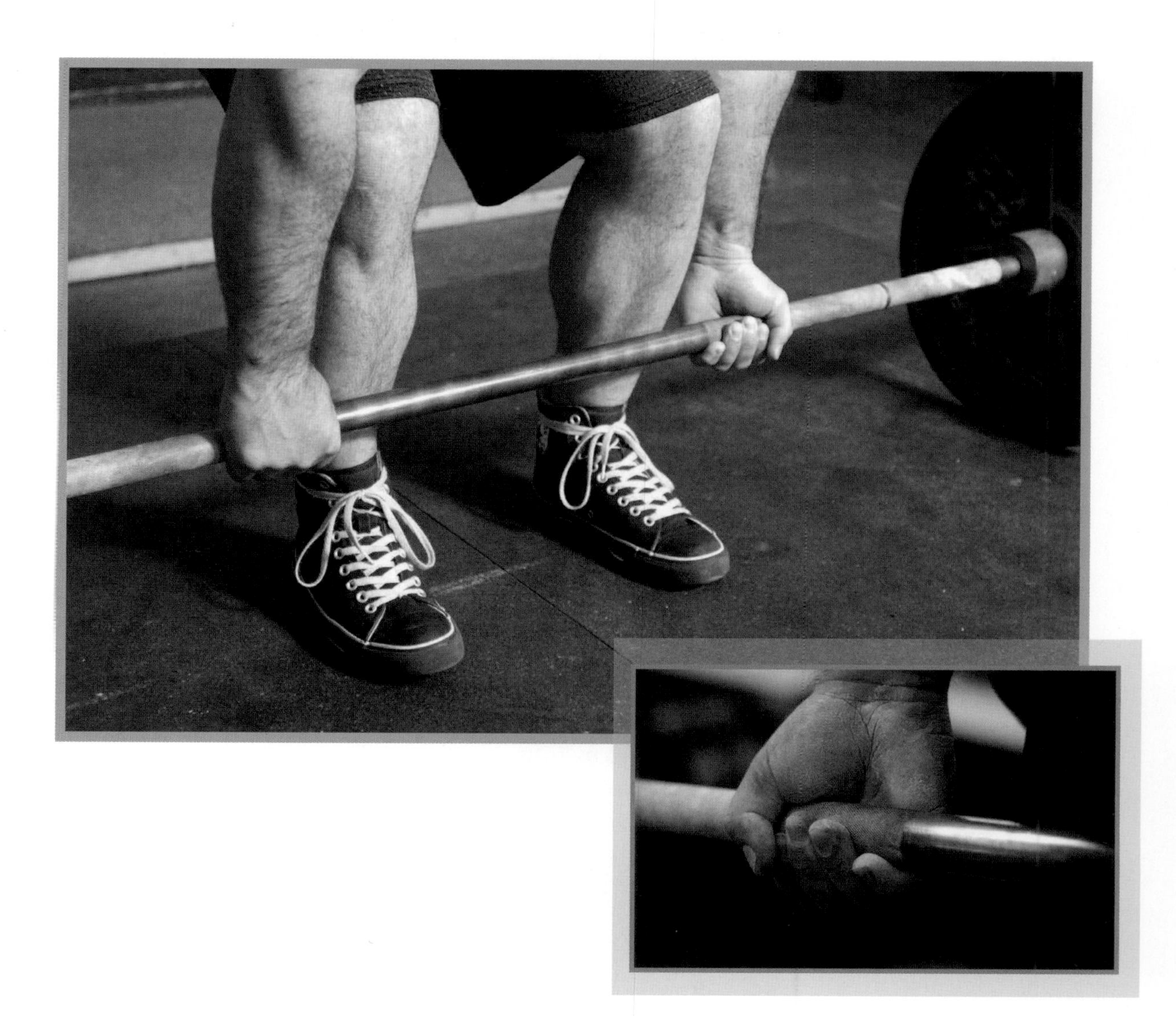

The Pull

Once you have pulled yourself into position, you have a very small window of opportunity to begin the pull before you lose the stretch reflex (only a second or so). Be sure not to lose the tension you built up when you initially pulled yourself down. Nothing makes me cringe more than watching a novice deadlifter violently snapping the slack out of their arms while starting a deadlift. The transition from pulling yourself down to pulling the bar off the floor should be seamless.

Keep your head up for the duration of the pull. Much like the squat, it helps to find a high focus point to stare at during the lift. As you pull, you want to keep the bar as close to you as possible. The further from your body it gets, the poorer your leverage will be. Almost all competitive lifters will apply baby powder to their legs so that the bar can slide up their thighs with minimal drag.

Once the bar clears the knees, lean back as much as you can. The weight will counterbalance you. Your hips and knees should lock out at about the same time. Overleaning at the top can cause your knees to unlock and place unnecessary stress on your back.

As you lock the weight out, it's a good idea to start letting out some air, but not enough so that you lose all your tightness. This will help prevent you from passing out from the pressure.

Once at the top of the lift, let your air out. If you are going to perform multiple reps, you can take another deep breath at the top, and hold it through the next rep. Otherwise, just put the bar back down in a controlled manner. Don't drop the bar. It's inconsiderate of other gym patrons, and depending on the equipment being used, can damage the weights, bar, or floor.

SUMO DEADLIFT

Muscles Targeted: Glutes, lower back, hamstrings, quadriceps, and upper back

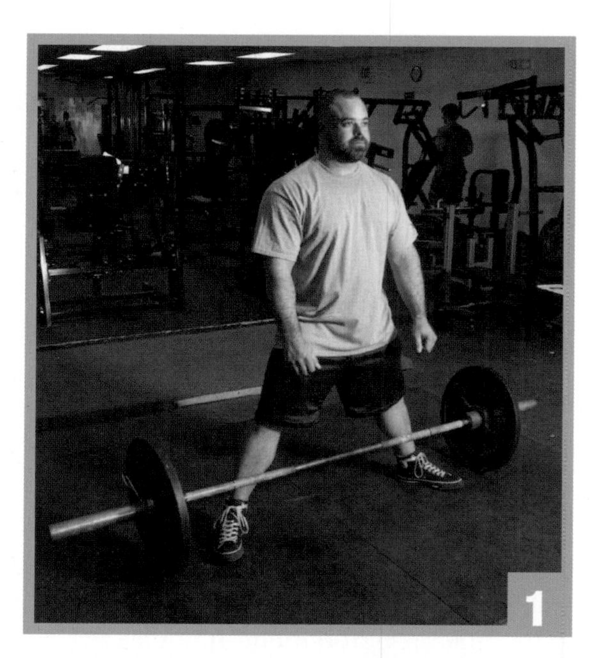

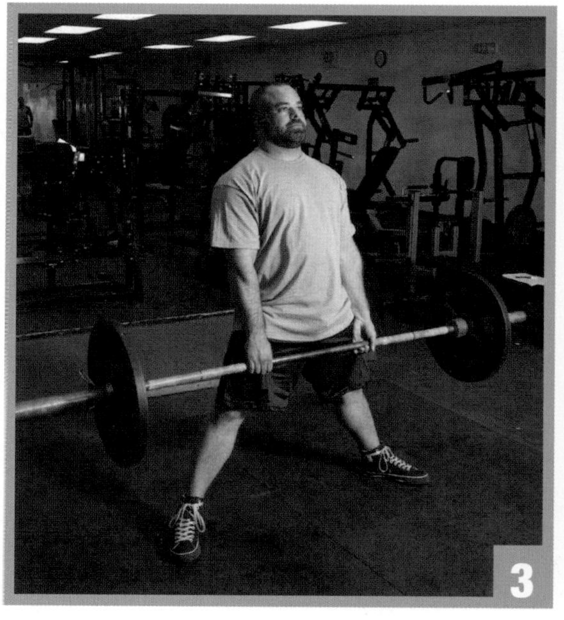

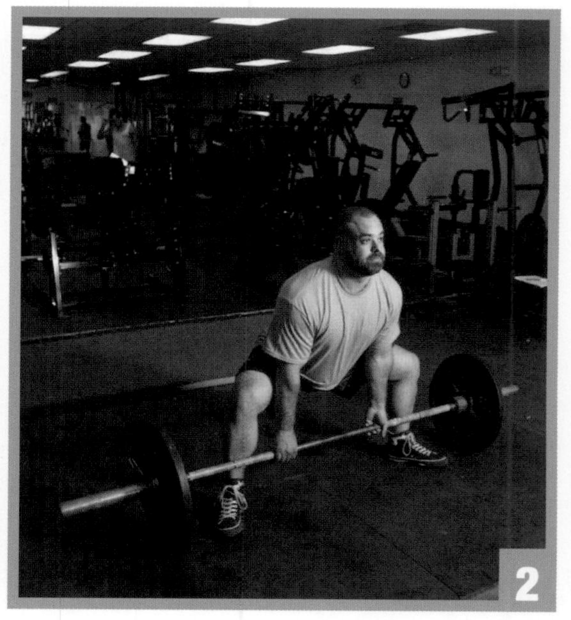

The sumo deadlift is a variation of the deadlift, often used in powerlifting competitions by lifters who favor it over the conventional deadlift. The sumo deadlift is a deadlift performed with a wide stance and with the hands gripping the bar between the legs.

In contrast to the conventional deadlift, which relies primarily on back strength, the sumo deadlift places the emphasis on the hips, allowing you to maintain a more upright posture, essentially turning the lift into a squat. With the exception of the stance, the majority of the cues for the sumo deadlift and conventional deadlift are exactly the same.

Powerlifters who favor the sumo deadlift over the conventional stance tend to be stockier, with stronger hips and legs relative to their backs. For the purposes of general strength training, alternating from the conventional deadlift to the sumo deadlift allows you to address weaknesses that may not be addressed sufficiently by using one or the other.

Set-Up

The sumo deadlift gets its name from the wide stance used, which mimics the stance taken by sumo wrestlers while preparing for a match. Your sumo stance will look much like your squat stance, although it tends to be a little wider, with your toes pointed out a little further.

The actual width of your stance will vary, but in most cases, you do not want your heels to be much wider than your knees at the starting position. While a super-wide stance will minimize the distance you need to pull, it can also disengage your hip flexors and give you stability issues at the top of the pull.

Grip the bar at shoulder width, exactly where you would grip the bar in a conventional deadlift.

Start the movement by taking a deep breath and pulling yourself down to the bar, just like you would with the conventional pull. Push your knees out much like you would with the squat. If you are wearing a lifting belt, push your belly into the belt and arch your lower back.

The Pull

Follow the same cues as you would for a conventional pull. Find a high focus point and keep your head up until the weight is locked. Keep your weight on your heels, and lean back as you pull. Do not overemphasize the lean at the top. Once you are in a standing position, the lift is complete.

Exhale at the top, and either put the bar down (if you are only performing one lift) or take another deep breath and return the bar to the starting position before beginning the next repetition.

DEFICIT DEADLIFTS

Muscles Targeted: Glutes, lower back, hamstrings, and upper back

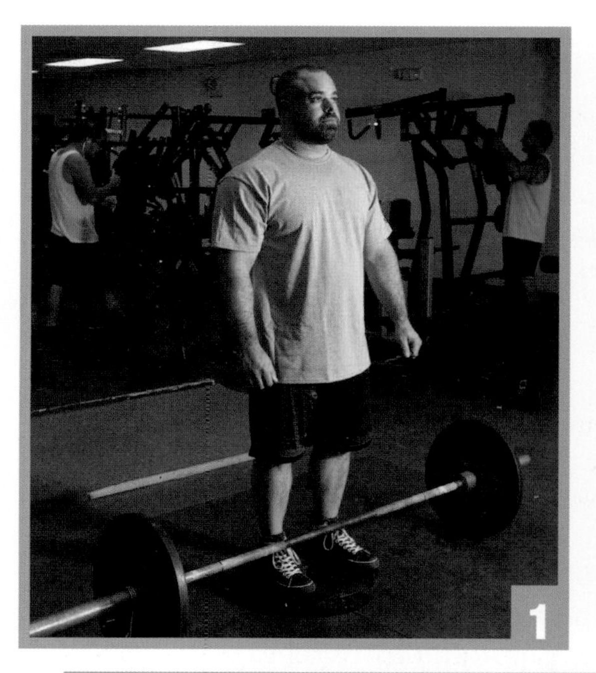
1

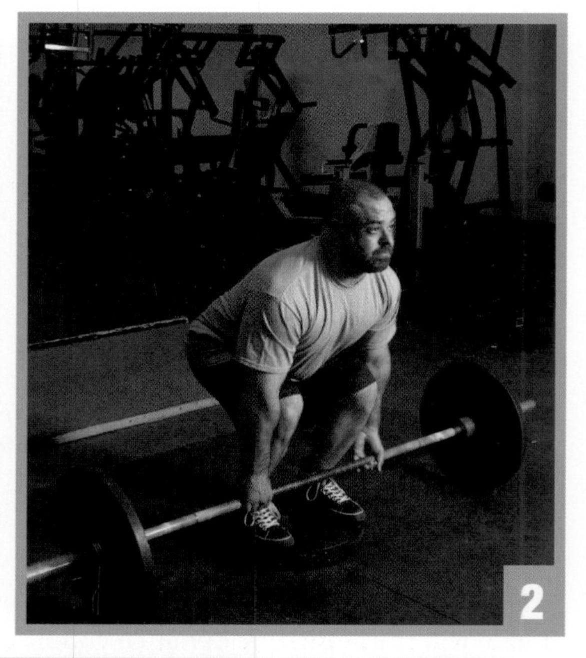
2

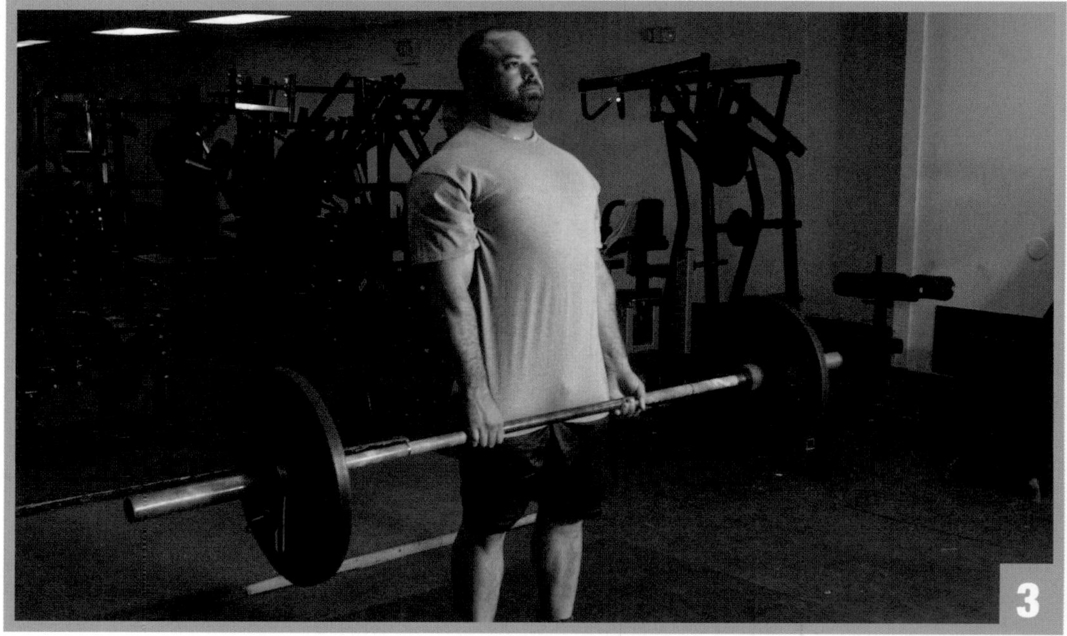
3

Since there is no lowering phase to the deadlift, you must have enough back strength to overcome the static inertia at the beginning of the lift. Bottom end strength is crucial to a big pull. If you find yourself missing deadlifts right off the floor, you probably have weak lower back muscles. The deficit deadlift works your back hard by requiring you to begin the lift at a lower point than you would in competition.

Set-Up

To set up for a deficit deadlift, you'll need some kind of low platform, anywhere between 1 and 4 inches. Most lifters will use rubber mats although in a pinch, an aerobics step will work. Set up the mats directly under the bar so that when you step onto it, your feet are just below the barbell. Your shins should be at about the same distance from the bar as they would be for the regular conventional pull.

The Ascent

As far as technique, try to pull exactly as you would for a traditional deadlift. Due to the awkward starting position, it's easy to get bent over at the start. Keep driving your head back and try to lean back against the weight.

Variations

If you don't have anything that will work as a platform, you can get the same effect by loading the bar with either 25- or 35-pound plates and pull from the floor. While it is possible to do deficit deadlifts with a sumo stance, I wouldn't use more than an inch-high platform. Deficit sumo pulls can really eat up your hips.

PIN PULLS

Muscles Targeted: Glutes, lower back, hamstrings, and quadriceps

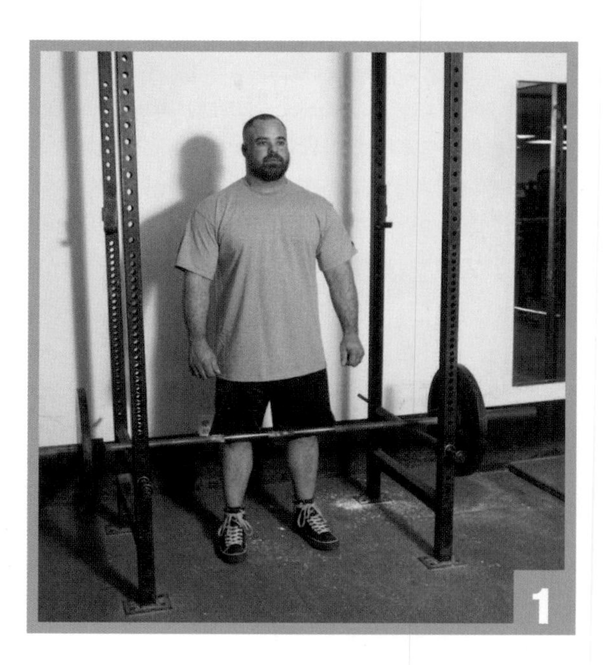
1

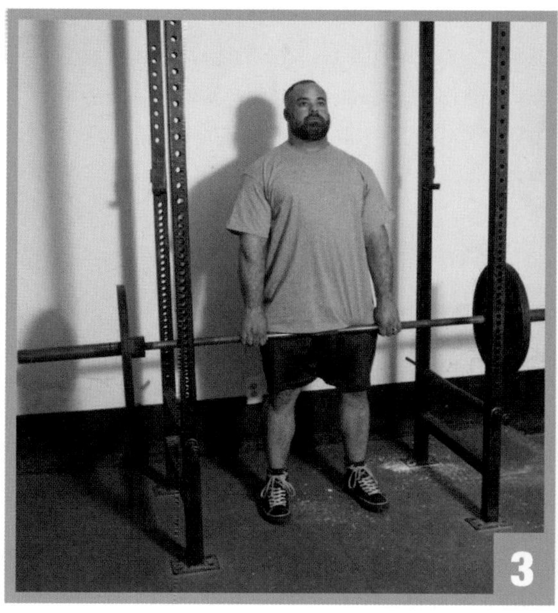
3

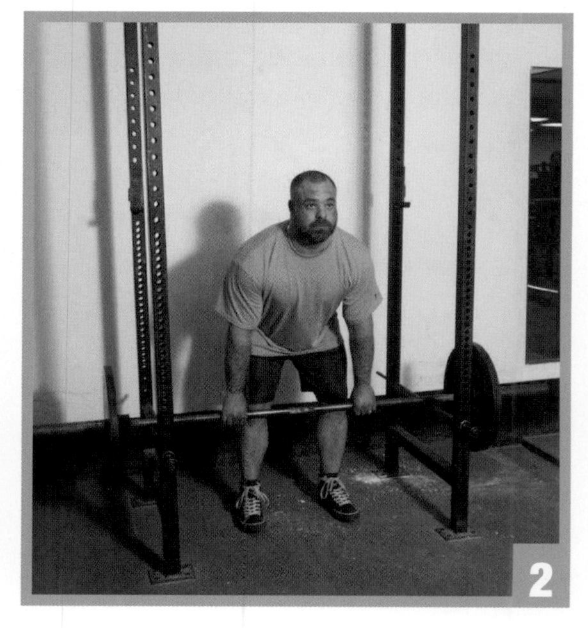
2

Sometimes a lifter will have a strong deadlift off the floor, but will lose it toward the top. This may be due to weak glutes, or an inability to transition the stress from their back to their glutes/ hamstrings at the midpoint of the lift. This is where pin pulls come in.

Much like rack presses in the bench press, pin pulls allow you to work the deadlift in a limited range of motion, allowing you to focus on different points of the movement and get your nervous system used to holding heavier loads.

Set-Up

Set the pins in the rack at the height you want to pull from. If you feel you need to work the transition point in the lift, set the pins at about knee height or below. If you want to simply overload the top of the lift, set them above the knee. High pin pulls are hard on the hands, so you might want to use a set of wrist straps. The goal of this movement is to overload the back, not the hands.

Set yourself up with your shoulder joints slightly behind the bar and arch your back before beginning the pull.

The Ascent

Think of the pin pull as a big hip thrust. Drive your head back and lean back right from the beginning. Generally, if you can break the bar off the pins, it's a matter of holding your position to make the lift.

Variations

One popular variation of the pin pull is the block pull. Rather than setting the bar up on the pins, you would lace the actual plates on mats or blocks. The biggest difference between the pin pull and the block pull is that you can roll the bar, making it more similar to a pull from the floor.

GOODMORNINGS

Muscles Targeted: Glutes, lower back, and hamstrings

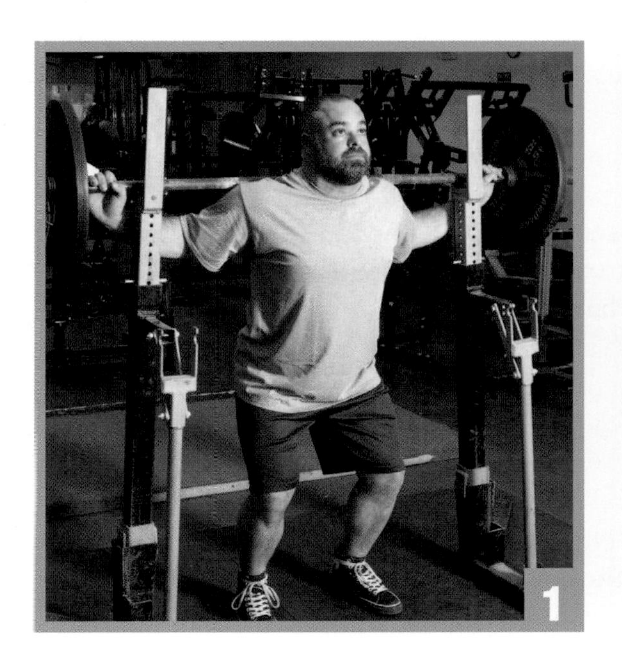

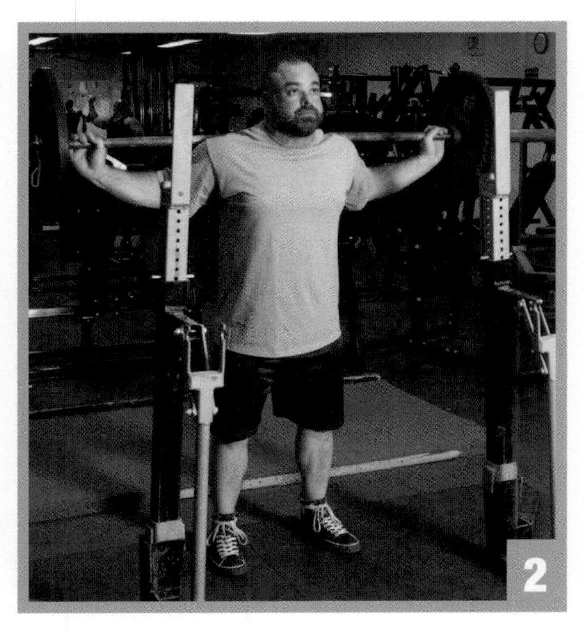

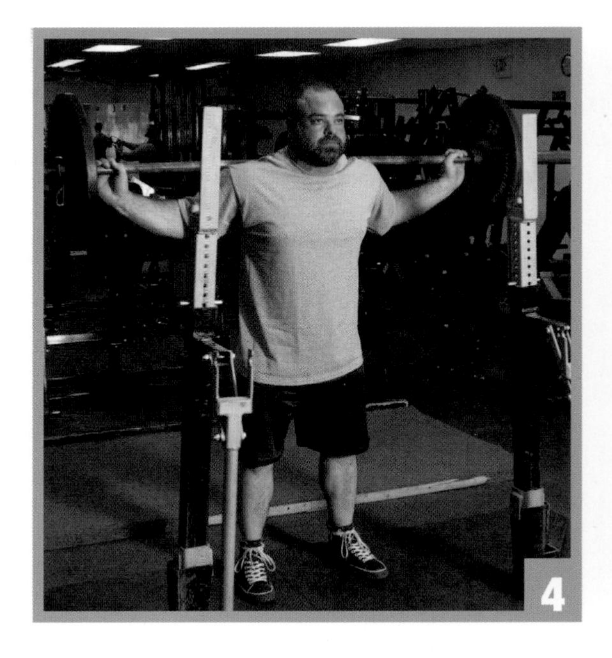

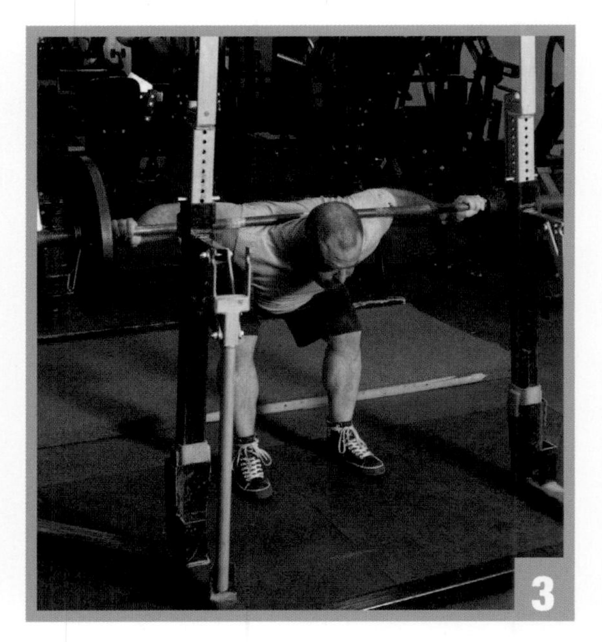

The goodmorning is an old-school back exercise, which is popular with serious lifters but hardly anyone else. This exercise looks like a cross between a squat and a bow. Goodmornings have largely fallen out of favor with the average gym goer because of concerns for the lower back. When performed correctly, they are a brutally effective tool for strengthening and thickening the lower back, hamstrings, and glutes.

Goodmornings are a particularly effective tool for bringing up a lagging deadlift because they load the same muscles, without being as taxing to the nervous system.

Set-Up

The set-up for the goodmorning is identical to the squat. The only difference is that your stance will generally be closer, at about shoulder width apart.

The Descent

To initiate the descent, push your hips back just as you would for the squat. Rather than bending the knees, continue pushing the hips back and tilt your upper body forward in a bowing motion.

Your legs should be straight, but with soft knees. If your hamstring flexibility is lacking, you might need to bend your knees a bit more. When your upper body is about parallel with the floor, it's time to reverse direction and come back up.

The Ascent

Once you've hit the bottom of the movement, Push your head back as you would in the squat and push your hips forward.

BENCH PRESS

Muscles Targeted: Pectorals, deltoids, and triceps

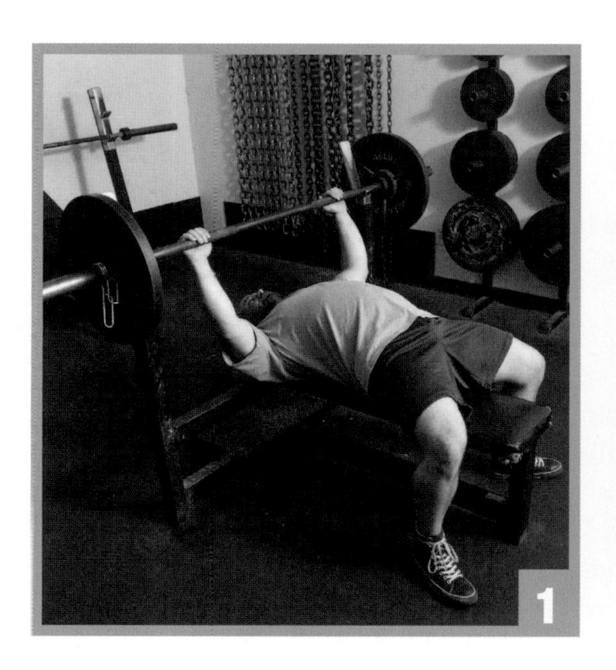

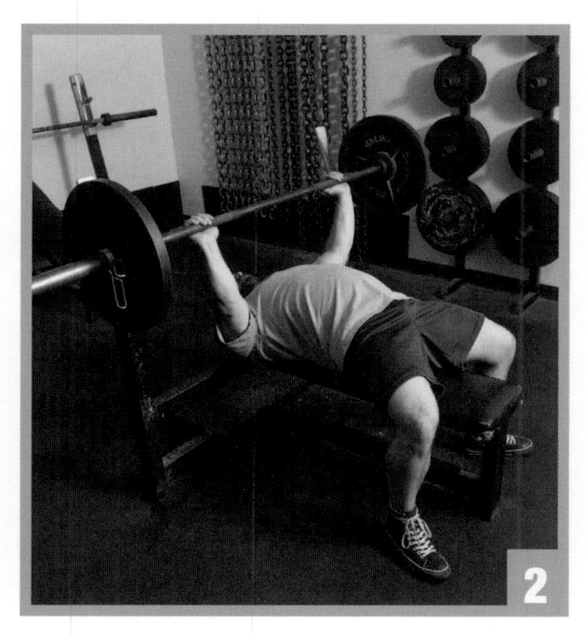

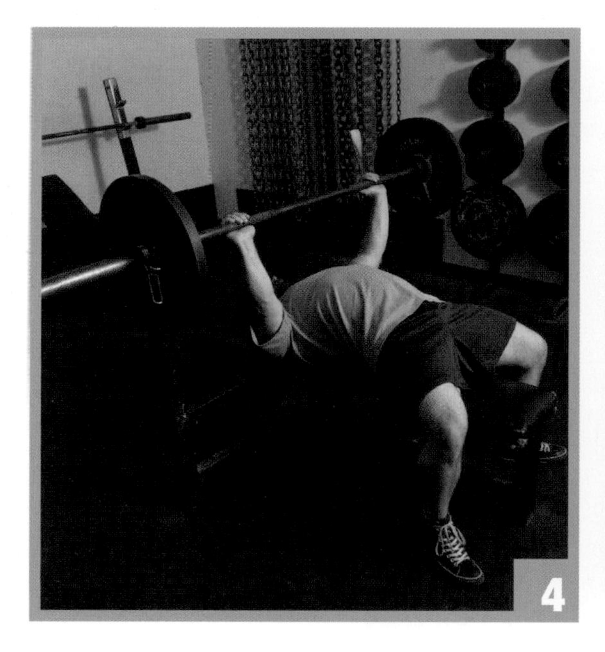

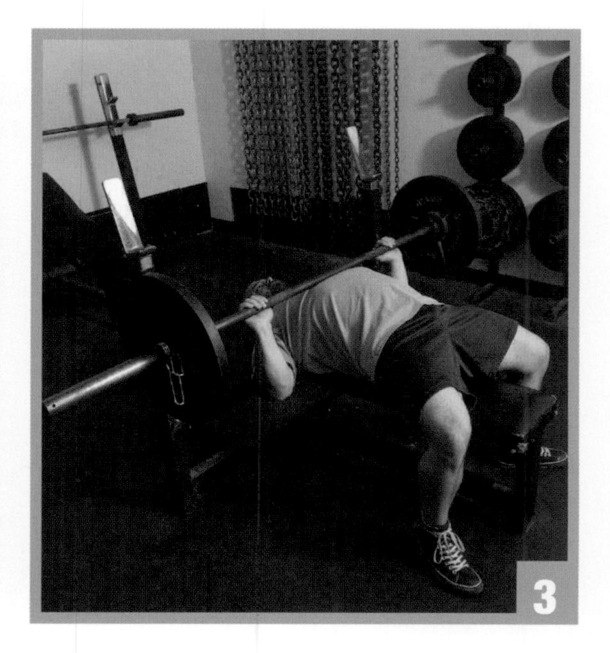

The bench press is by far the most well known of the power lifts among casual fitness people and nonlifters. Even people who have never seen a bench press performed have probably heard the phrase "How much ya bench?" at one time or another.

The bench press is easily the single most popular lift among bodybuilders, even though most lifters perform it incorrectly. The most glaring mistake made with the bench press (and it's made by the vast majority of gym goers) is with regard to elbow position.

Most exercisers are taught to perform the lift with their elbows out at a 90-degree angle from the body, with the goal being to build the pectoral muscles. However, the problem is that this position places the shoulders in a relatively unstable position, which, when combined with heavy weights, increases the risk of shoulder or pectoral injuries.

Pro powerlifters who practically live and die by their bench press understand this, and bench with their elbows closer to the body. While this technique differs from what is commonly taught, it's actually a much more natural movement. As an example, imagine yourself trying to push a heavy door open. Without ever being taught, you would be far more likely to keep your elbows close to your torso than you would be to flare them out.

A correct bench press takes advantage of this more natural, stronger position.

Set-Up

A successful bench press starts before the bar is even in your hands. In order to stabilize a heavy weight from a lying position, you must be able to remain as tight as possible on the bench. Once you are properly set up, a strong man should have difficulty pushing you off the bench.

There are a couple of ways to actually get on the bench. Some lifters prefer to set their lower body first from a sitting position, then arch back into a lying position. Others will lie down first, then simultaneously lock their upper body and lower body into position. Either method works, so try them both, but below is an overview of what you're looking for in a proper set-up.

Legs

Keeping your chest up and your head neutral, lower yourself to the bar by bending Most casual lifters vastly underestimate the importance of the legs in the bench press. It's not uncommon to see lifters in bodybuilding gyms even benching with their feet off the floor. Others shift or even kick their feet spastically as the weight becomes difficult, which as you might imagine, doesn't help.

For a strong, stable foundation, set your feet wide, with your feet directly under your knees. Throughout the lift, maintain stability by driving your knees out, as you would in a squat. Driving your knees out serves a dual purpose of tightening up your lower body, while preventing you from lifting your butt off the bench.

Lower Back

A really common technique for the bench press is to keep your back flat on the bench, with some instructors going so far as to take their clients feet off the floor and place them flat on the bench.

Despite what many trainers still say, however, benching with an arch in your lower back is not only safe, but it's perfectly natural. If you look at a picture of the human spine from the side, you'll notice a distinct curvature at the lumbar vertebrae. This is the natural shape of the spine and there is no benefit in trying to eliminate it.

You can see for yourself by standing with your back against a wall. Even when standing up straight with a neutral (not arched) back, you'll notice a space between your lower back and the wall from about your mid-upper-back to your buttocks.

In powerlifting competitions, athletes will actually *emphasize* their arch, in order to cut down the distance from chest level to arm's length, creating a more efficient lift.

Upper Back

When most casual lifters miss a weight in the bench press, it's because they did not keep their upper back locked in throughout the lift. You can usually tell when a lifter is trying to bench with a loose upper back because they will have trouble getting the weight moving off their chest, and the barbell will often pitch to one side.

Locking in your back properly starts even before the unrack. To practice this, lie on the bench with your arms straight up as if you are holding a barbell. Now squeeze your shoulder blades together as if you are actually trying to grip the bench with them. Combined with the correct leg position, it should be very difficult to move from the bench when you dig in and tighten up.

Belly

Much like with the squat, keeping a full tight belly will stabilize you during the lift. A loose weight lifting belt can be a great teaching tool for this, but unless you are very serious about increasing your bench press numbers, a belt is not really necessary for the bench press.

Personally, because I am small compared to the weights I'm using (I've officially benched tripled my body weight and routinely handle that in training), I need all the support I can get and use a tight, stiff belt.

Grip

As far as grip width, the sweet sport for the bench press will be somewhere between pinky and middle finger on the ring, although some benchers with very strong triceps can use a narrower grip. A maximum-width grip (pointer finger on the ring) will be very wide for most lifters, and can put the shoulders and pectorals at risk for injury.

Some lifters prefer to grasp the bar with their thumbs around it because they feel it is safer. Others will use a false grip (no thumb) because it allows them to maintain a more natural stroke. Use whichever you feel more comfortable with.

The Unrack

While most lifters take a casual, even rushed approach to the unrack, it's actually a critical step in performing the bench press properly.

Some lifters prefer to get set on the bench before they touch the bar. Others, myself included, actually use the bar for leverage during the set-up, with their upper backs deep into the pad. To use the barbell to aid your set-up, lie down on the bench, take your grip, then pull yourself up to the bar, making sure to pinch your shoulder blades together tightly. Keep them pinched together while you carefully lower yourself onto the bench.

By far the most common mistake when unracking the bar is to lose tightness in the upper back (that is, assuming it was tight enough to begin with). When you reach for the bar, make sure to keep your shoulder blades together and avoid allowing your elbows to flare out. You should also be close enough to the uprights to reach no more than a few inches past where you will ultimately start the lift from.

When you take the bar out of the rack, either by yourself or with the aid of a hand-off, you should not need to lift the bar more than an inch or so to get it out. A good handoff will involve much more lateral than up-and-down movement. I routinely tell my training partners to hand the bar "out" to me rather than "up and out." This is why the best benches are made with a shallow lip on the j-hook. Before you lower the bar, your elbows must be locked.

When you finally have the bar at arm's length, you'll need to reset your shoulders one more time. To do this, try to pull the bar as far down as you can while keeping your elbows locked. I've found that taking a deep breath at this point helps me set my shoulders. Others will hold their breath from the handoff to the completion of the lift. In either case, you should hold your breath from the start of the lift to the finish.

The Descent

Another common mistake in the bench press is to lower the bar with the elbows perpendicular to the body. Because of the structure of the shoulders, this position puts you at an increased risk for pectoral/shoulder injury and also limits the amount of weight you will ultimately be able to lift.

Instead, lower the bar while keeping your elbows at about a 45-degree angle from your body. Since you must always keep the bar over your elbows, this will also mean that the bar will touch your chest at the bottom of your sternum rather than the middle.

Benching with tucked elbows requires thick, strong lats because you will physically be mashing your upper arms against them for support during the descent. This is why great benchers, almost without exception, have large, thick backs.

To maintain upper-back tightness during the lift, try to push your chest up toward the bar. When the bar touches your chest, you can either touch-and-go, or come to a brief pause before pressing the weight back up into lockout. In competitive powerlifting, a pause is required, although for general strength training purposes, either is fine. If you find yourself failing at the bottom of the lift, the paused bench is great for building power out of the bottom of the lift.

If you choose to touch-and-go, make sure you are not bouncing the bar off your chest.

The Ascent

Initiate the lift by pressing the weight back up to arm's length. In order to remain tight on the bench, drive hard with your legs throughout the entire lift. To get the leg drive you need without lifting your butt off the bench, drive your knees out like you would in the squat.

A great cue for keeping your upper back tight is to think about driving your back into the bench against the weight, rather than pressing the weight up. About halfway into the press, open your elbows a bit to put you in a better position to lock the weight out.

Hold the bar at arm's length for a brief pause, then reset your upper back on the bench before beginning your next rep.

Variations

The bench press can also be performed on either an incline or decline bench. On an incline bench, you will touch the bar higher on your chest, just above the nipple line. On a decline bench, you will touch the bar lower, at about the solar plexus (just above the abdominals). Since changing the angle at which you're pressing will affect the leverage of the lift, you will need to record separate personal records for each variation.

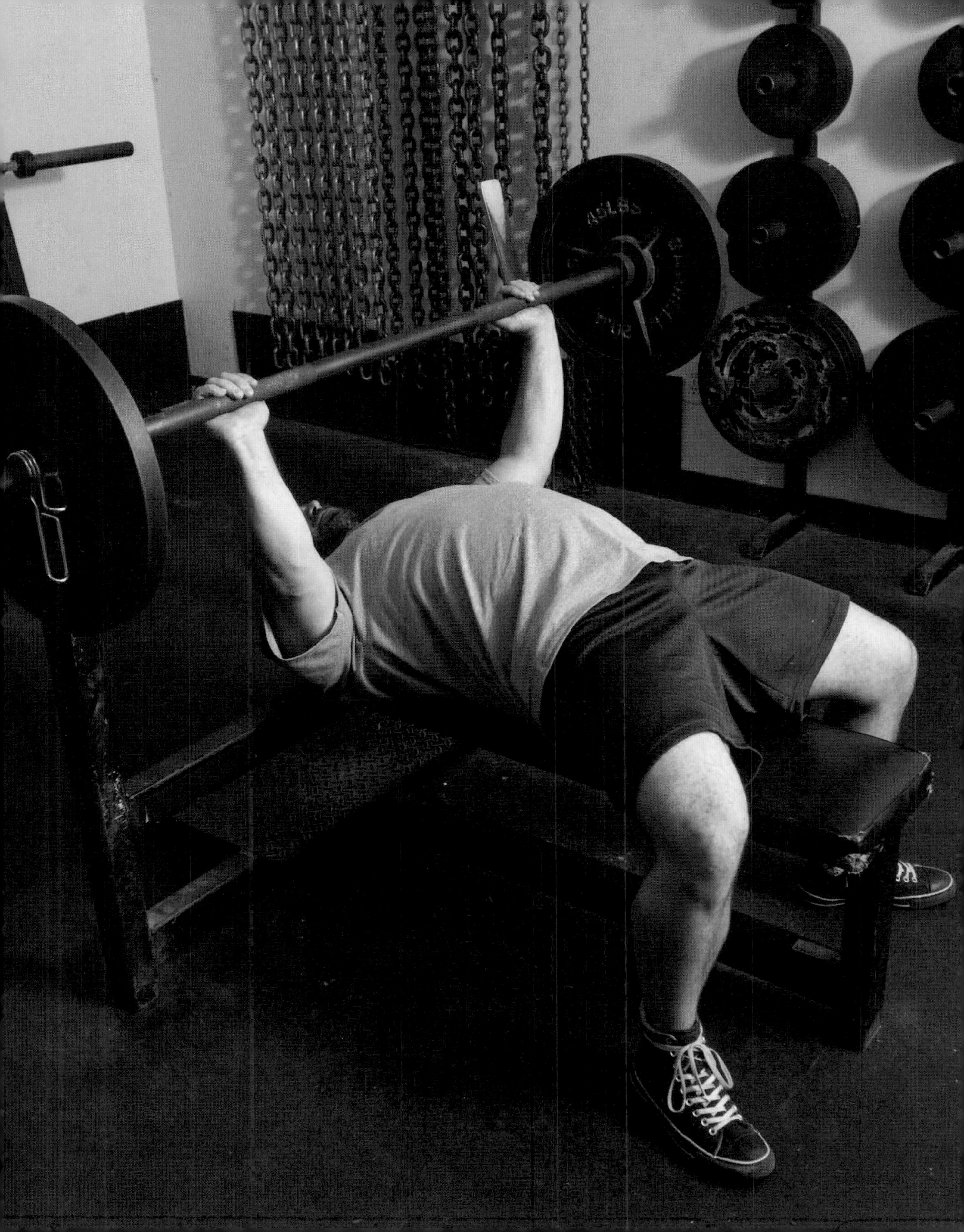
45LBS

CLOSE GRIP BENCH PRESS

Muscles Targeted: Pectorals, deltoids, and triceps

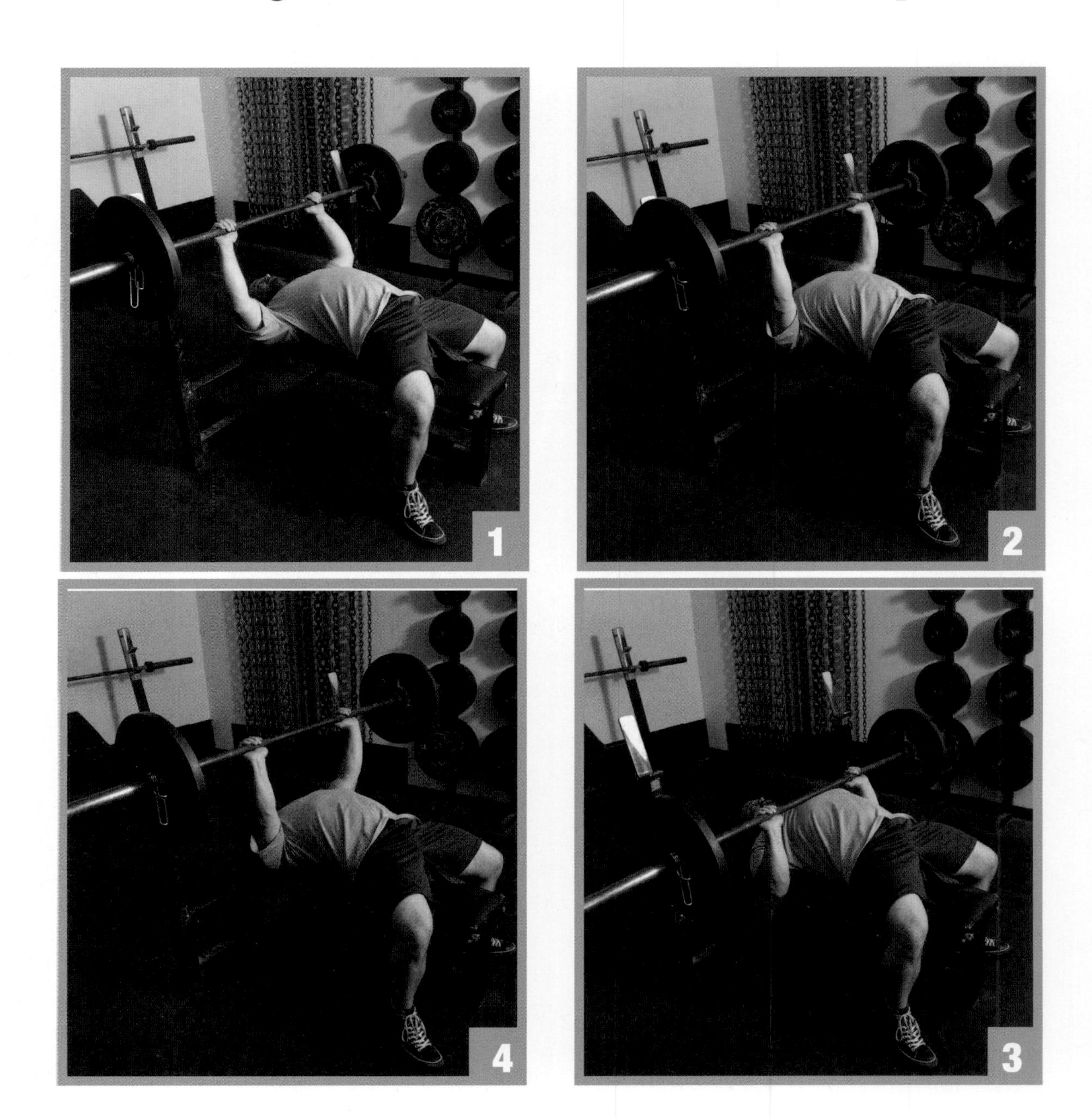

While the bench press is a great movement for building serious upper body strength, the lift can admittedly be tough on the shoulders.

The best way to minimize shoulder and pectoral stress in the bench is by benching with a close grip. In fact, many bench press superstars will do little wide grip raw benching, if they do it at all.

Set-Up

Setting up the close grip bench press is exactly like setting up for any other bench press, the exception, of course, being the grip width. Since the close grip creates a longer bench stroke, you will probably raise the uprights on the bench so you can unrack the weight comfortably.

I consider a close grip to be anything in between the lines on a standard power bar; however, the closest most lifters will be able to go is placing the pointer finger on the border between the center knurling and the smooth. Any closer and your torso will actually force your elbows out, negating the favorable position the close grip is supposed to give your shoulders.

The Unrack

Unracking the bar is actually easier in a close grip bench press than it is in a wide grip bench press. This is because you do not have to fight as hard to keep your elbows in position (tucked and not flared out). As soon as the bar is over your chest, pull your shoulder blades back hard before breaking your elbows.

The Descent

Unlike with the wider grip bench press, you should not have to work too hard to pull your elbows in. They should naturally track that way. If you are keeping your elbows in with the bar over your elbows, the bar should touch right on the lower chest/upper ab area fairly effortlessly. Generally when a lifter has trouble tucking their elbows correctly, it's due to years of practicing poor bench technique, and it may take a few weeks, or even months, to really correct.

The Ascent

A close grip bench press tends to travel in a straighter line than a typical bench press, which may have a bit of an arcing motion from your chest toward the rack because you will not be flaring your elbows, just press straight up to lockout.

Variations

Close grip bench presses work great as a max effort lift, or as an assistance movement. The close grip bench press can also be performed on either an incline or decline bench. Since changing the angle at which you're pressing will affect the leverage of the lift, you will need to record separate personal records for each variation.

BOARD PRESS

Muscles Targeted: Pectorals, deltoids, and triceps

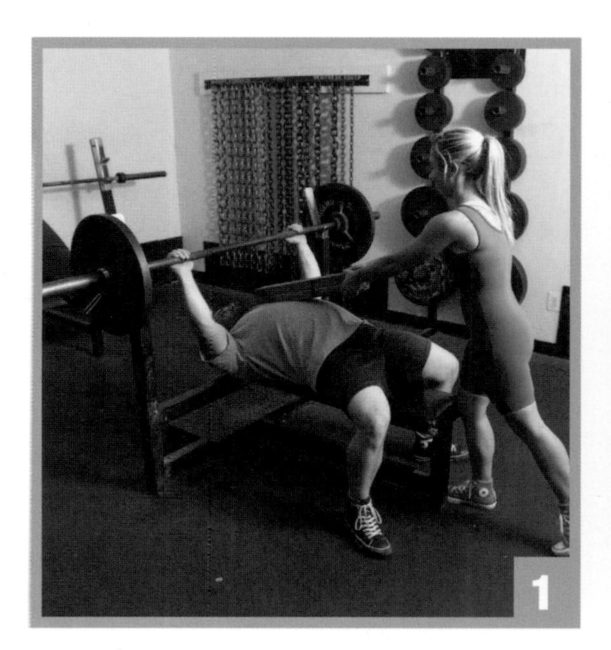

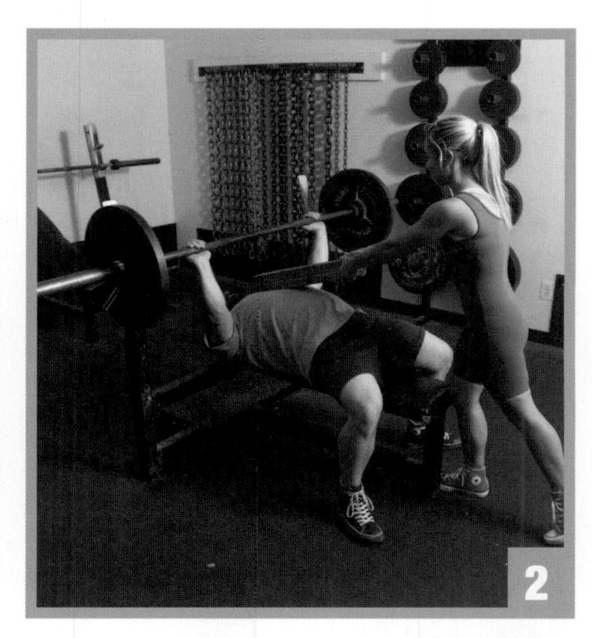

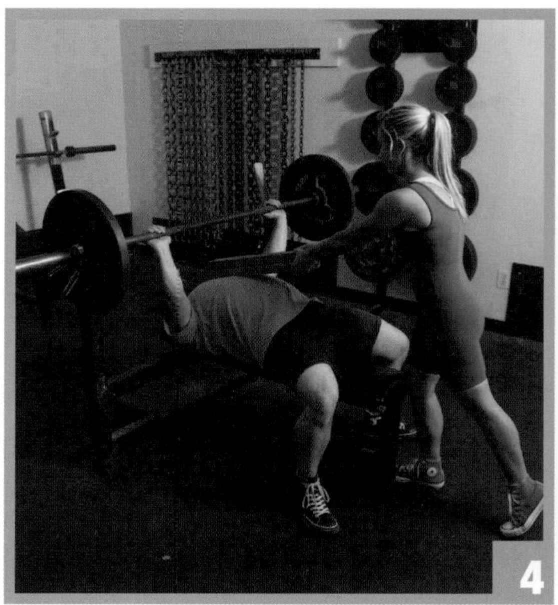

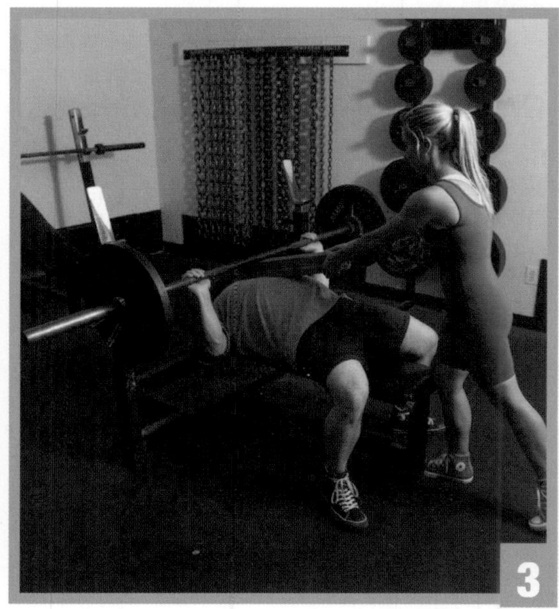

When you first start taking your lifting seriously, you shouldn't worry about specific movements as much as getting stronger overall. As you become more in tune with your own strengths and weaknesses, however, you'll most likely start to see consistent sticking points in the bench.

A sticking point is a point in the lift where the bar stalls, causing you to miss the lift. A sticking point can either be technical or physiological (and sometimes mental). Whatever the reason, the board press is an effective tool for strengthening these weak points.

The board press is performed by laying anywhere from one to five stacked boards on your chest while benching (although most recreational lifters won't ever need more than two). Instead of touching your chest, you settle the weight on the board before pressing it back up. The board press differs from a traditional bench press in two important respects:

- Much like the box squat, you know exactly how far the bar is traveling on each rep, making the process of addressing a sticking point simple
- The board allows you to momentarily take the load off your musculature, requiring you to start from a dead stop, improving your explosive strength from whatever point in the lift you're trying to improve

Set-Up

Set up for the board press exactly as you would for the raw bench press with the addition of the board. While in a pinch, you can hold the board to your chest with a band or bungee cord, but the best option is to have a training partner hold it firmly to your chest.

The Unrack

Same as a raw bench press.

The Descent

Most mistakes in the board press come when the bar actually touches the board. You should not bounce or touch-and-go from the board. Instead, allow the weight to settle on the board before pressing it back up to lockout. This will build your ability to strain through your sticking point. While you should be allowing the board to take some of the weight, do not relax your torso. Stay tight on the bench.

The Ascent

When the bar has stopped completely, press it back up to lockout. Because the bar will be at a full stop, press it back up as explosively as possible.

Variations

You can use a wide, medium, or close grip. Make sure you record separate personal records for each grip as well as each board.

PIN PRESS

Muscles Targeted: Pectorals, deltoids, and triceps

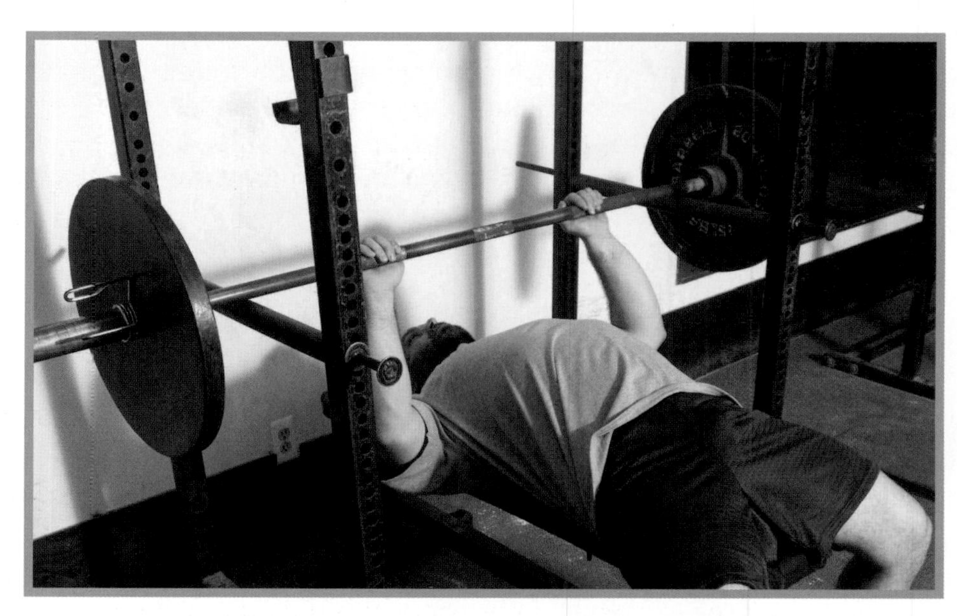

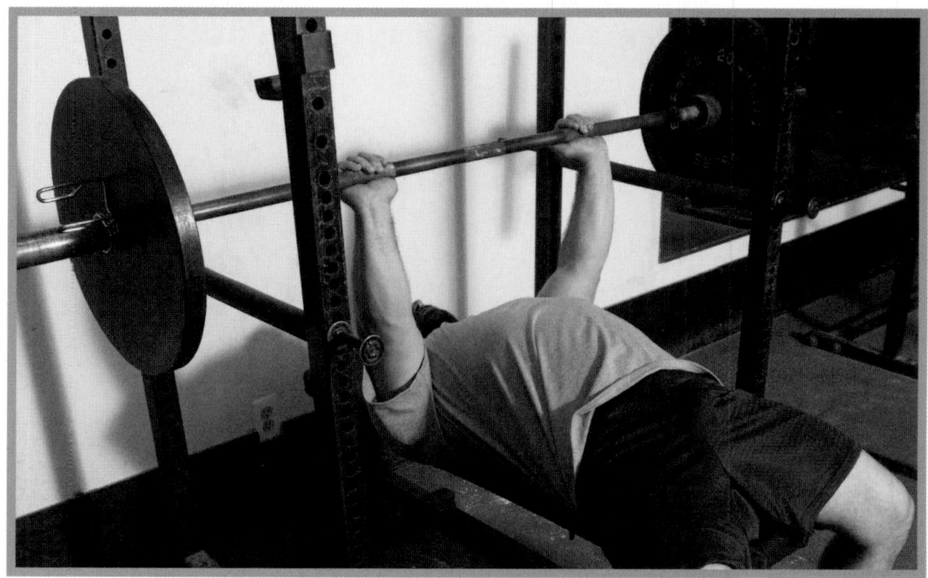

The pin press is another method to work specific sticking points in the bench press. The pin press differs from the board press in that you are starting the movement from the bottom, in a true dead stop.

To execute the pin press, set the pins in the rack to anywhere within the top half of your bench range of motion and lay the bar over them. Lie down under the weight and press the bar the rest of the way to the top

The pin press is a tough movement, designed to build grinding strength and get you used to heavier weights. Since you're pressing from a completely deloaded state, this can be a very hard movement on your joints, especially your shoulders. I do not recommend doing pin presses any lower than halfway into your stroke. Personally, I've always done them for top-end lockout work only.

This movement is for heavy weights only. There is no point in ever going below five reps with it.

Set-Up

Unlike most other forms of benching, you do not need to unrack the weight before beginning the lift. In fact, the unrack *is* the lift. Instead of setting up with the bar over your forehead as if you are about to take a handoff, set yourself up so that the bar is where it would be relative to your body just before you lock it out.

Before pressing it off the pins, make sure your shoulder blades are locked together and your body is as tight on the bench as possible. If you do not nail the initial press, you will rarely be able to recover and finish the lift.

The Ascent

Press the weight up, pressing as hard as you can.

Variations

You can perform the pin press with either a close or traditional bench press grip, and take advantage of various rack heights. The higher the rack height, the more you will be focusing on triceps/lockout strength and the more weight you will be able to handle.

FLOOR PRESS

Muscles Targeted: Pectorals, deltoids, and triceps

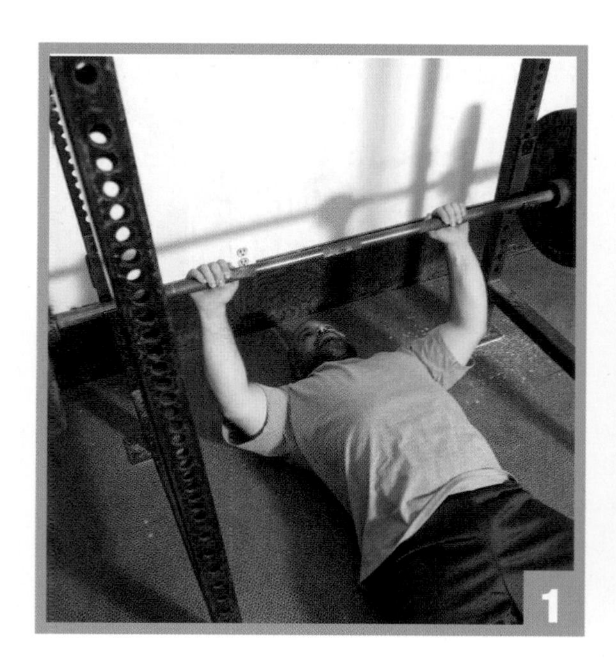

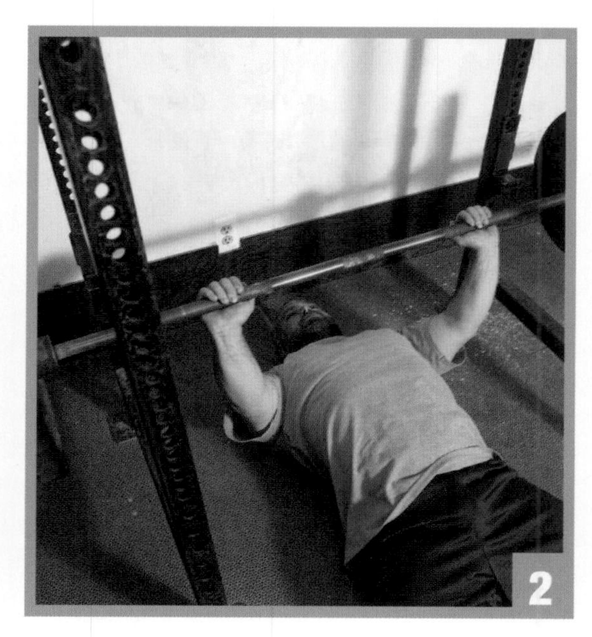

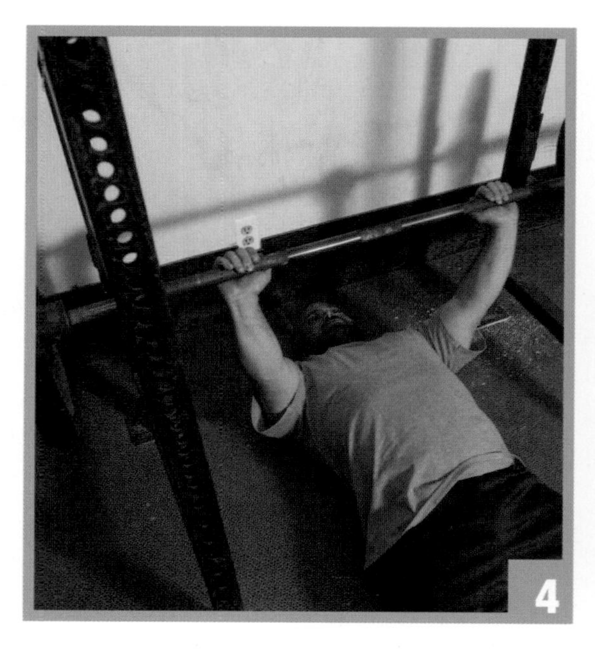

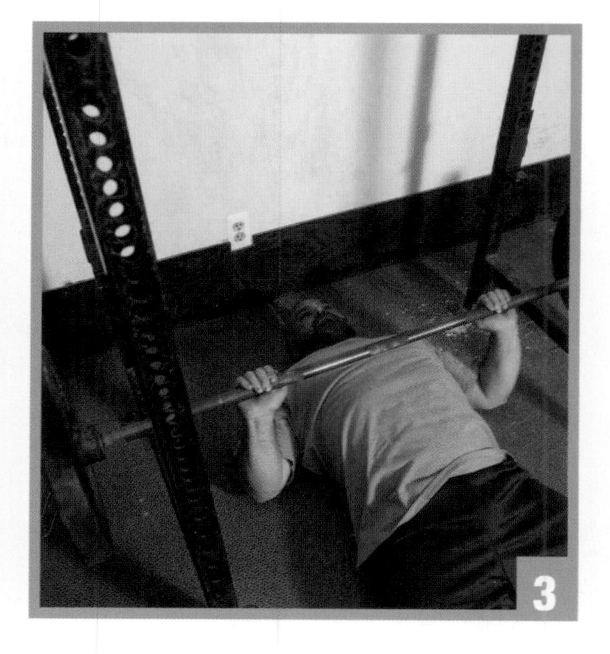

The floor press is an odd-looking movement to most casual gym goers because it's basically a bench press without the bench. Instead of being performed on a bench, the floor press is performed lying on your back, on the floor with a rack set about a foot and a half from the floor.

The floor press helps build brute pressing strength because it eliminates the lower body from the lift, thus doing away with strong leg drive and extreme arching. It's also valuable as another partial rep bench movement because most lifters' elbows will settle on the floor before the bar reaches their torso.

Set-Up

Setting up a floor press actually feels kind of strange, especially if you've been working hard to learn proper bench form. At first you won't know what to do with your feet. You may find yourself kicking and jockeying to find a comfortable position. Your upper body should be set just like it would be for any other bench press, with your shoulder blades squeezed together as if you are trying to grip the floor with them.

The Unrack

If you're getting a handoff from a training partner, make sure the partner knows what he or she is doing when handing off to you. The bar will be much lower for her or him than with a traditional bench press. The first instinct may be to pull the bar too high, which can screw up your set-up.

The Descent

Lower the bar in exactly the same path you would use for a traditional raw bench press, including trying to push your chest and belly up to the bar. Control your speed on the way down so that your triceps settle on the floor instead of plopping down to it. Hitting the floor too hard can injure your elbows and wrists or cause you to dump the bar. Never bounce your elbows off the floor. Instead, allow your upper arms to settle just enough to lose momentum before pressing the weight back up.

The Ascent

From the bottom position of the floor press, drive your head back and press the bar from the bottom just as you would for a standard bench press.

Variations

The floor press can be performed with dumbbells for repetition work, as well as with a barbell for heavy/max effort training. If you're careful with the lowering phase, you can even use the floor press for speed work. The fat bar works particularly well on the floor press because the greater surface area reduces the stress on your wrists.

OVERHEAD PRESSES

Muscles Targeted: Deltoids and triceps

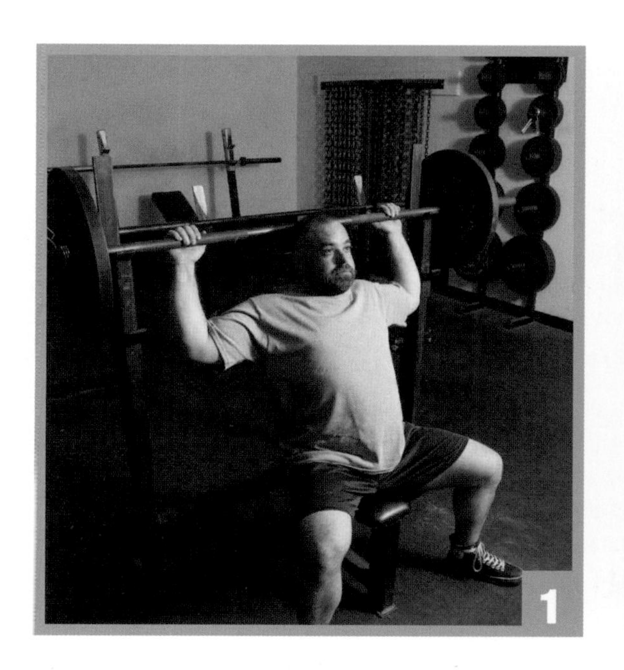

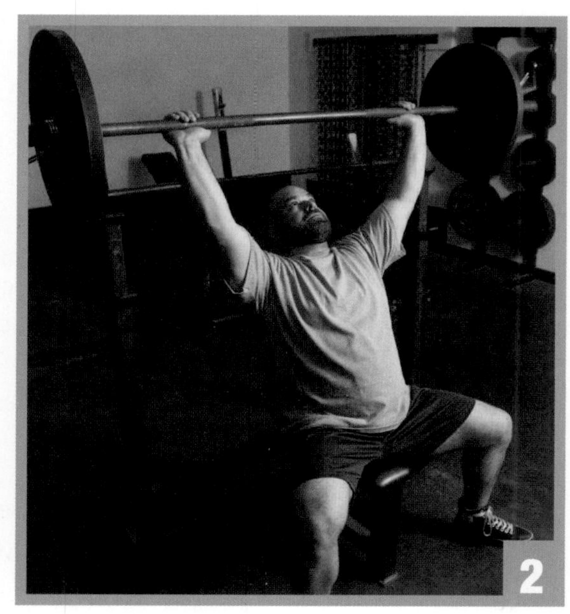

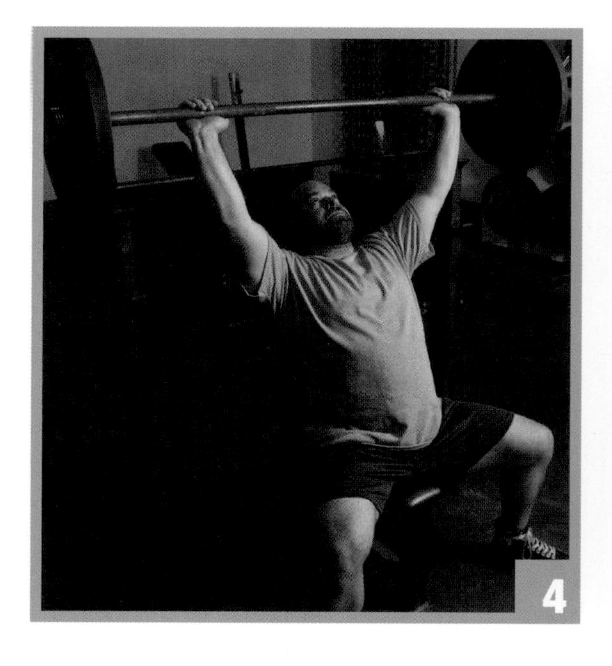

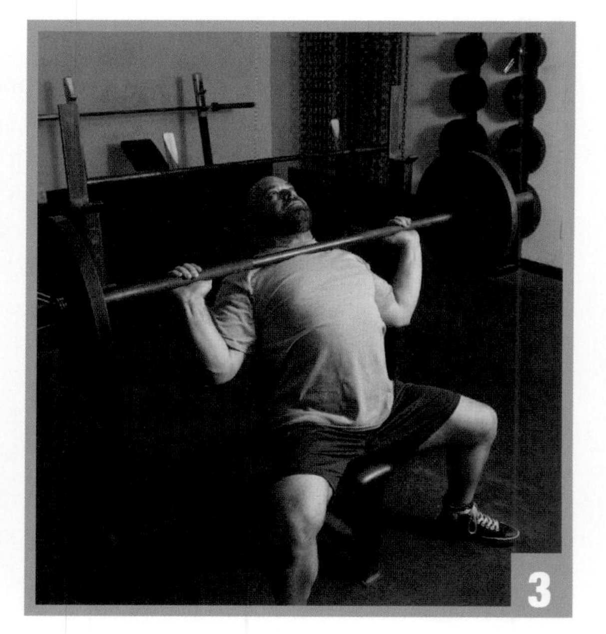

Shoulder strength is a critical component of upper body power, and no exercise builds shoulder strength quite like the overhead press. If performed while standing, overhead presses will also help strengthen your entire body as a unit, because you must rely on your lower body to transfer energy from the floor to the bar.

Set-Up

You can start the lift from either the bottom or the top. Starting at the top is easier, because you have the eccentric portion of the lift to build elastic energy. Generally the standing overhead press will be started from the bottom and walked out of the rack like a front squat.

A seated press starts at the top, with the lifter taking the weight from the racks like a bench press. If you are performing the overhead press while seated, make sure that the rack is not too far behind you, which could put too much stress on your shoulders. A handoff is preferable.

You can take either a thumbs-around or thumbless grip. I prefer the thumbless grip because it makes it easier for me to keep my elbows in close to my body and reduces the stress on my shoulders.

For the seated shoulder press, you can either lean back on an upright bench or perform the exercise unsupported. Leaning back will allow you to use more weight, while going at it unsupported will do more to strengthen your midsection.

Once you have the weight overhead, lift your head and chest and depress and retract your shoulder blades to lock yourself in.

The Descent

Lower the weight in a controlled manner while keeping your elbows tucked somewhat, rather than flared out. While this exercise can be performed behind the neck, few lifters have the shoulder flexibility for this. I always recommend lowering in front of your head, to just below.

The Ascent

When the bar descends below the chin, reverse the direction and press straight up to lockout.

Variations

You can perform shoulder presses with varying degrees of incline, as well as special bars (such as a fat bar) and dumbbells.

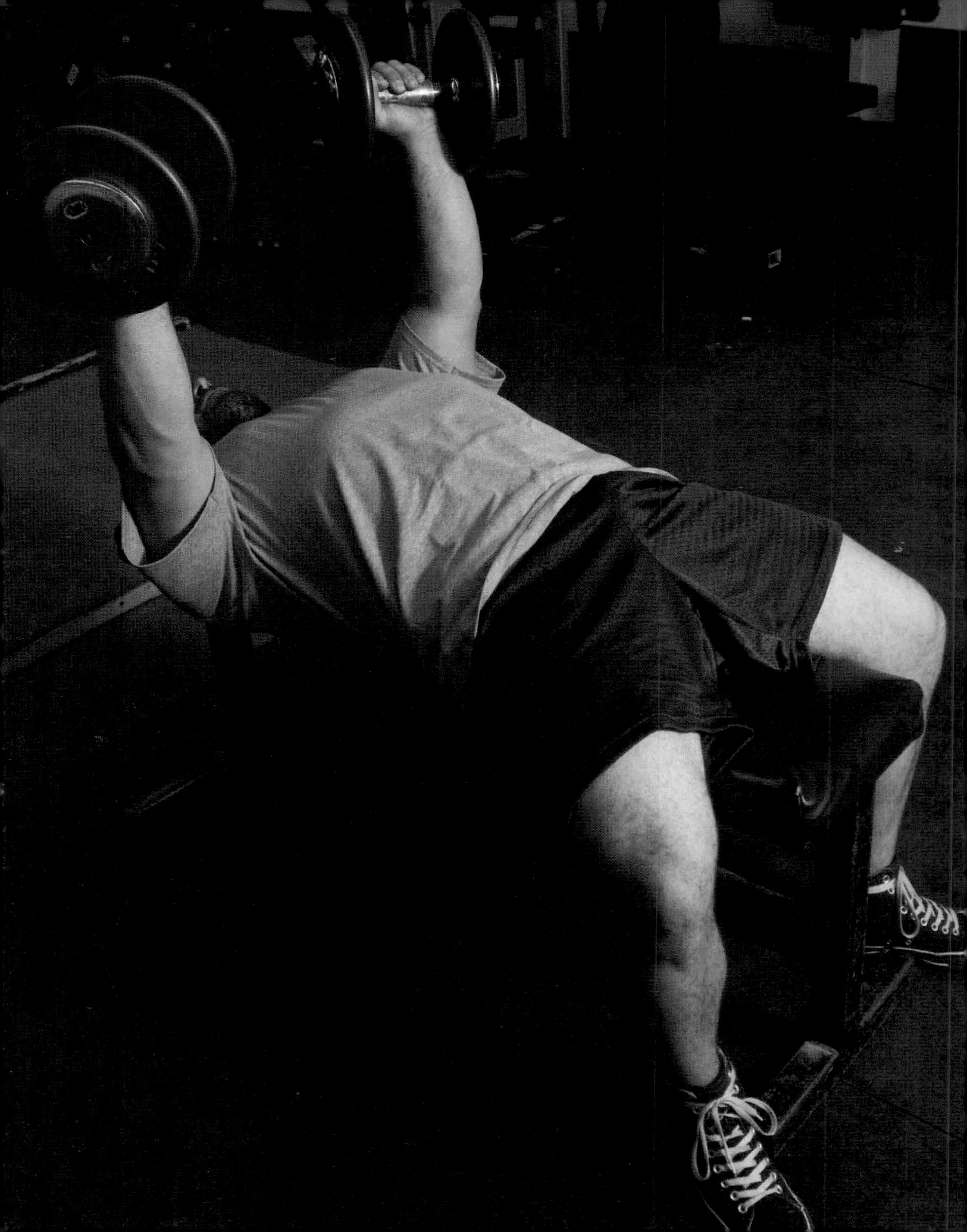

ASSISTANCE EXERCISES

Unlike special exercises, which are intended to stimulate your nervous system, assistance exercises are designed to strengthen and develop your musculature.

When used in conjunction with either special or competitive lifts, assistance exercises are used to more thoroughly train relevant muscles as well as bring up lagging ones.

With the exception of extra or feeder workouts, assistance exercises should generally be performed after special or competitive lifts because you should be fresh when attempting maximal or near maximal lifts.

While special exercises can often be used for assistance exercises, assistance exercises are rarely acceptable as special exercises. The reason for this is that they are often not safe to perform maximally and often do not have a movement pattern that is similar enough to the competitive lifts.

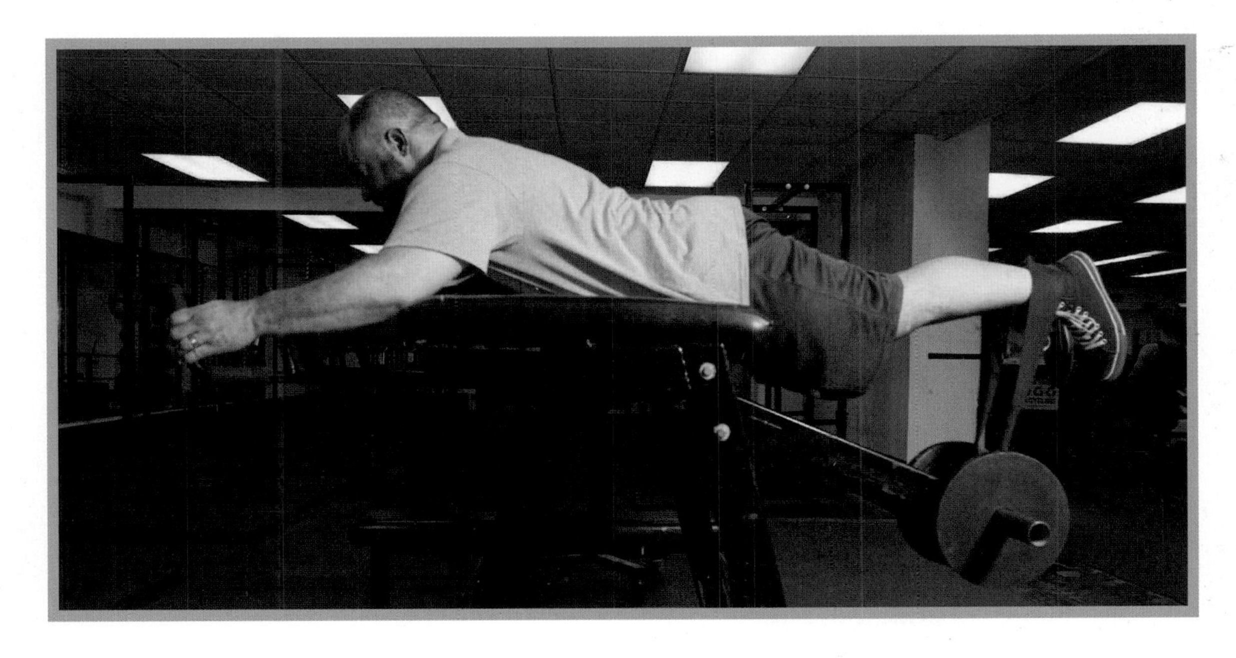

BACK EXTENSIONS

Muscles Targeted: Hamstrings, glutes, and lower back

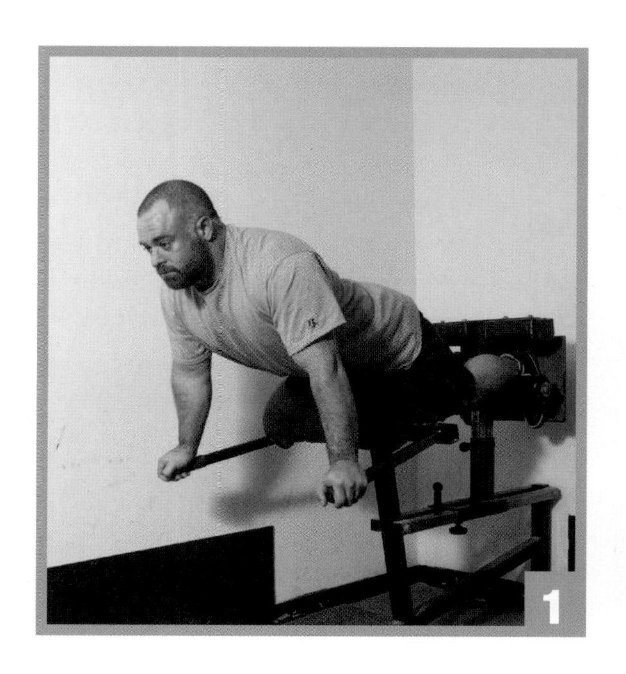

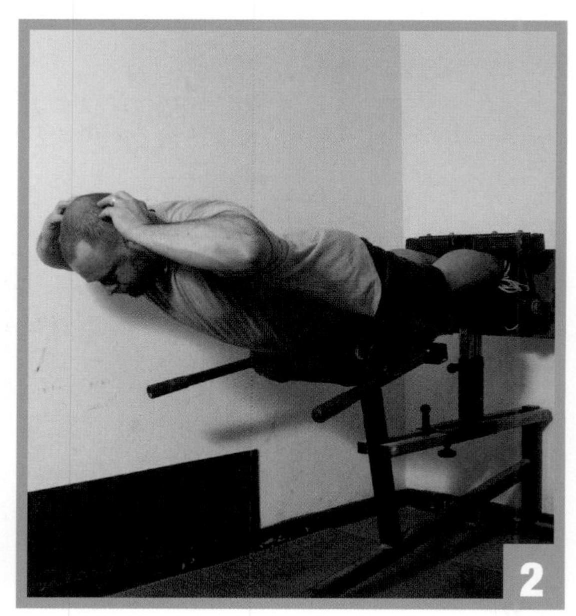

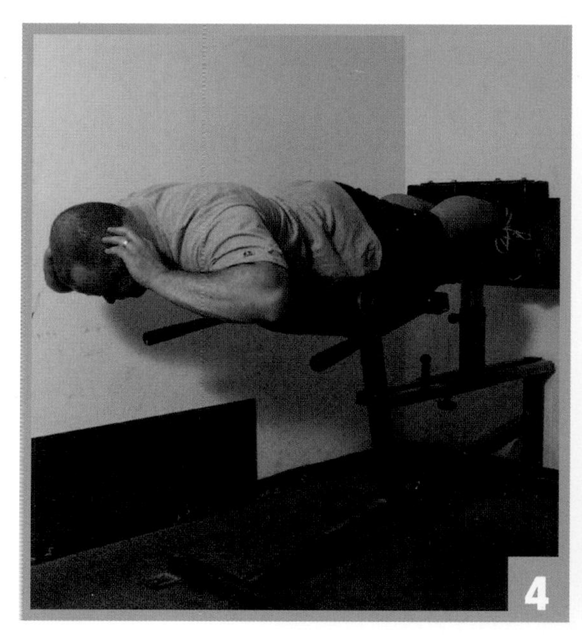

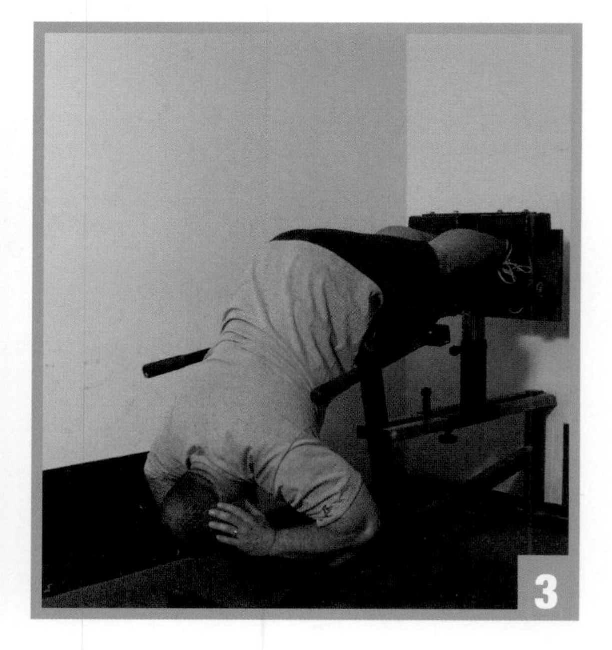

The back extension can be found in almost any commercial gym. Although the more comfortable 45-degree models are more popular, the older style 90-degree ones are harder, and in my opinion, more effective. You can use a glute-ham bench for these as well.

Set-Up

Climbing onto a back extension bench for the first time can be a little scary because there is nothing supporting your upper body, and you might get the sensation that you will fall off. As long as your feet are securely anchored, you are perfectly safe. Start by placing your feet on the foot plate while supporting your weight with your hands on either the pad, or side handles. Your feet should be slightly closer than shoulder width, and the pad should be firmly against the back of your legs, just above the heels. Make sure that the pad extends to just below the crease of your hip, so you have full range of motion. If it is not, get off and adjust the thigh pad height.

The Exercise

Keeping your legs straight, bend over at the hips until your hips are at about a 45-degree angle, then reverse direction until your back and torso are straight.

Variations

You can increase difficulty by holding a weight to your chest or draping an anchored band or chain around your neck.

GLUTE-HAM RAISES

Muscles Targeted: Hamstrings, glutes, lower back, and calves

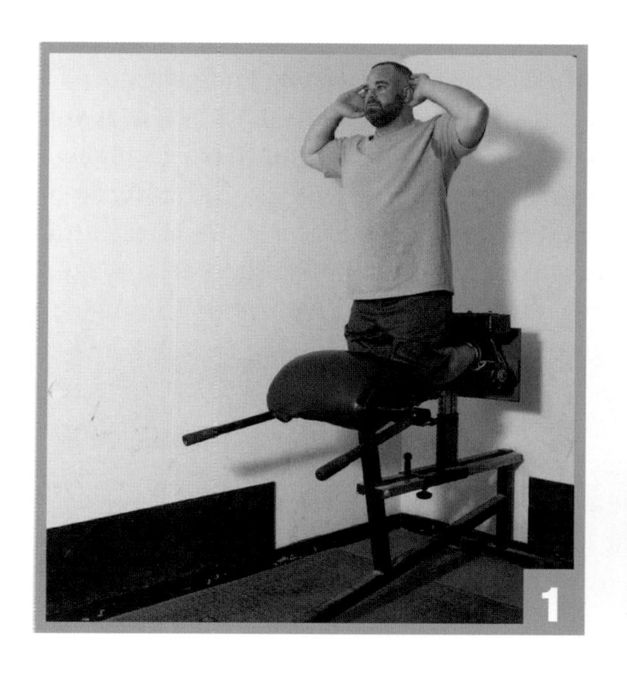

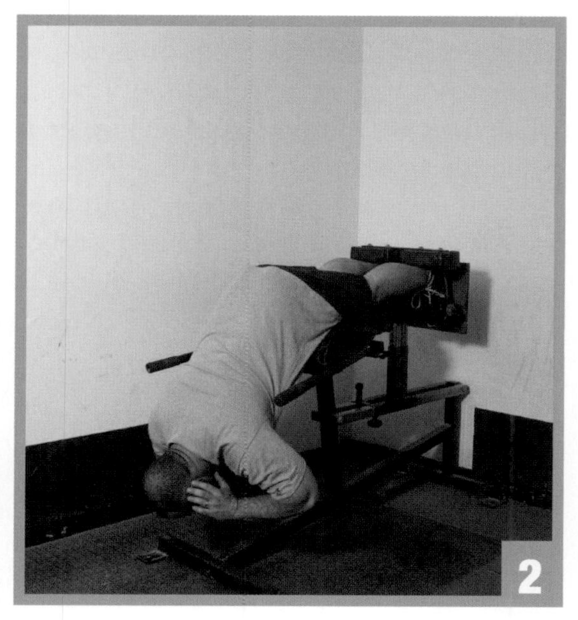

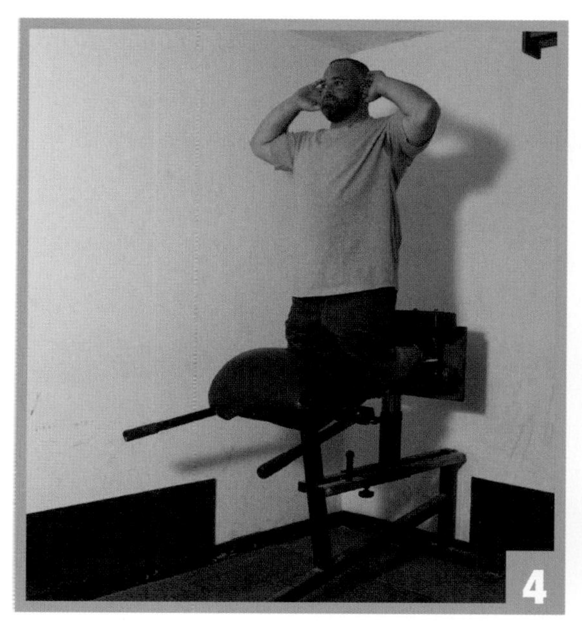

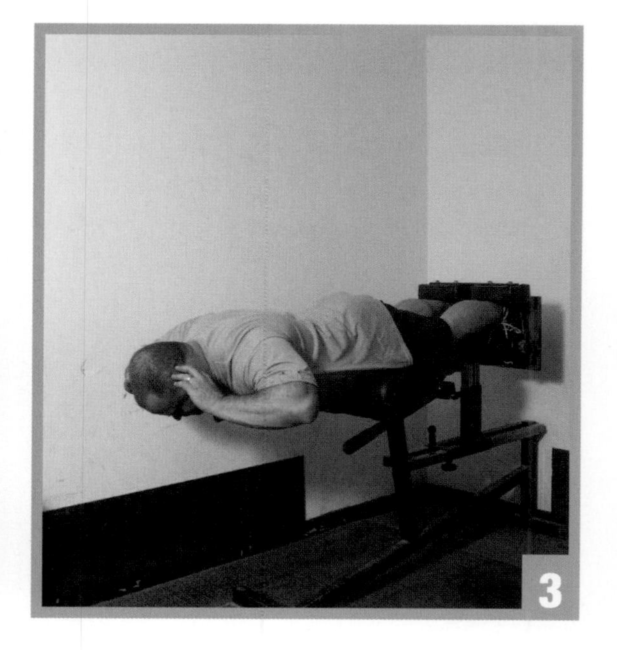

To the average gym patron, glute-ham raises look nearly indistinguishable from a back extension, with the main difference being a rounded, rather than flat, pad. If you do happen to spot one in a commercial gym, you are more likely to see members doing sit-ups on it than an actual glute-ham raise.

Set-Up

To get into position, Place your feet flat against the plate, with the round pad against your quadriceps. There will usually be handles on either side of the round thigh pad to hold yourself up with. The start position may be uncomfortable at first but most lifters get used to it.

The Exercise

The first phase of the exercise looks just like a standard back extension. However, rather than stopping when your back is straight, continue the movement by bending at the knee and pulling yourself up with the strength of your hamstrings.

This exercise is remarkably effective because unlike the back extension or hamstring curl, the glute-ham raise works the hamstrings at both the hip and knee joints.

The combination of hip extension and knee flexion makes this exercise very effective, and very difficult. Many gyms do not even have a glute-ham raise machine because the members would not know how to use it.

Variations

To make the glute-ham easier, you can prop the front of the machine up on a platform or block. To make it harder, prop the back up. You can also increase difficulty by holding a weight to your chest.

STRAIGHT LEG DEADLIFTS

Muscles Targeted: Hamstrings, glutes, and lower back

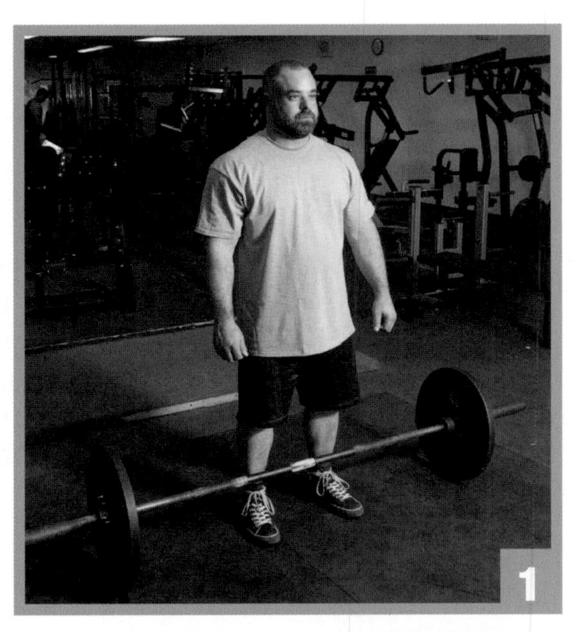

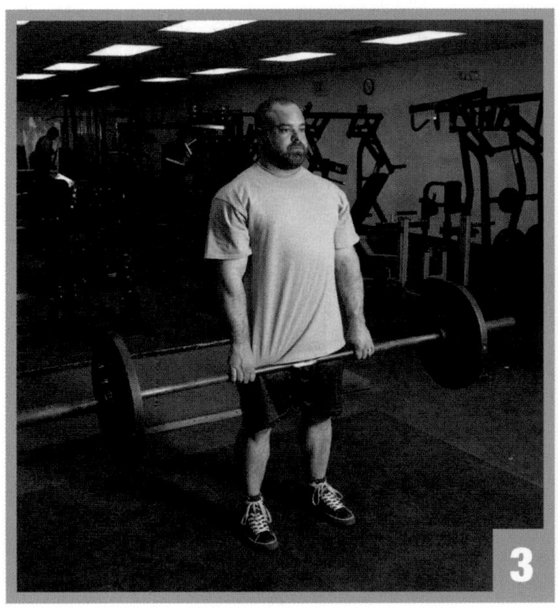

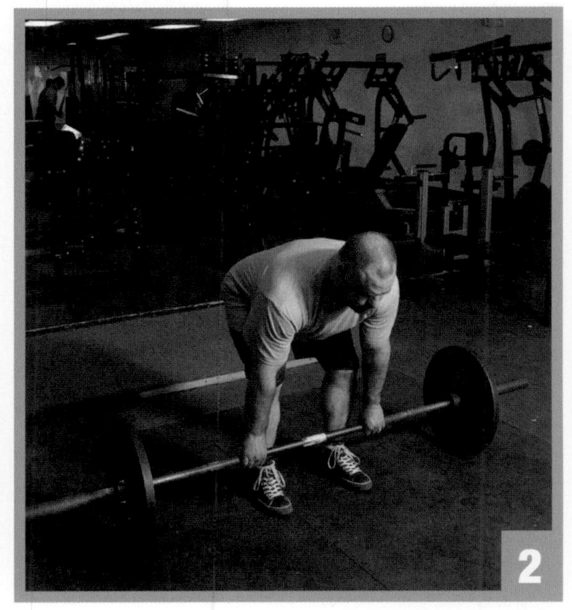

The straight leg deadlift is exactly what it sounds like: a deadlift with minimal knee-bend.

Set-Up

The starting position is a lot like that of a conventional deadlift, with the difference being that you would keep your hips high, and your knees only slightly bent. Although you can start the first repetition from the floor, I generally recommend starting out of a rack, to reduce the risk of a hamstring pull. Set the bar in the rack at about mid-thigh height. Take a shoulder width grip and lift the bar out of the rack by pushing your hips forward. Take a couple of steps back and take a narrow stance (feet about 8 to 12 inches apart).

The Exercise

Lower the weight by pushing your hips back and using a bowing motion. Your back should remain neutral and your knees should be slightly bent. You can either touch the weight to the floor before standing back up, or let it settle momentarily like a conventional deadlift. The dead stop is superior for gaining strength, while the touch-and-go version is used primarily for gaining muscle mass. Lift the weight by standing up and pushing your hips forward. Avoid allowing your back to round, and keep your spine neutral throughout the set.

Variations

The straight leg deadlift can be performed with either a barbell or dumbbells. Straight leg deadlifts can also be performed standing on mats, or as a partial movement out of the rack.

CABLE PULL-THROUGHS

Muscles Targeted: Hamstrings, glutes, and lower back

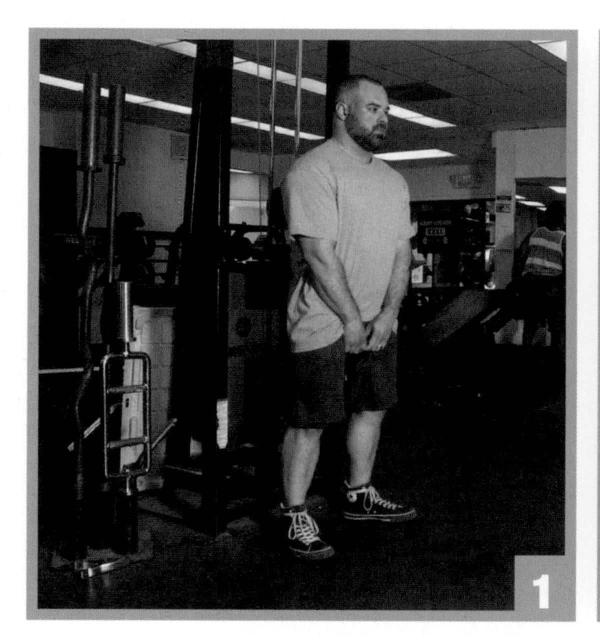

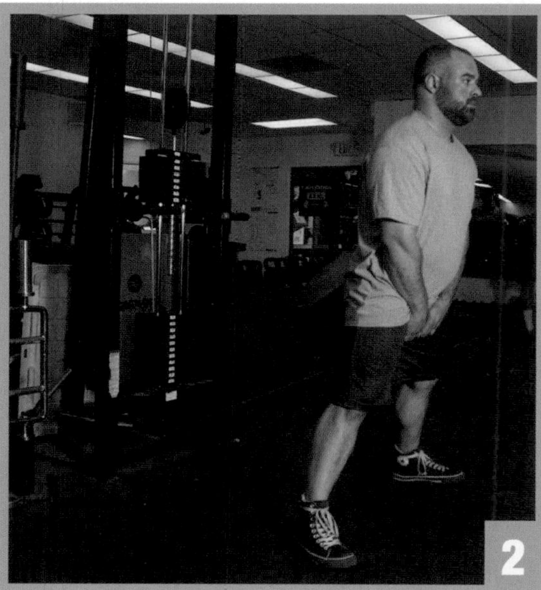

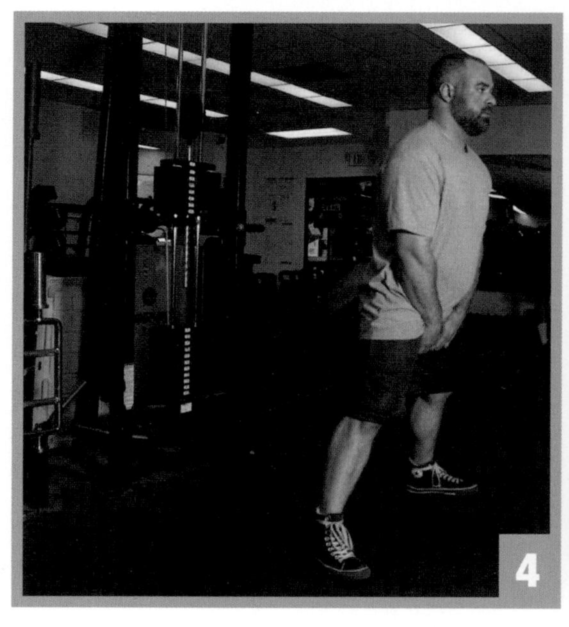

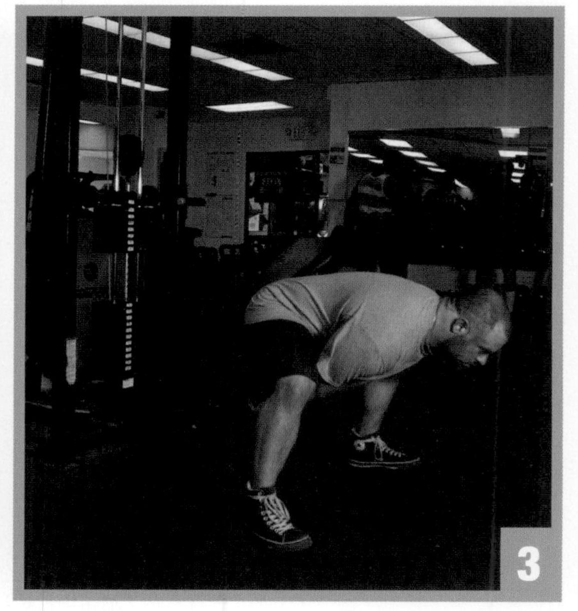

The cable pull-through is an odd-looking cable exercise, although it's very effective at building posterior chain strength. For lifters who lack access to special machines like the reverse hyper and glute-ham bench, the cable pull-through is a great replacement, requiring only a low cable pulley, which is found in most gyms.

Set-Up

Attach either a rope handle or single handle to the end of the cable. Standing up, facing away from the pulley, hold the handle with both hands so that you are straddling the cable. If using the single cable handle, you may only have room to grasp the handle with three fingers, leaving the pinky off. Walk forward a few steps and take a slightly wider than shoulder width stance. You may need to lean forward slightly to prevent the resistance from pulling you back.

The Exercise

Keeping your knees slightly bent and your back neutral, bend forward at the hip. Your arms should remain relaxed, and the pull of the resistance should cause a slight stretch in the hamstrings.

Variations

In addition to the low cable, pull-troughs can also be performed with an elastic resistance band.

DUMBBELL BENCH PRESS

Muscles Targeted: : Pectorals, deltoids, and triceps

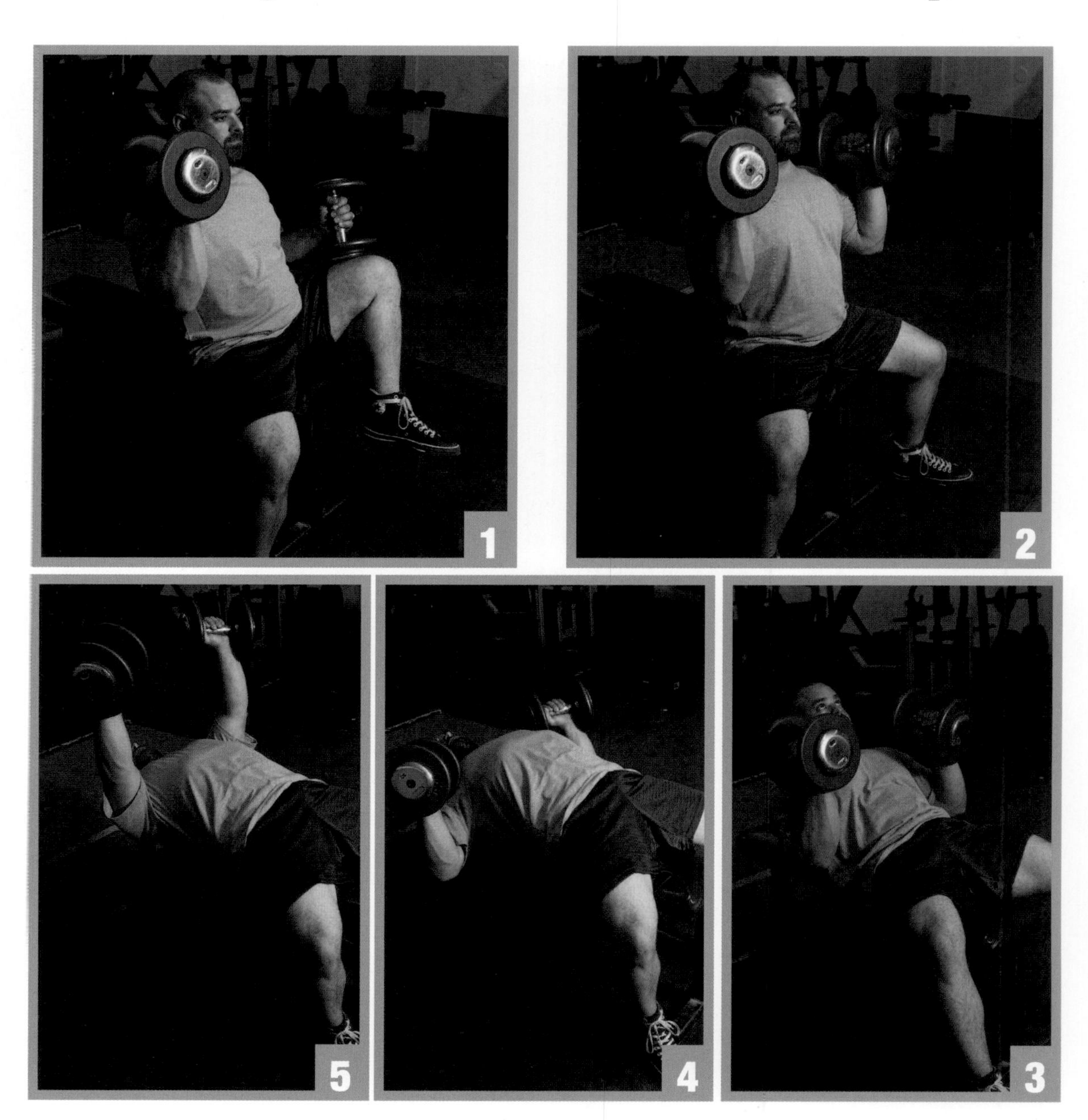

The dumbbell bench press is a bench press variation typically used as an assistance exercise, but rarely as a main lift due to the inherent instability of dumbbells versus barbells. Used in the 8 to 15 rep range, however, they are an excellent exercise for building strength and stability in the bench press, especially off the chest.

Set-Up

The biggest challenge of the dumbbell bench press can be getting into the start position with a pair of heavy dumbbells. Start by sitting on the end of the bench, with the ends of the dumbbells resting on your thighs. To get into the start position, lay back on the bench while simultaneously "kicking" the dumbbells to arm's length by lifting the knees.

You should now be lying on the bench, on your back, with the dumbbells at arm's length, and your feet flat on the floor.

The Exercise

Keeping an overhand grip (palms of your hands toward your knees), lower the dumbbells until your hands are level with your torso. At the bottom position, your hands should be in the same spot that they would be for the barbell bench press–in line with the bottom of your sternum. Once you reach the bottom position, press the dumbbells back into lockout. Unless the dumbbells are particularly large, you should not touch them at the top.

Variations

Dumbbell bench presses can also be performed on an incline or decline bench. As with the barbell bench press, your bottom position will vary—with your hands in line with the top of your chest on an incline bench, and in line with the top of your abdominals on a decline bench. Dumbbell bench presses can be performed with a parallel grip (palms facing each other), which places more stress on the triceps and alleviates stress on the pecs. Dumbbell presses can also be performed in an alternating fashion, where you complete 1 rep on one side while holding the opposite dumbbell at arm's length, then repeating on the opposite side. This variation challenges stability and coordination.

DUMBBELL OVERHEAD PRESSES

Muscles Targeted: Deltoids and triceps

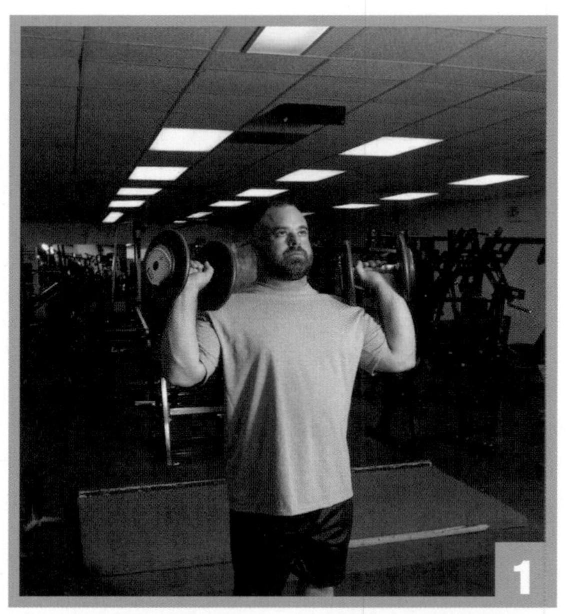

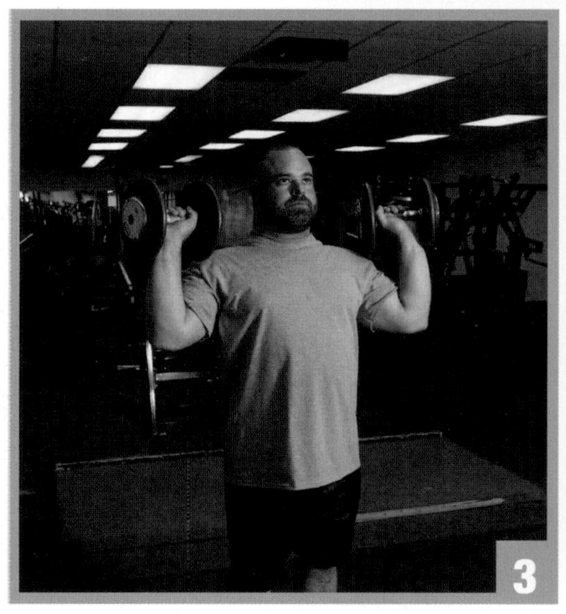

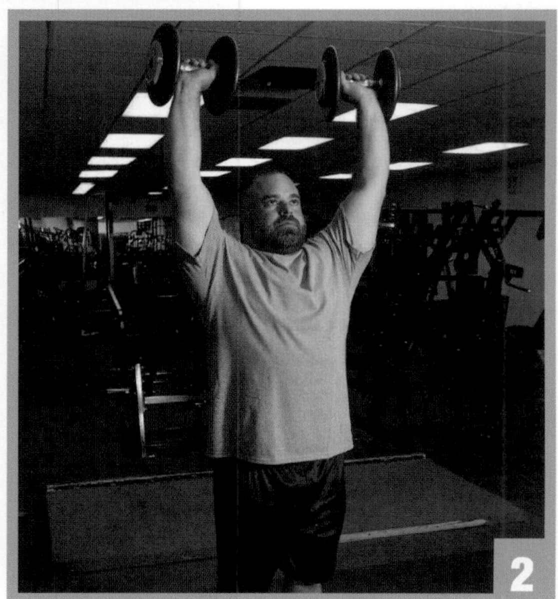

Like the dumbbell bench press, the dumbbell overhead press is a variation typically used as an assistance exercise, but rarely as a main lift due to the inherent instability of dumbbells versus barbells. Also like the dumbbell bench press, they are excellent for building strength in the barbell lift, especially out of the bottom position.

Set-Up

Like the dumbbell bench press, the biggest challenge of the dumbbell overhead press can be getting into the start position with a pair of heavy dumbbells. Start by sitting on the end of the bench, or on the back-supported bench with the ends of the dumbbells resting on your thighs. To get into the start position, kick the dumbbells to shoulder height where you will start the press.

To start the movement, you should be sitting upright, holding the dumbbells at shoulder height with your palms facing forward. Keep your feet flat on the floor for additional support.

The Exercise

Press the dumbbells into lockout. At the top position, the dumbbells should be directly over your shoulders. Unless the dumbbells are particularly large, you should not touch them at the top.

Variations

You can perform dumbbell overhead presses on a bench either with or without a back support. A bench with the support will make the movement easier, but a bench without support will provide more of a challenge to your back and torso. Dumbbell overhead presses can be performed with a parallel grip (palms facing each other), which places more stress on the triceps and alleviates stress on the shoulders. Dumbbell presses can also be performed in an alternating fashion, where you complete 1 rep on one side while holding the opposite dumbbell at arm's length, then repeating on the opposite side. This variation challenges stability and coordination.

BENT-OVER ROWS

Muscles Targeted: Latissimus dorsi, trapezius, biceps, spinal erectors, and rhomboids

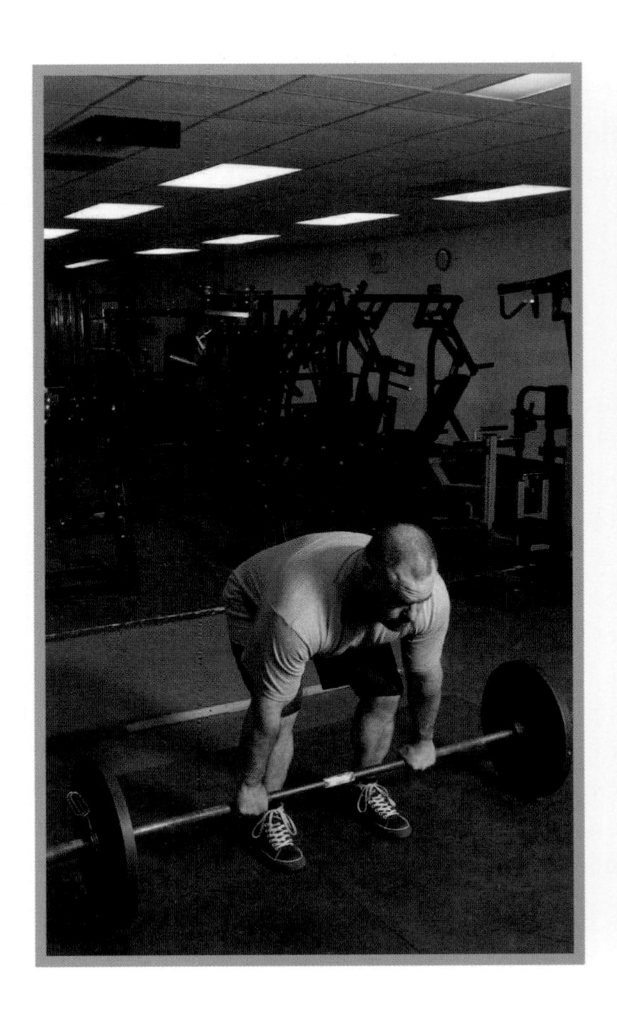

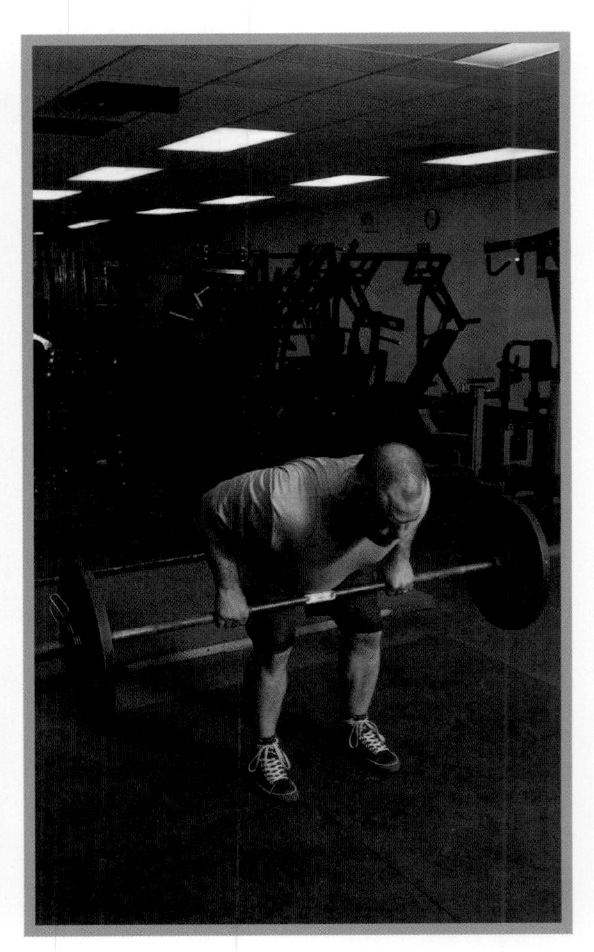

If your goal is to get as strong as possible, your mid-back region can never be too strong. The bent-over row is a great tool for strengthening your entire back. Due to the bent-over position, you need to use your lower back muscles to maintain your posture while your lats, rhomboids, and trapezius pull the weight toward your torso.

Bent-over rows work best in the 5 to 8 rep range. If you notice a lot of trouble keeping your posture, reduce the weight until you can maintain a neutral back.

Set-Up

Set the bar in the rack at about mid-thigh height. Take a shoulder width grip and lift the bar out of the rack by pushing your hips forward. Take a couple of steps back and take a shoulder-width stance. Bend forward at the waist at about a 45-degree angle to the floor allowing your arms to hang straight down.

The Exercise

Keeping your back neutral, pull the barbell toward your upper abdominals.

Variations

You can perform bent-over rows with barbells, dumbbells, and a reverse grip. You can also do these rows from a hang, or with a dead stop on the floor between reps. Since the object of rowing exercises is to strengthen your back, it is acceptable to use lifting straps on your top sets.

STANDING T-BAR ROWS

Muscles Targeted: Latissimus dorsi, trapezius, biceps, spinal erectors, and rhomboids

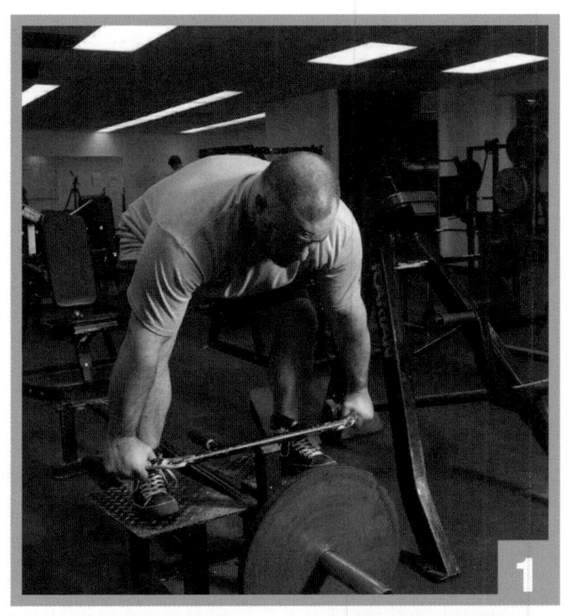
1

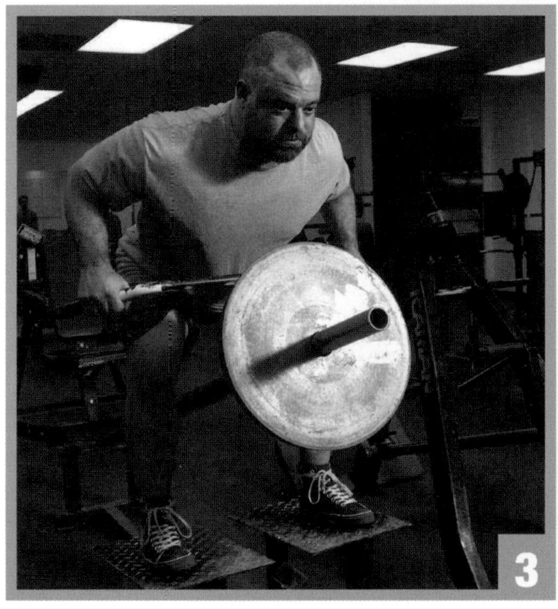
3

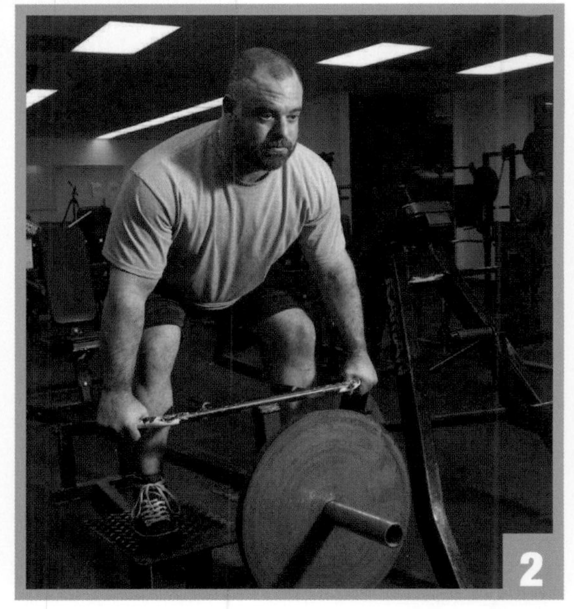
2

Set-Up

The standing t-bar row is a variation of the bent-over row using a simple lever. While plenty of gyms have a machine for this, you can also do the same thing with either a Core Blaster or by sticking one end of a barbell in the corner of the gym and placing a v-grip around it (not recommended with good bars). If you do use the corner, fold up a towel and place it in the corner to protect the walls from the barbell.

The Exercise

Keeping your back neutral, pull the v-grip toward your upper abdominals.

Variations

As with the barbell bent-over row, you can do this exercise with a dead stop, or from a hang position. Always start the pull by squeezing your shoulder blades together. This will teach you to keep them tight during a heavy bench or squat.

CHEST-SUPPORTED ROWS

Muscles Targeted: Latissimus dorsi, trapezius, biceps, and rhomboids

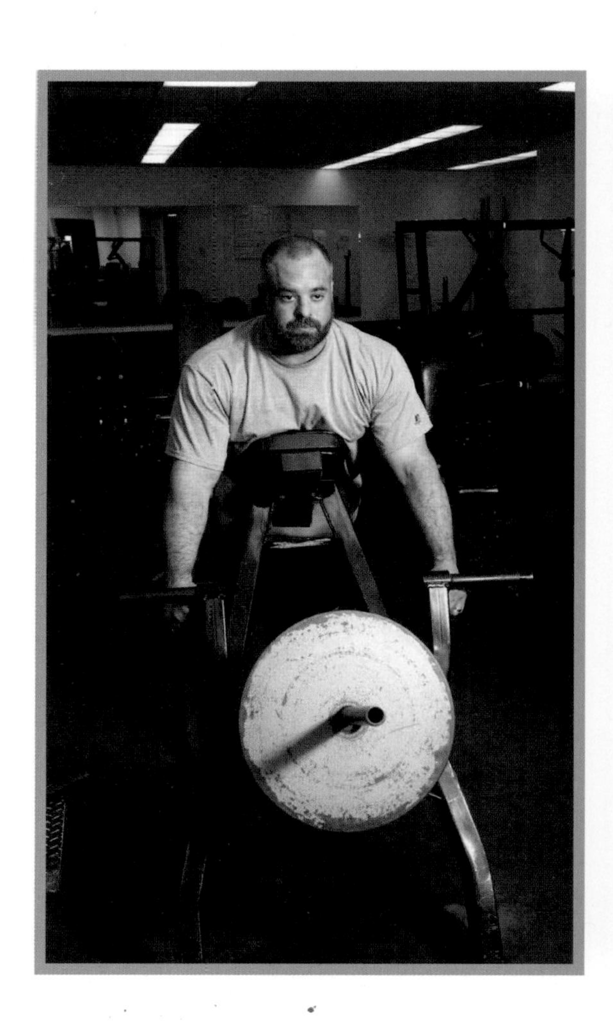

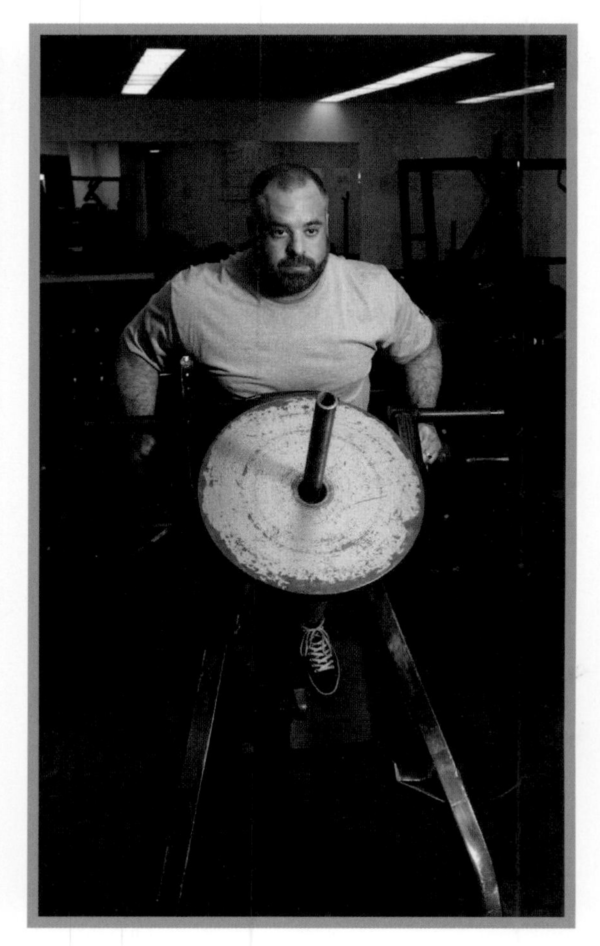

Chest-supported rows allow you to train the basic pulling movement without being limited by your lower back strength. Think of the chest-supported row as a bench press in reverse. There are numerous versions of the chest-supported row. If you are limited by equipment, you can do them with dumbbells or a barbell while laying over an adjustable bench. Some gyms have a variation of a t-bar row with a bench for you to lie on. Just about any commercial gym will have a selectorized chest-supported row machine, which is outlined in the machine exercise section. Any of these will work.

Set-Up

For the chest-supported t-bar version, adjust the height of the foot platform (if possible) so that the handles are in line with your mid-chest at the top of the movement. Load your desired weight on the sleeve at the end of the lever, then lay on the bench with your hands grasping the handles. Pull the bar out of the rack and hold it at arm's length. Before beginning the exercise, pull your shoulder blades together.

The Exercise

Pull the handles toward your chest, pausing for a beat at the top, before lowering the weight back to the starting position.

SEATED CABLE ROW

Muscles Targeted: Latissimus dorsi, trapezius, biceps, spinal erectors, and rhomboids

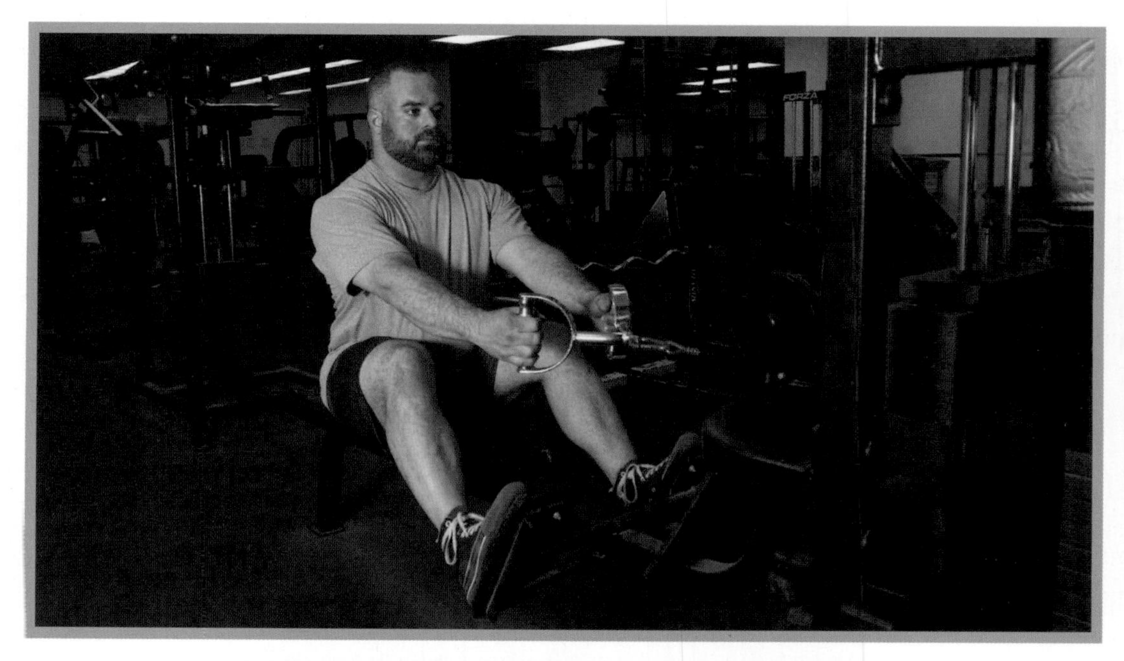

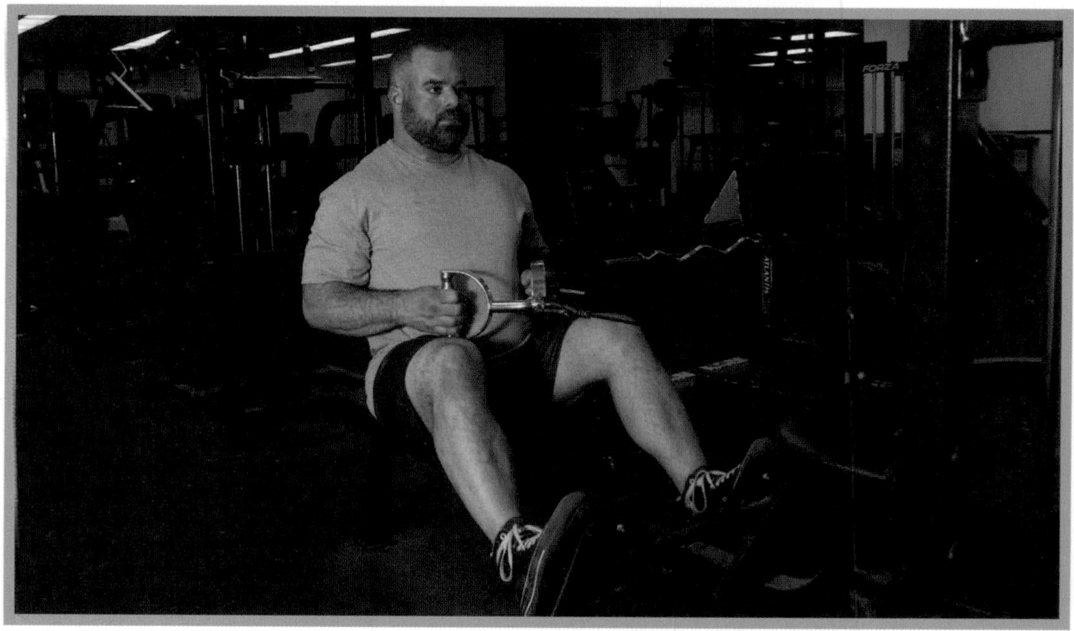

Even the most basic gyms have some kind of low pulley for the seated cable row. While not as hard on your back as the bent-over row, the seated cable row does place some stress on your spinal erectors because you need to maintain the chest-up posture.

Set-Up

Select your desired weight on the stack, then sit on the bench, facing the pulley. You should be sitting far back enough on the bench that you should need to bend forward slightly to grasp the cable attachment. Once you've got the attachment in your hands, lean back slightly until your torso is perpendicular to the bench. Lift your chin and chest, and pull your shoulder blades together.

The Exercise

Pull the handle toward your upper abdominals. As you pull the handle toward your torso, pay particular attention to your shoulder blades. Keep them tightly pulled together, which will teach you to keep them that way while squatting or benching.

Variations

You can do these with a wide grip, narrow grip, overhand grip, underhand grip, or the v-grip.

PULL-UPS

Muscles Targeted: Latissimus, trapezius, biceps, and rhomboids

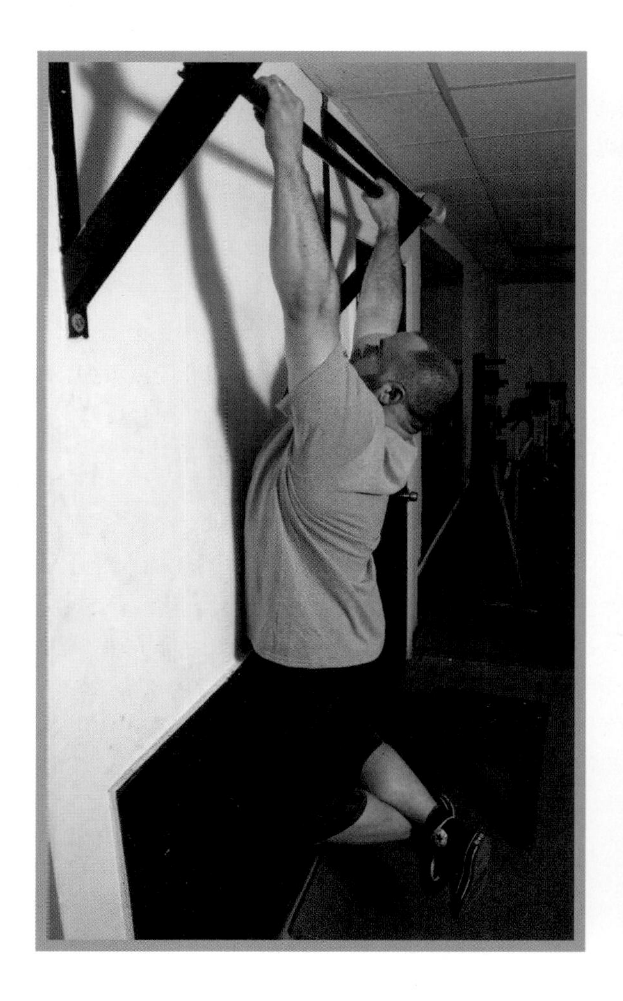

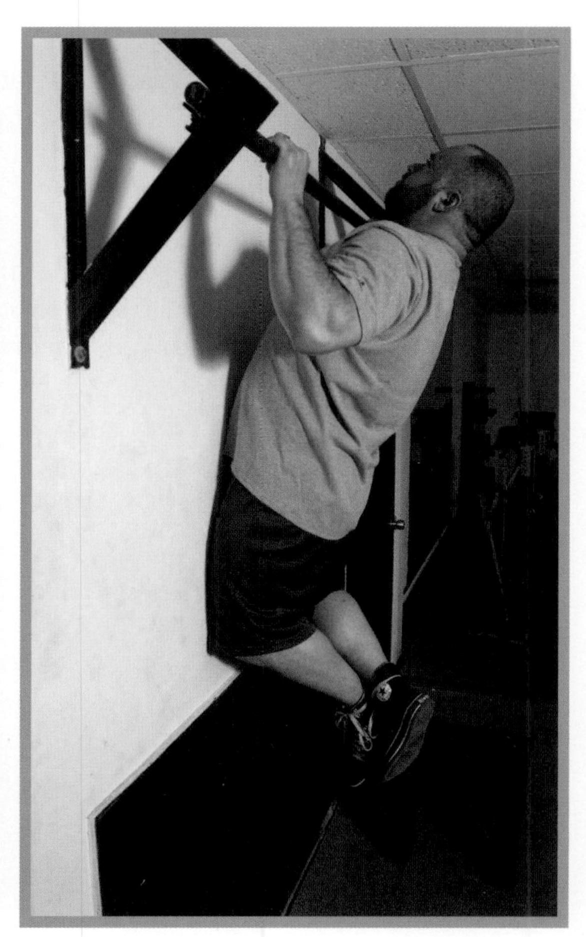

Pull-ups are a simple and very effective way to increase pulling strength. They are particularly good for those strapped for equipment or space because all you need is a sturdy bar or beam that will support your weight.

Although pull-ups are a very common exercise, it's actually quite rare to see them performed correctly. Most of the pull-ups you see are either partial reps, or kip-ups, which are essentially a "cheating" pull-up where the legs are kicked for momentum. The reason for this is simple: pull-ups are hard!

Set-Up

You can either jump or use a step to reach the pull-up bar. Take an overhand grip, slightly wider than shoulder width. Before starting the pull-up, make sure you are hanging still, and not still swinging from getting into position. At the starting point, your arms should be completely straight

The Exercise

Pull yourself up, lifting your chest toward the bar as you pull. Use as little momentum from your lower body as possible. When your chin clears the bar, you have done a complete rep.

Variations

If you are not good at pull-ups, you can do a modified version with your knees cradled in a band suspended from the rack or bar. You can also use an assisted pull-up machine at a commercial gym, which is explained in the machine exercise section. If you are getting more than 10 to 12 reps at a time, you can make them harder by hanging weights from a belt, or draping chains around your neck.

Pull-ups can be performed with an overhand grip, underhand grip, wide grip or parallel grip.

TRICEPS PUSHDOWNS

Muscles Targeted: Triceps

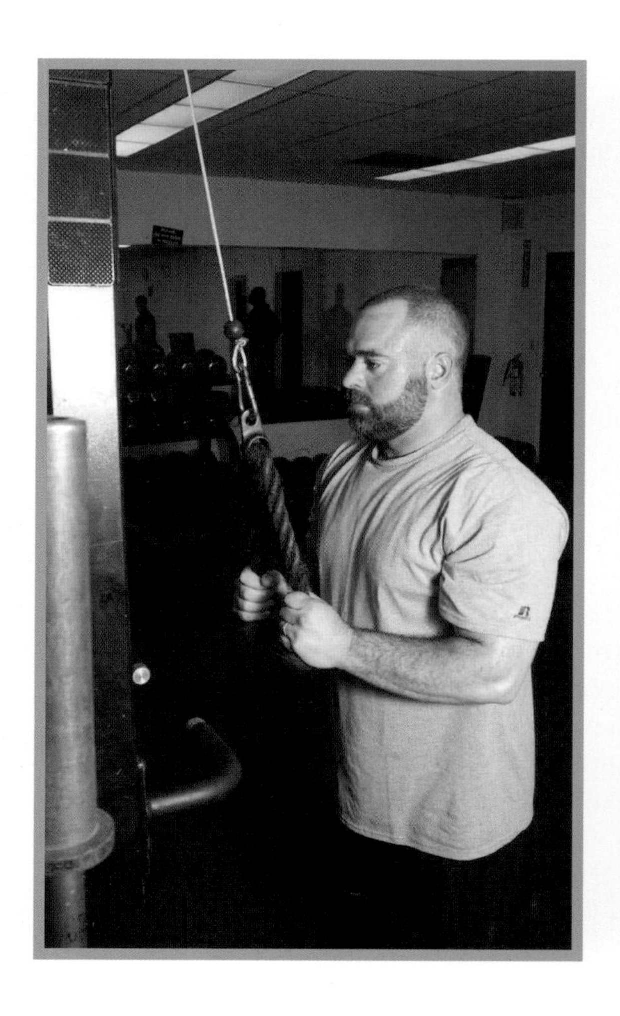

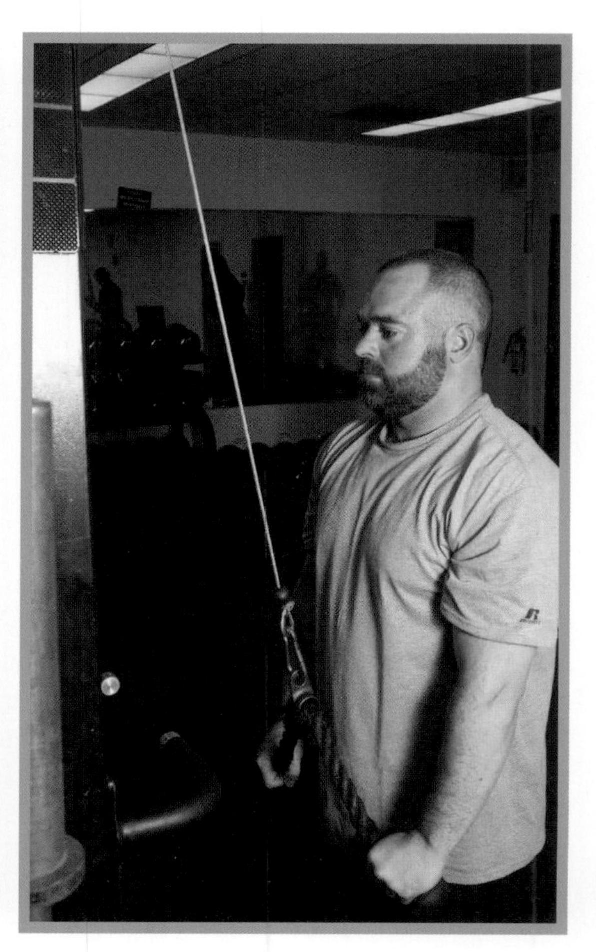

The triceps pushdown is one of the most popular assistance exercises for the triceps, primarily because it's one of the easiest to do. All you need is a cable set-up or a resistance band to loop over a rack, bar, or anything sturdy.

Set-Up

Start by grasping the band, rope, or handle with your arms at your sides and your elbows at 60 to 70 degrees.

The Exercise

Extend your elbows, keeping them at your sides.

LYING TRICEPS EXTENSIONS

Muscles Targeted: Triceps

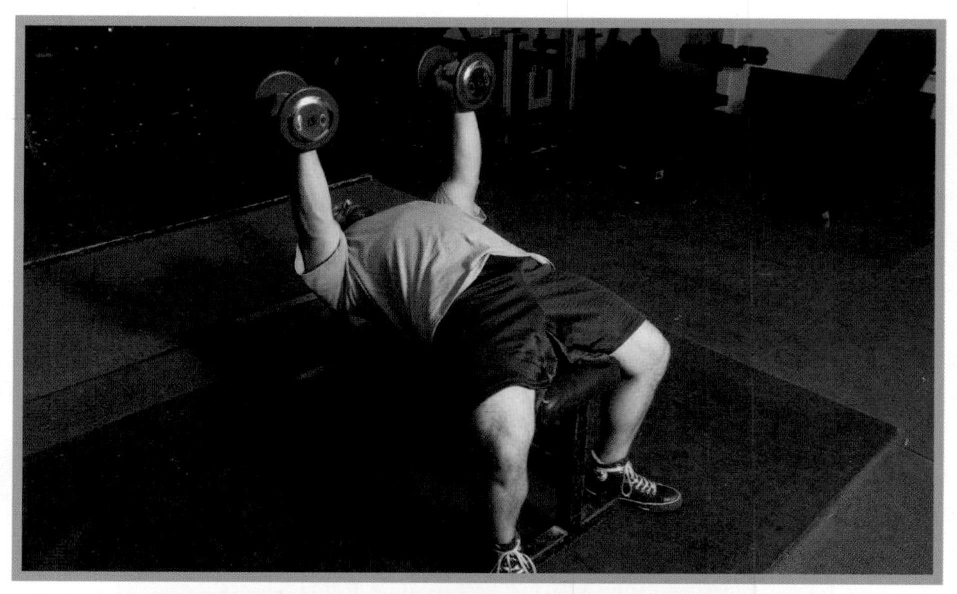

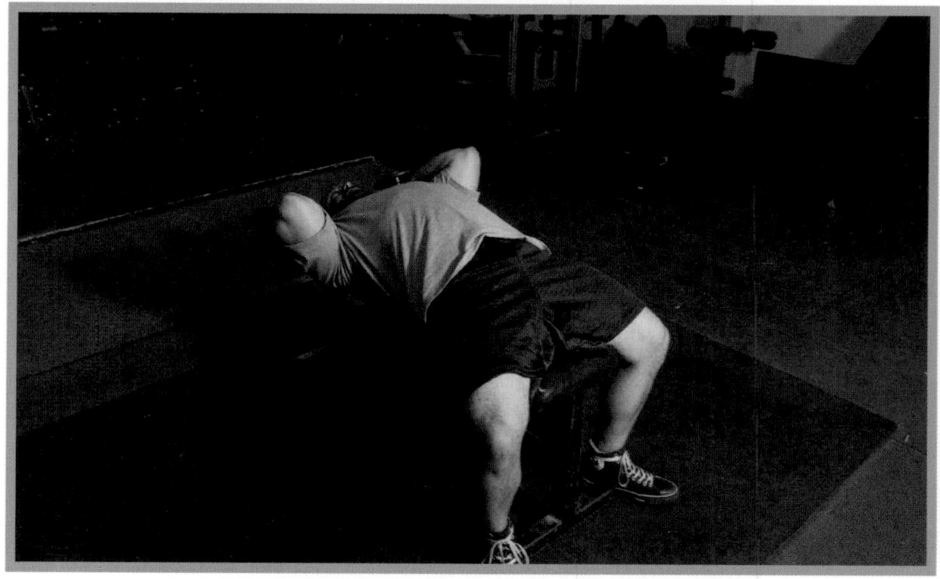

Set-Up

Select your desired dumbbells and sit on the end of the bench. Lie back, using your knees to help kick the dumbbells into the start position. You are ready to go when you are lying on your back, with the dumbbells at arm's length above you.

The Exercise

Without allowing your elbows to flare out, bend them until the dumbbells are right beside your head. When your elbows pass 45 degrees of flexion, reverse direction and lock the weights out.

Variations

There are tons of variations of this simple movement. You can use almost any style of bar, dumbbell, or kettlebell. You can add bands by wearing them around your back or looping them around the bench. You can use chains on the ends of the barbell. You can strictly bend your arms to lower the dumbbells, or eliminate the negative rep by rolling your arms back with your arms bent, then straightening your arms to lift the weight.

You can even perform lying triceps extensions on the floor, letting the dumbbells or barbell settle on the floor between reps.

SHOULDER RAISES

Muscles Targeted: Anterior, medial, or posterior deltoids, and rhomboids

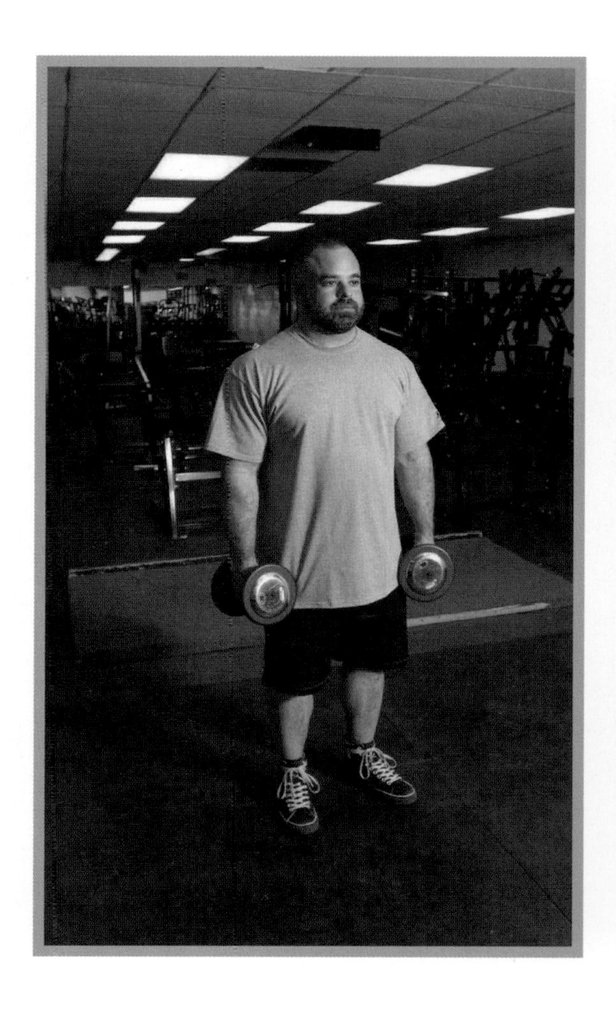

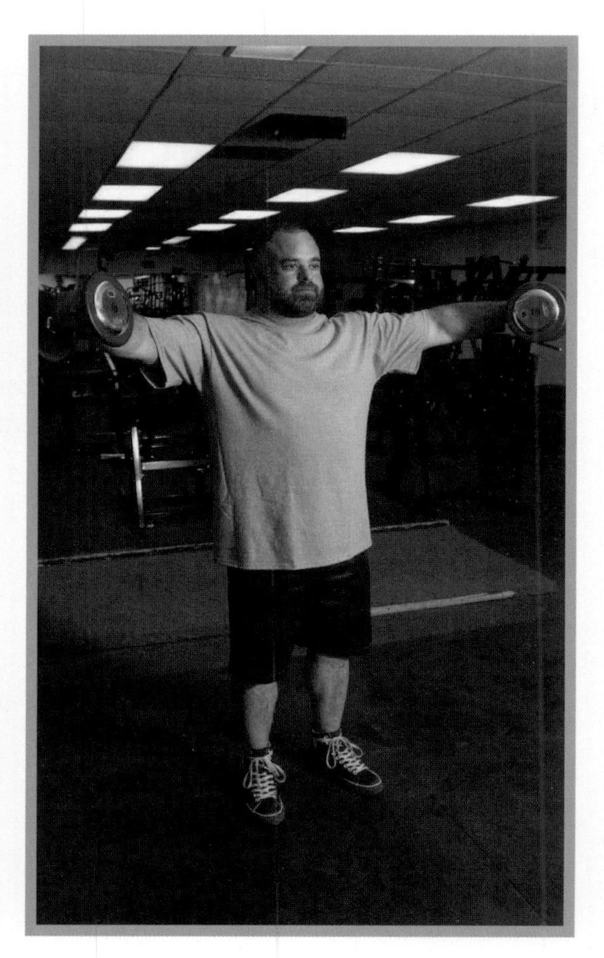

Shoulder raises are a simple and effective exercise for the shoulders.

Set-Up

Select two dumbbells and stand straight up, holding the dumbbells at your sides like suitcases.

The Exercise

Lift your arms out to your sides like a bird flapping its wings (only slower). When the dumbbells are at shoulder height, reverse direction and lower them back to the starting point.

Variations

Most often performed with dumbbells, there are three major variations of the shoulder raise:

- The lateral raise, which targets the medial (middle) deltoid (described above).
- The front raise, which targets the anterior (front) deltoid. To execute the front raise, lift the dumbbells with a forward arm movement, instead of out to the sides.
- The reverse fly, which targets the posterior (rear) deltoid. The reverse fly is particularly important for the bench and squat because it strengthens the rhomboids as well as the read deltoid, which helps you maintain position in the squat and bench. This variation requires you to lay face down on a slightly inclined bench. You'll lift the dumbbells in a similar manner to the lateral raise, but your body position will focus the stress on your rear deltoids.

BICEP CURLS

Muscles Targeted: Biceps

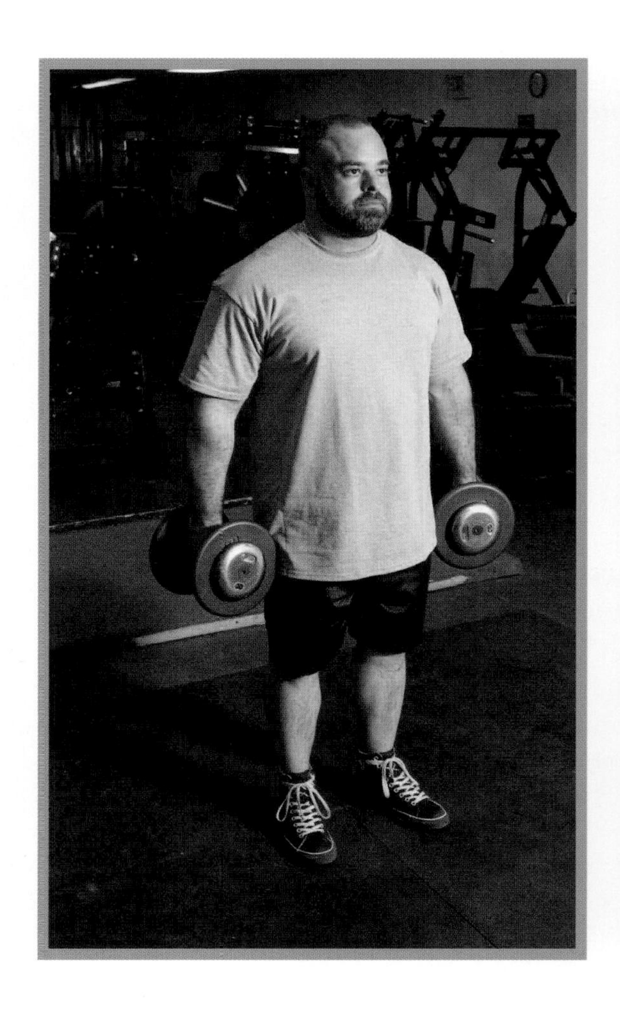

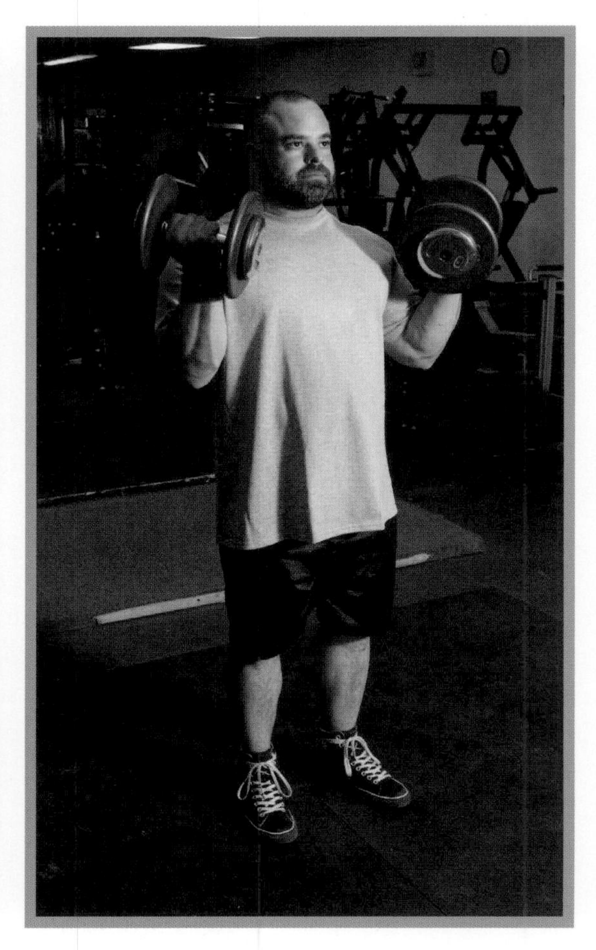

The biceps curl is a simple but often over-complicated arm movement. There are enough variations of the biceps curl to fill their own book.

Biceps curls are probably the most popular exercise in the weight room, which for most exercisers is completely disproportionate to their importance in terms of overall body strength. Of course, some curling is a good thing because it will balance your triceps work and prevent elbow problems, but most lifters already get plenty of biceps work from all the rowing exercises they do.

The Exercise

Just grab a weight and curl it. Do this a few times a month, whenever you remember.

FACE PULLS

Muscles Targeted: Rear deltoids and rhomboids

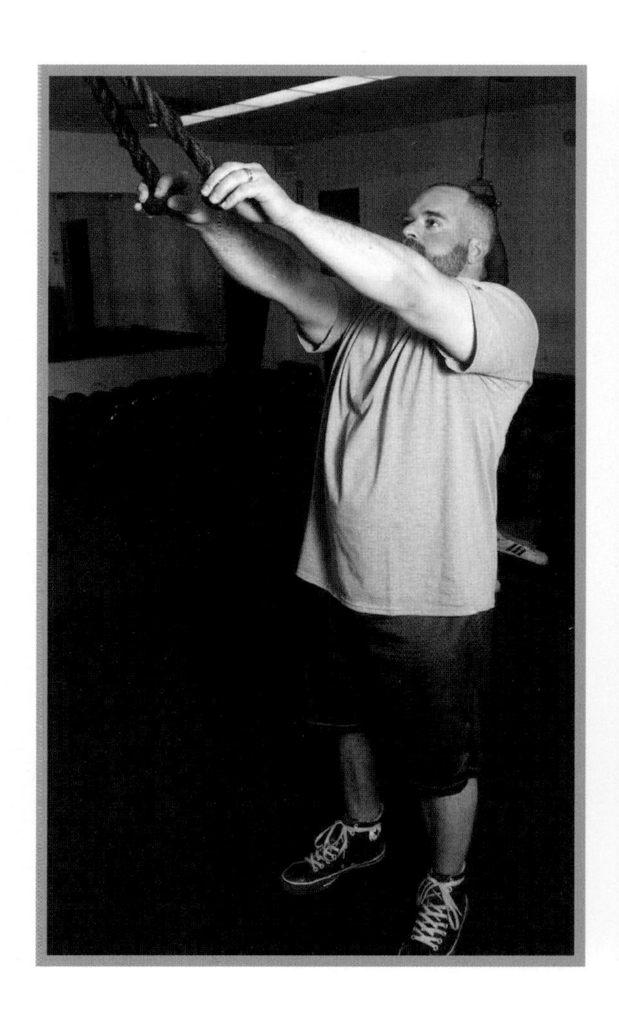

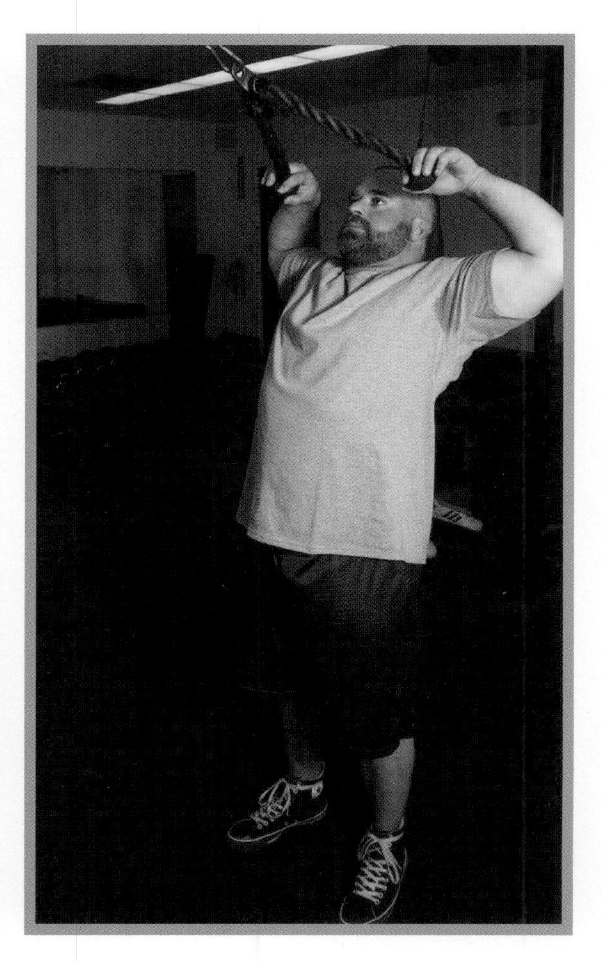

Face pulls are another good exercise to strengthen the upper back and help prevent some shoulder issues.

Set-Up

Attach a rope attachment to a high pulley. Grasp the rope with an overhand grip. Take a few steps back until you are supporting the weight with your arms outstretched.

The Exercise

Pull the rope toward your face, keeping your elbows high and allowing your shoulders to externally rotate as you reach the end of the motion. Pinch your shoulder blades together as you pull the rope toward your face.

REVERSE HYPERS

Muscles Targeted: Hamstrings, glutes, and lower back

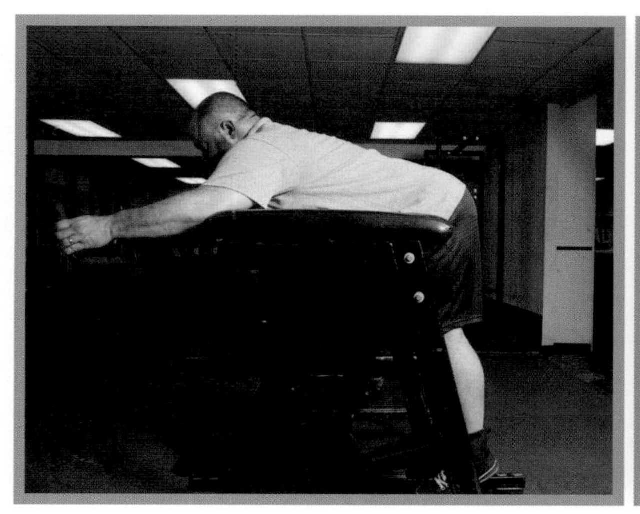

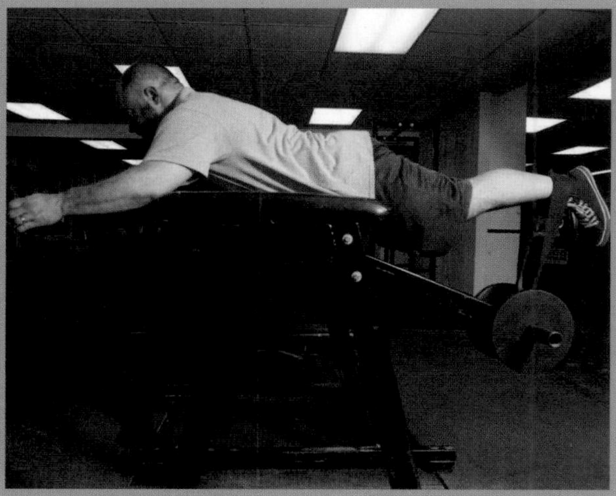

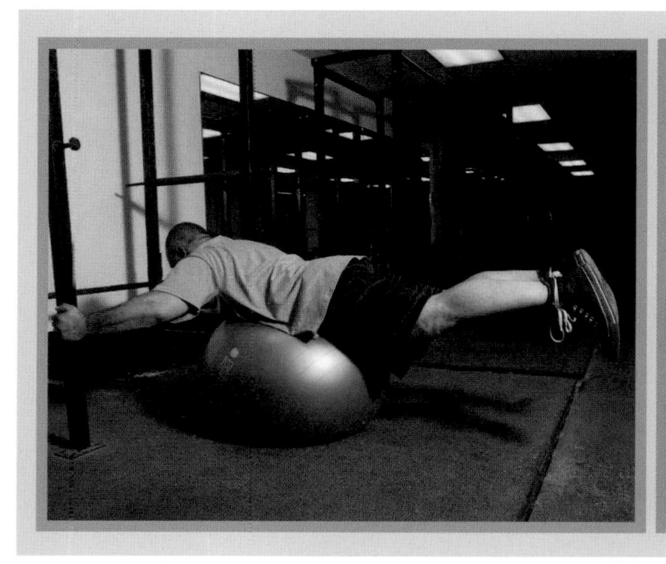

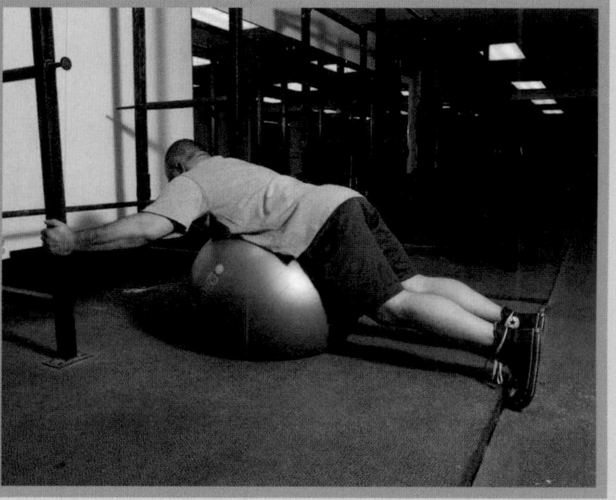

The reverse hyper is a popular assistance exercise among powerlifters for lower back strength and health. It's a great way to strengthen the back without compression. Serious gyms have a machine dedicated to this lift. In absence of this machine you can lay backward on a glute-ham or hyperextension bench.

Set-Up

Lay face-down on the pad with your legs hanging off so that your hip is at a 45-degree angle. The end of the pad closest to your feet should be just far enough above your hip to allow your legs to move freely. If you are on the machine version, loop the strap around your ankles. Some models have a roller at the bottom rather than the strap. In this case, place your ankles between the rollers.

The Exercise

Raise your legs until your body is completely straight. Allow the strap to pull your legs back down, stretching and applying traction to the back. Make sure that at the top of the movement you squeeze your lower back and glutes. You want to pump blood into the lower back to allow it to recover from all the heavy training.

Variations

You can do reverse hypers either by allowing the pendulum to swing or by strictly controlling the movement. The swinging movement puts more emphasis on tractioning the spine while the strict motion is more for strengthening the spinal erectors. I generally recommend the more controlled version because swinging the pendulum tends to allow for sloppier technique.

If you do not have access to a reverse hyper machine, you can replicate the movement by lying face down on a stability ball and holding something sturdy, like a rack. For resistance, you can hold a dumbbell between your legs, wear ankle weights, or just use your body weight and perform the movement slowly, focusing on contracting your lower back and glutes at the top of the movement.

CRUNCHES

Muscles Targeted: Rectus abdominis

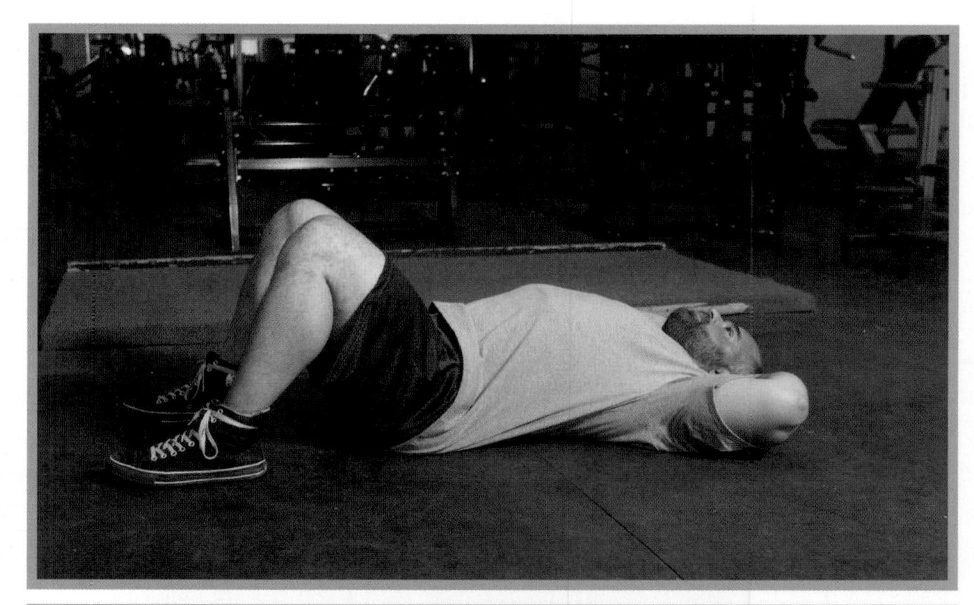

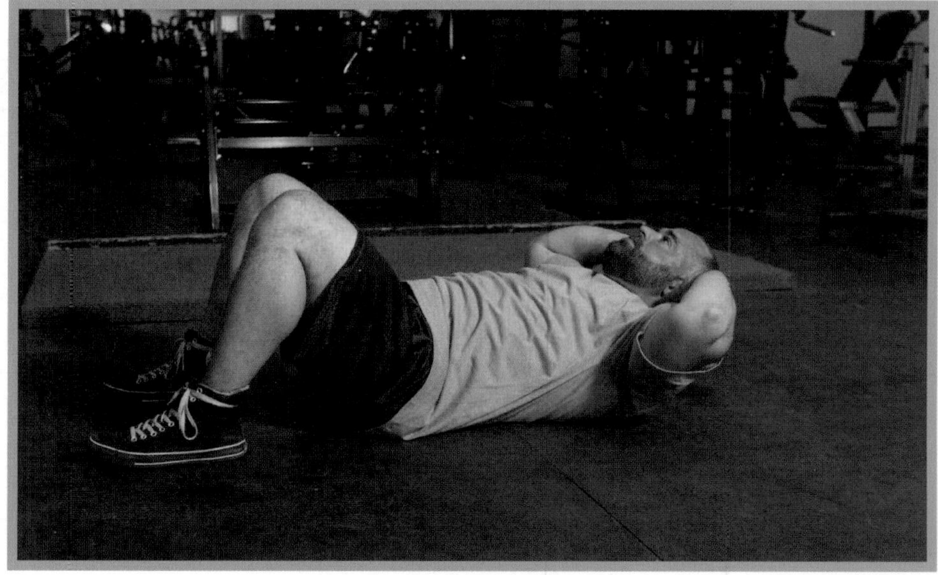

Crunches are easily the most popular abdominal exercise there is, and while they're often looked at as the stuff of aerobics classes, they do have a place in a strength training program if performed correctly.

Set-Up

Lie on the floor or on a mat, on your back, with your knees bent and your feet flat on the floor. Leaving your hands at your sides is the easiest variation, with hands on the chest being slightly harder, and fingertips at the ears being the hardest.

The Exercise

Keeping your face toward the ceiling, curl your torso up while contracting your abdominal muscles. This should be a slow, deliberate movement with no momentum to aid you.

Variations

You can make crunches more difficult by placing a weight on your chest or holding it behind your head. You can also place a medicine ball on your belly and practice pushing the ball up with your abs on each rep. This simulates how you will use your abdominals during the power lifts.

PULLDOWN ABS

Muscles Targeted: Rectus abdominis and obliques

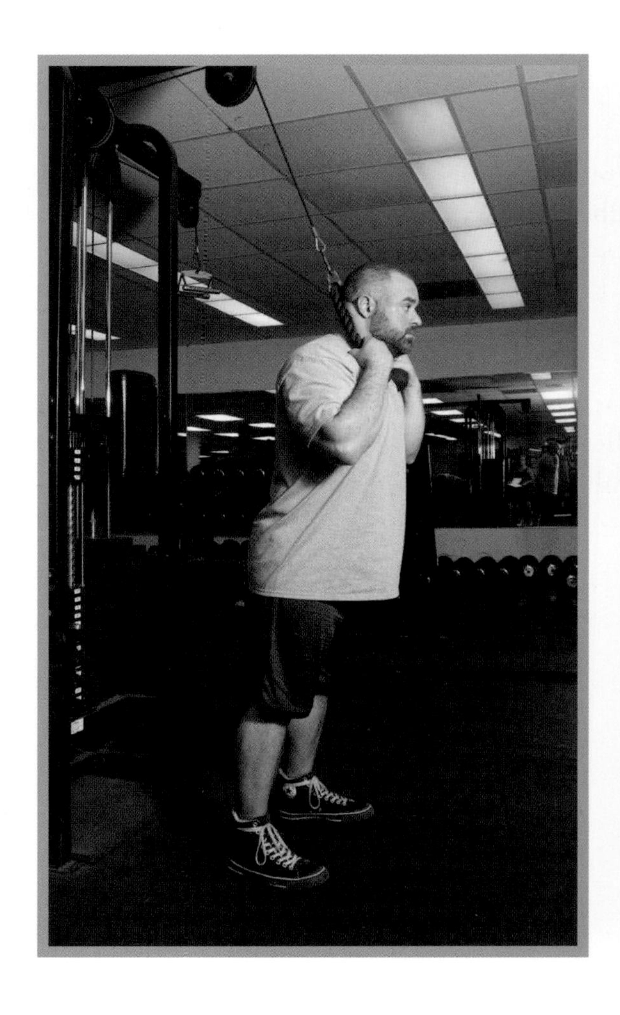

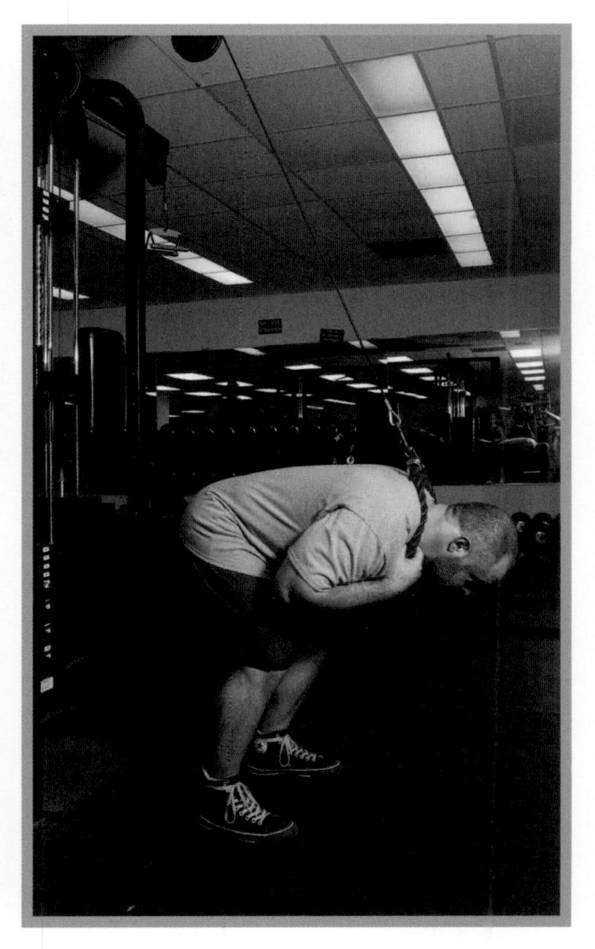

This is a wildly popular abdominal exercise for powerlifters because it's easy to perform, and it trains the abdominal muscles from a standing position. You can do it with a high pulley or with a resistance band. If you use the pulley, you can use either the rope attachment or the ab straps you can usually find on most gym pull-up bars.

Set-Up

Hold the cable attachment/band so that your head is between the ropes/bands.

The Exercise

With your gut full of air, pull the rope/band down toward the floor with a strong abdominal contraction. You should not be just flopping over and using your body weight to do the movement. If you are not out of breath after a set of 10 (even light ones), you are not doing it correctly.

Variations

You can also hold the band/cable to one side and do a standing side bend. This will strengthen your obliques and improve overall torso strength.

INCLINE BENCH SIT-UPS

Muscles Targeted: Rectus abdominis

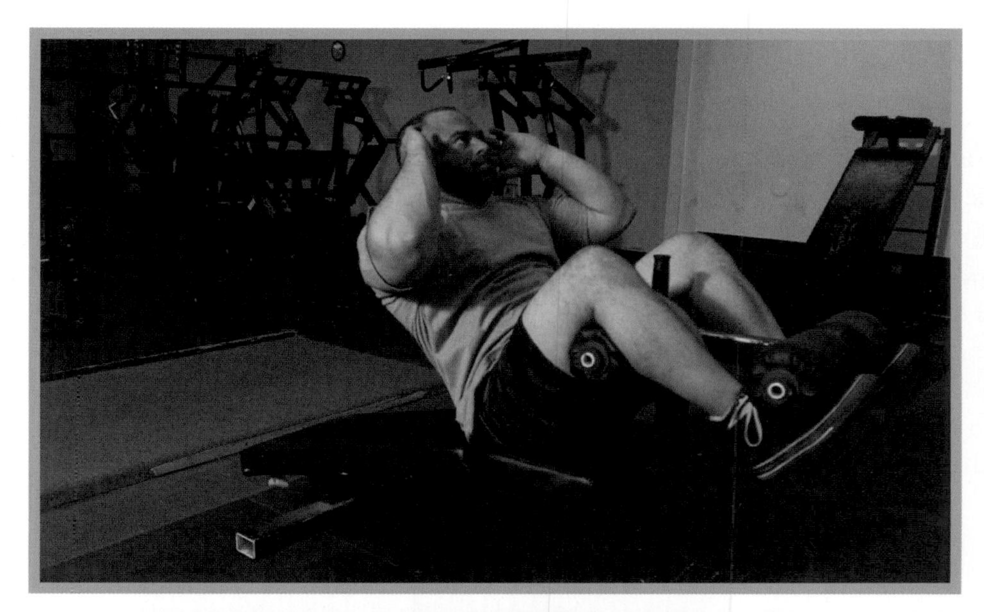

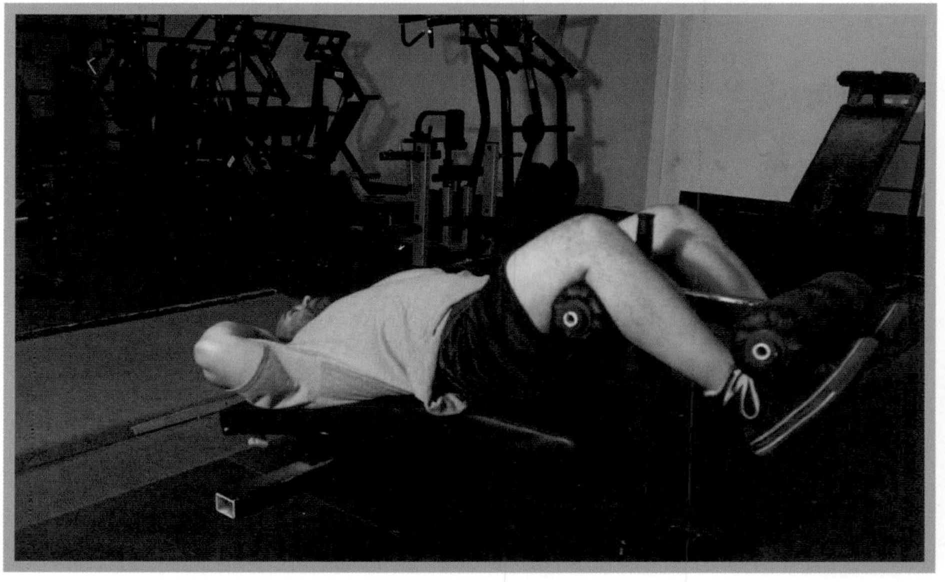

Incline bench sit-ups are another mainstay in most gyms and weight-rooms.

Set-Up

Set your bench to the desired decline (if the bench is adjustable) and secure your feet in the pads. Start the movement sitting all the way up, looking straight ahead. Place your hands either across your chest (easier) or with your fingertips at your ears (more difficult).

The Exercise

Without moving your hands, lean back on the bench until your upper back touches the bench at the bottom position. Make sure that you are only touching, not settling. Sit back up, pulling yourself up with your abdominals and hip flexors.

As with the pulldown abs, you should be pushing your gut out, not sucking it in. For higher rep recovery workouts, do these with body weight. For more strength gain, hold a weight to your chest or use an extreme incline.

SPREAD EAGLE SIT-UPS

Muscles Targeted: Rectus abdominis

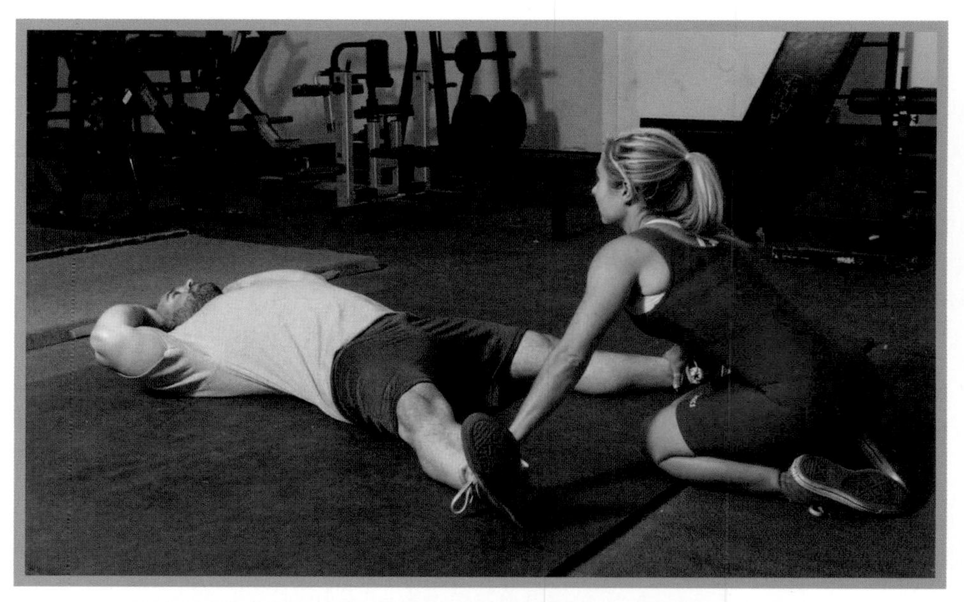

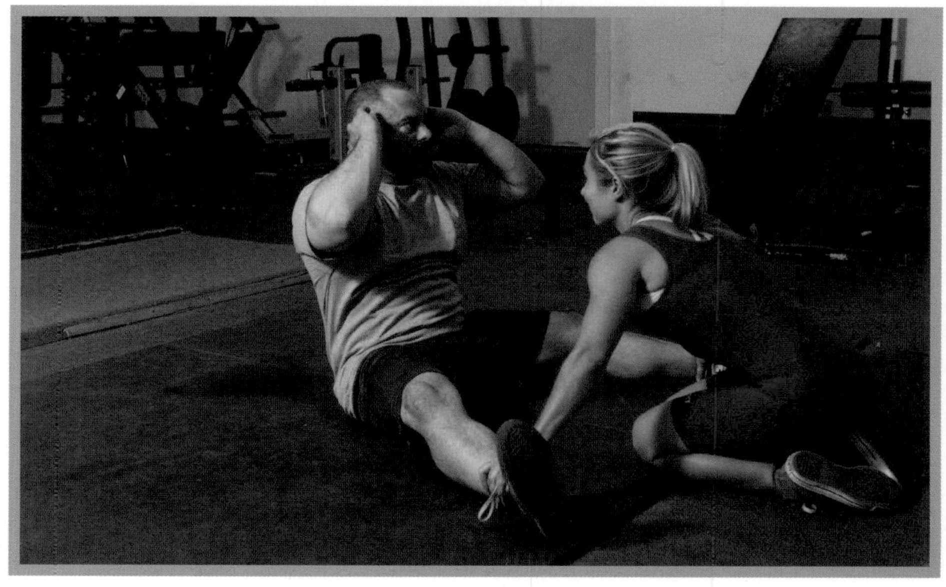

The point of the spread eagle leg position is to disengage your hip flexors, putting more stress on your abdominal muscles to complete the movement. Make these tougher with a weight on your chest. These are harder than they look!

Set-Up

Start by sitting on the floor, with your legs straight and set wide into a "v." You'll need to anchor your feet, which you can do with a rack, or you can just have a training partner hold your feet.

The Exercise

From a lying position, sit up, until your torso is perpendicular to your legs. Keep your head and chest up for the entire exercise.

GLUTE-HAM BENCH SIT-UPS

Muscles Targeted: Rectus abdominis

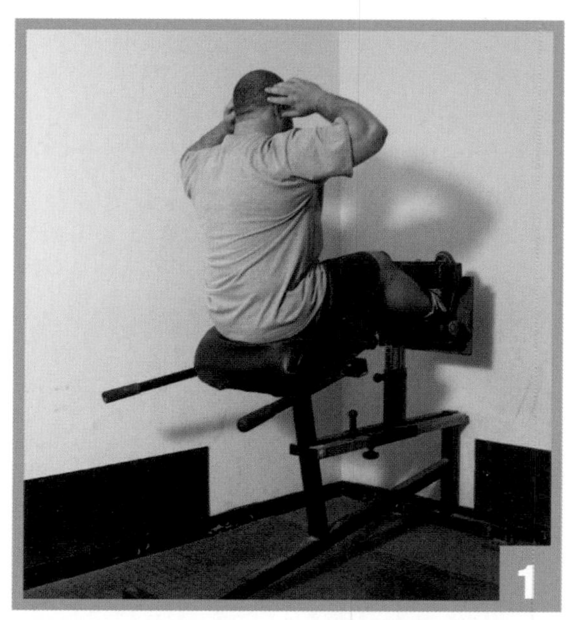

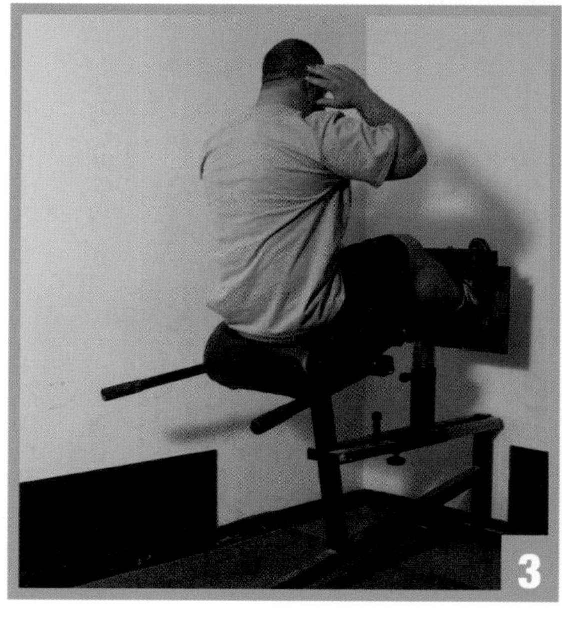

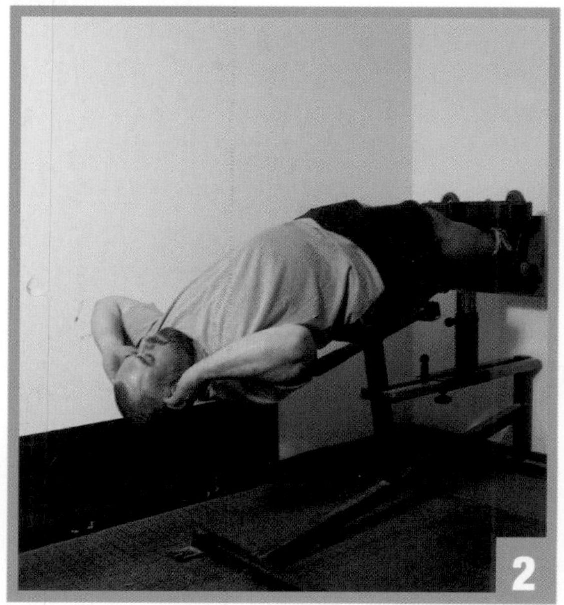

This is great way to add versatility to a glute-ham bench if you have access to one.

Set-Up

Hook your feet into the pads face up, with the pad against your hamstrings.

The Exercise

Lean all the way back so that your upper body is almost perpendicular to the floor before sitting back up.

Variations

You can make glute-ham bench sit-ups tougher with either a weight on your chest or band tension.

STABILITY BALL SIT-UPS

Muscles Targeted: Rectus abdominis

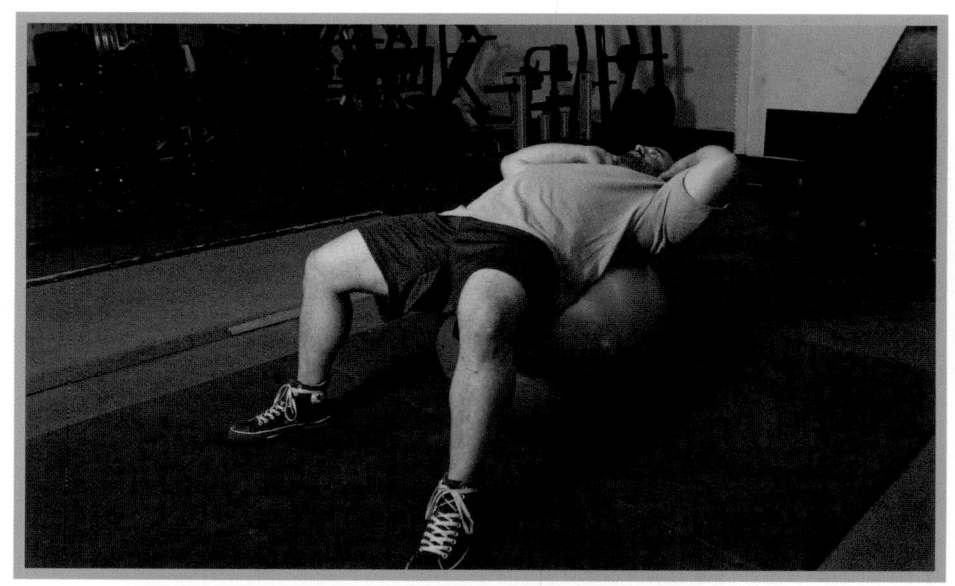

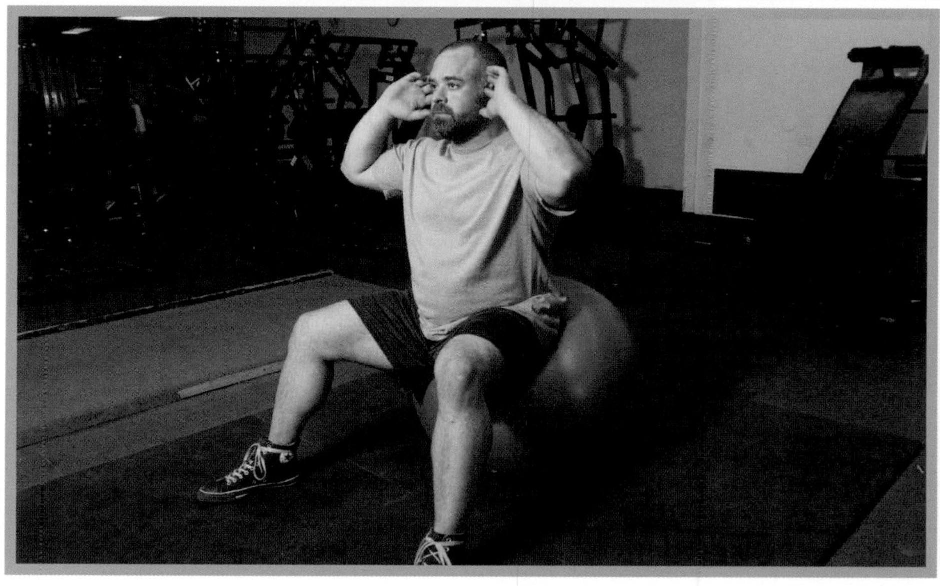

This one is a staple in most aerobics classes, but performed correctly, it will strengthen your abdominals for serious lifting.

Set-Up

Sit on the ball, then roll forward until the ball is against your lower back and supporting your body weight. Keep your hands either across your chest or with your fingertips at your ears.

The Exercise

Lean back as far as you can without flopping over the ball. Without moving your hands for momentum, sit up until you are facing forward.

Variations

You can make this exercise tougher with a weight on your chest, or by anchoring a band behind you. If you do these weighted or with the band, you will probably need to hook your feet under a rack, or have a training partner stand on them

SIDE BENDS

Muscles Targeted: Obliques

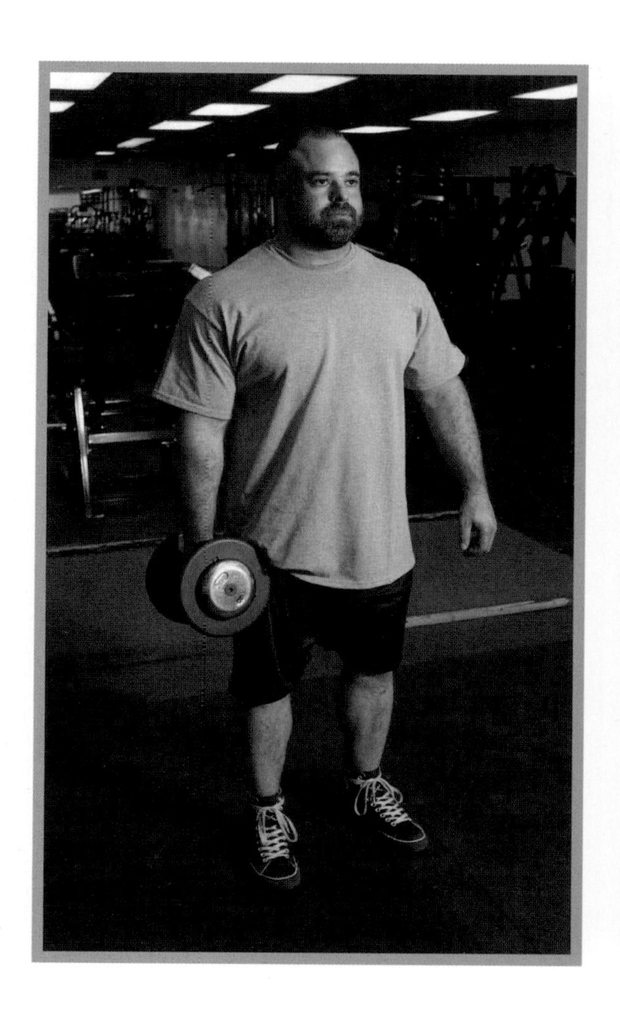

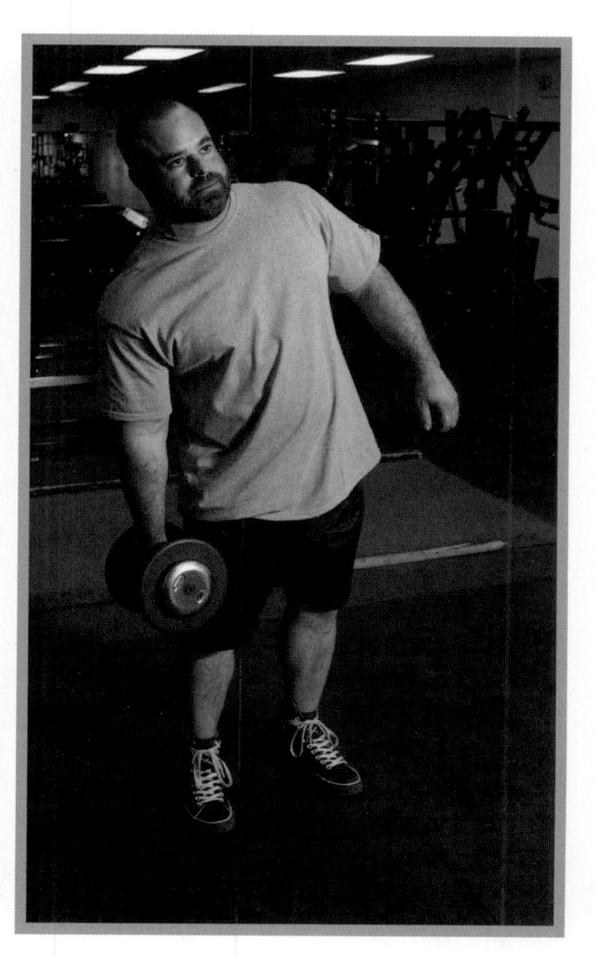

Side-bending movements are effective at building lateral strength and stability in the torso.

Set-Up

Hold a dumbbell in one hand and stand straight up.

The Exercise

Without bending backward or forward, bend at the waist to the opposite side from the dumbbell, then straighten back up.

Variations

You can do side bends with either a dumbbell, low cable, or low anchored resistance band. Do not make the beginner mistake of holding a dumbbell in each hand. This will counterbalance you and will put little resistance on the muscles you are trying to target.

PLANK

Muscles Targeted: Transverse abdominis, rectus abdominis, and obliques

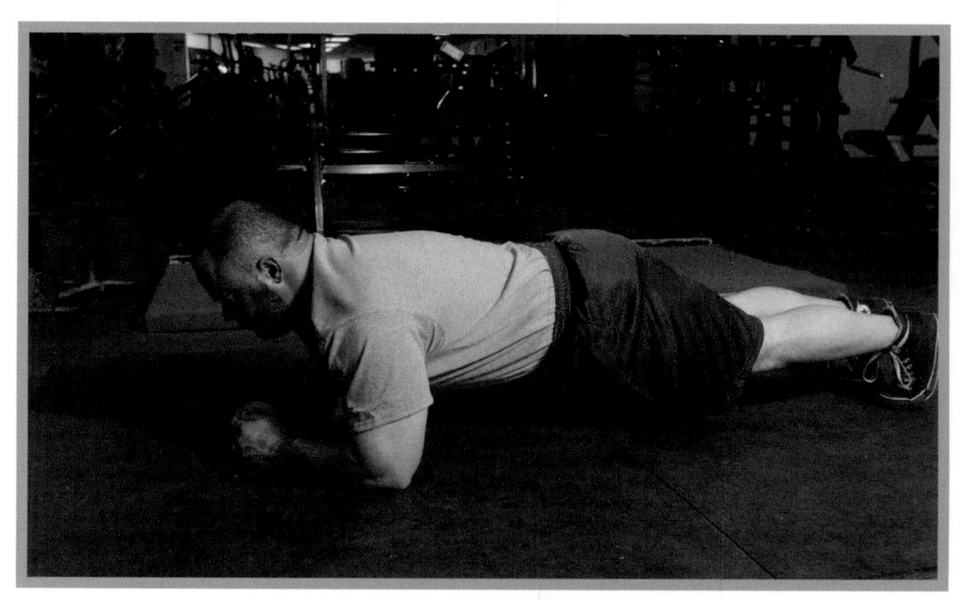

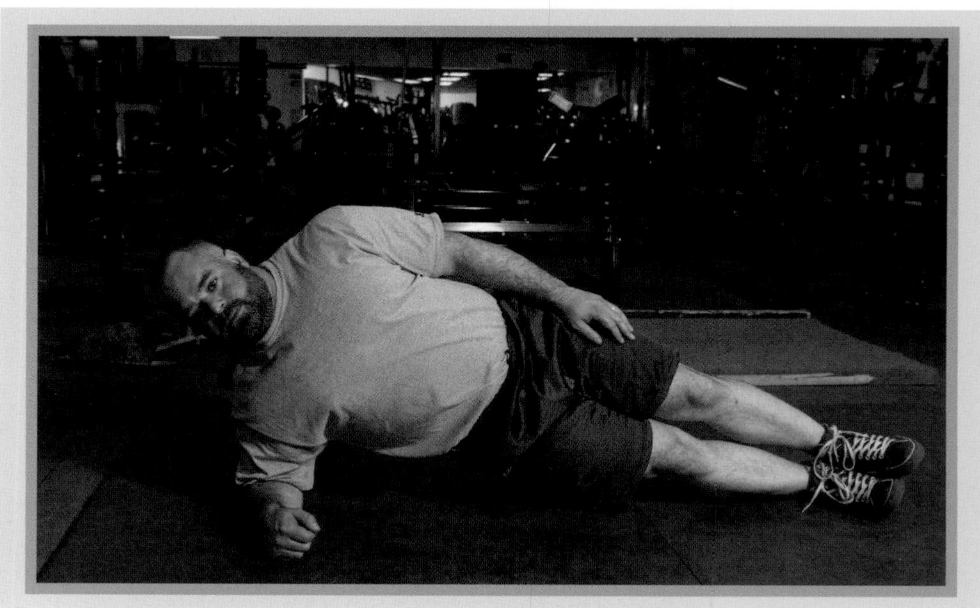

The plank is an effective exercise for building core stability and endurance.

Set-Up

Lie down on the floor, face down, with your forearms on the floor underneath your torso.

The Exercise

Lift your body off the floor, so that only your forearms and toes are in contact with the floor. Your body should be stiff and straight. Maintain this position for time, rather than repetitions.

Variations

Planks can also be performed on your side, to more directly target the obliques, and improve lateral stability. To perform a side plank, place one forearm on the floor, then lift your body so that one forearm and the side of your foot are on the floor. Keep your body straight for the duration of the plank.

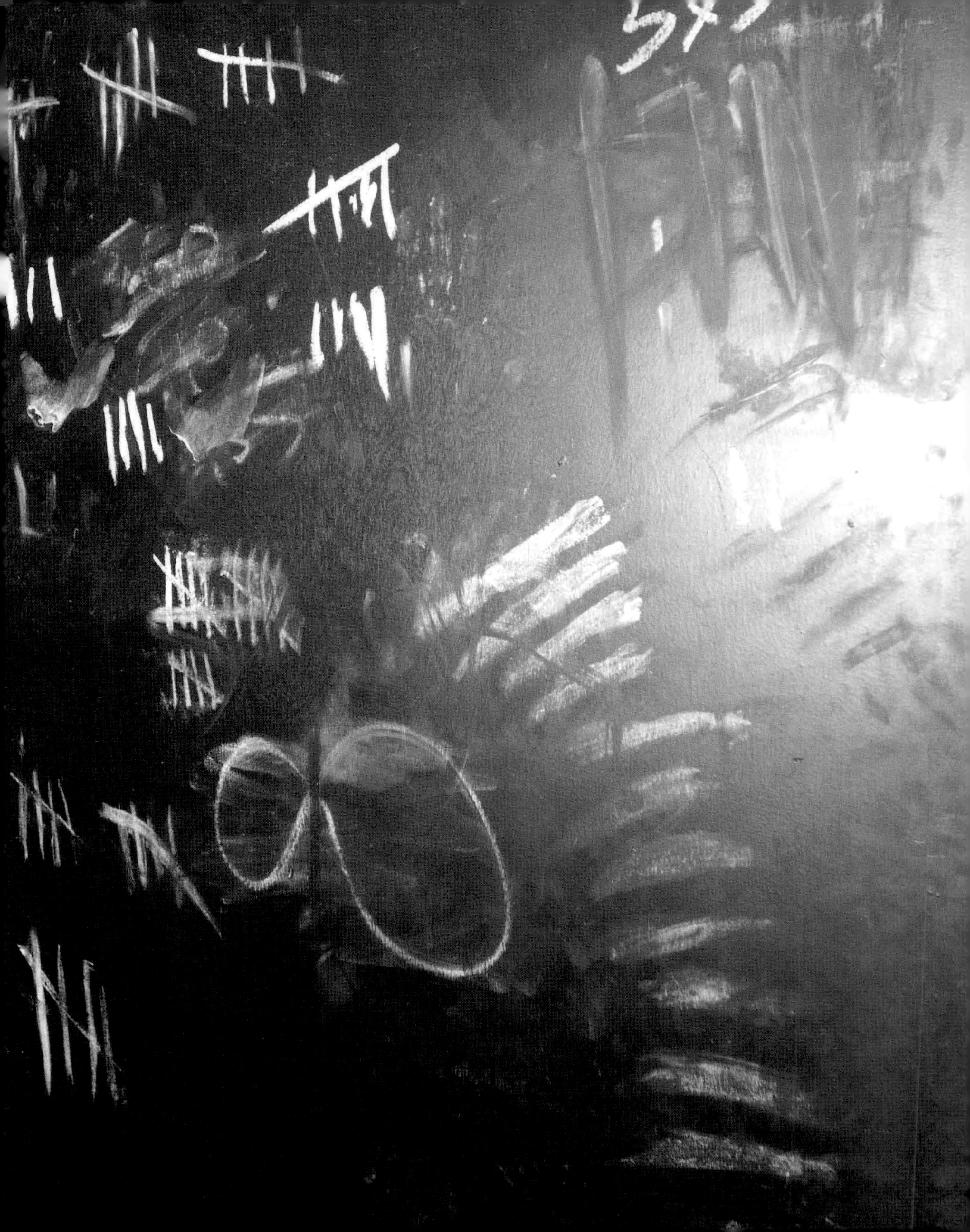

THE PROGRAMS

I've been involved in strength and fitness for over two decades, and the single biggest difference I've seen between those who continuously progress and those who do not, is the level of planning. Much as in any other setting, those who follow a plan tend to be more successful than those who just "wing it".

In the previous chapter, I described your exercises as the car, and your programming as the roadmap. Just as you would not want to stray from your map (or GPS) while driving in an unfamiliar city, you will not want to deviate too much from your programming when you are new to strength training. As you gain experience, you will learn when and where to make adjustments to what's on the page, but for now, follow everything as closely as you can.

Properly programmed training will not call for you to break personal records day in and day out, but will instead tend to have an ebb and flow. For more motivated individuals, the temptation will often be to keep piling on the weights, but remember that progress is measured in months and years, not days and weeks. Some workouts will be less challenging than others, in order to allow for recovery. Resist the urge to push too hard at the onset, so you can enjoy continuous progress in the long-term.

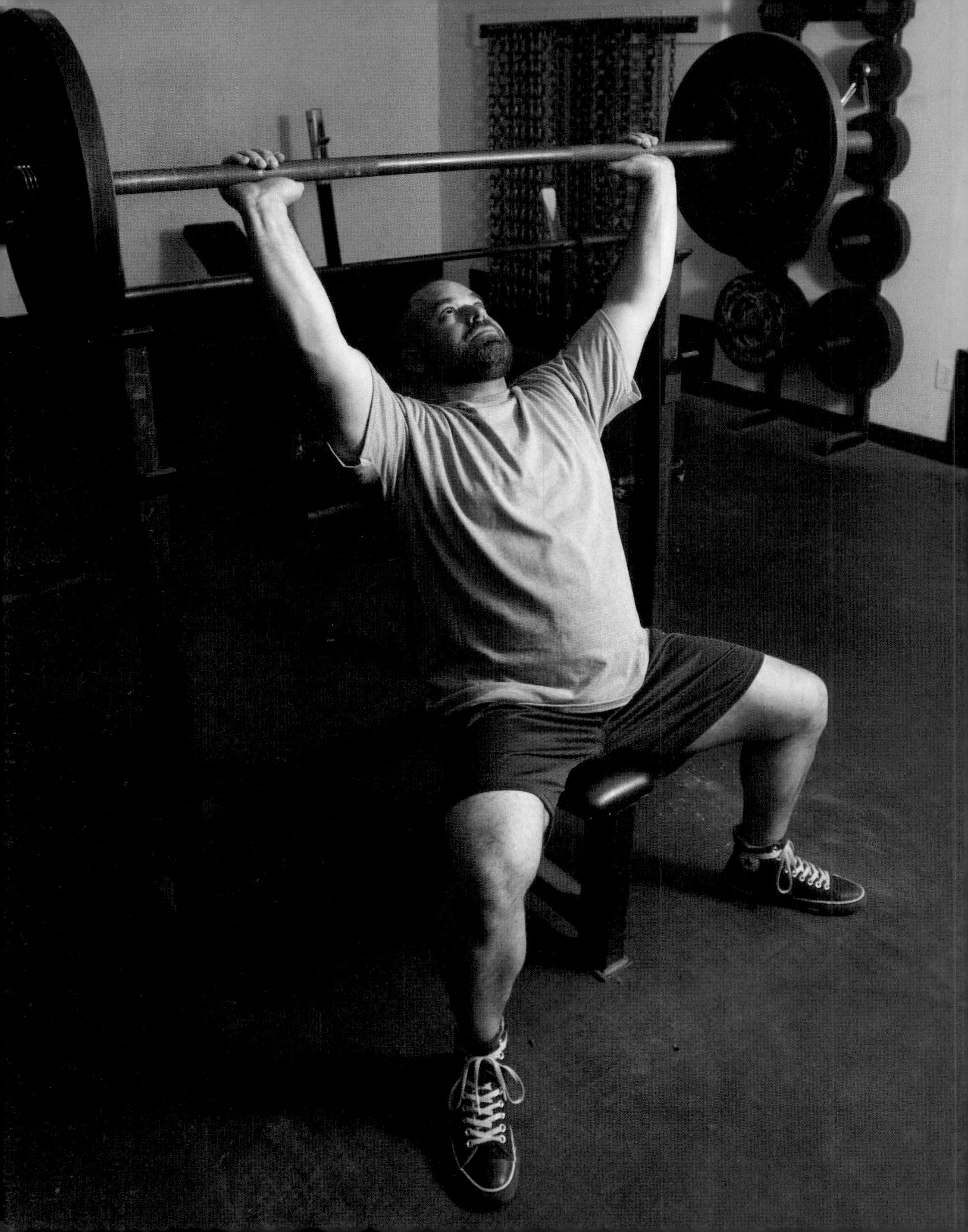

INTRODUCTORY CYCLE

This cycle is for total novices who have never lifted weights before (or who have in the past, but have not lifted in a long time). The introductory cycle is the only one in this book that revolves around machines. While free weights are generally superior for building strength, machines will allow you to get into the habit of training and will prepare your tissues for the hard work to come, in a less intimidating, more "plug and play" format.

You'll notice that all of the programs included in this book call for training 3 days per week. The exact days are up to you, but I would recommend having at least one rest day in between each training day to allow recovery. A schedule like Monday, Wednesday, and Friday in the gym with Tuesday, Thursday, Saturday, and Sunday off is a typical schedule.

While technique is *always* important, starting on machines will allow you to introduce the basic pressing and pulling movements while minimizing the risk of mistakes. This cycle is designed to be used for only 4 weeks. Following a month of machine training, you should be ready to start incorporating the barbell lifts.

On the days where you are prescribed 15 reps of each exercise, you should have the weight at about 60 percent to 65 percent of your 1 rep max. On the days where you are prescribed 10 reps, you should use a weight around 70 percent to 75 percent.

If you do not know what your 1 rep max is, this is no problem. As long as you are getting the prescribed number of reps, but wouldn't be able to do much more, you are right in the range you need to be in. Since there is an inverse relationship between resistance and repetitions, you should be able to handle more weight on the 10 rep days, as opposed to the 15 rep days.

While this introductory period is recommended, it is not absolutely essential. If you do not have access to machines for some reason (for example, if you are training at home), you can go ahead and skip to the Beginner cycle. If you do decide to skip ahead, do it with caution. Make conservative increases in weights, pay extra attention to technique, and most of all, listen to your body. A little bit of soreness is normal following training, but overall, you should feel good. If your muscles are especially stiff, or sore to the touch, dial the weights back a bit until your body adjusts to the new stimulus.

WEEK 1

DAY 1	DAY 2	DAY 3
3 sets of 15 reps each:	**3 sets of 15 reps each:**	**3 sets of 15 reps each:**
Machine Leg Press	Hack Squat	Machine Leg Press (45 degrees)
Chest Press Machine (Overhand Grip)	Smith Machine Push-up	Chest Press (Parallel Grip)
Machine Lat Pulldown (Wide Grip)	Assisted Pull-up (Wide Grip)	Machine Lat Pulldown (Parallel Grip)
Machine Overhead Press (Wide Grip)	Smith Machine Overhead Press	Machine Overhead Press (Parallel Grip)
Machine Row (Parallel grip)	Smith Machine Inverted Row	Machine Row (Wide Grip)
Back Extensions	Incline Bench Sit-ups	Back Extensions
Crunches	Reverse Hypers	Crunches

WEEK 2

DAY 1	DAY 2	DAY 3
3 sets of 10 reps each:	**3 sets of 10 reps each:**	**3 sets of 10 reps each:**
Machine Overhead Press (Overhand Grip)	Smith Machine Overhead Press	Chest Press (Parallel Grip)
Lat Pulldown (Wide Grip)	Assisted Pull-up (Wide Grip)	Lat Pulldown (V-Grip)
Machine Leg Press	Hack Squat	Leg Press (45 degrees)
Chest Press Machine (Overhand Grip)	Smith Machine Push-up	Machine Overhead Press (Close Grip)
Machine Row (Parallel grip)	Smith Machine Inverted Row	Machine Row (Wide Grip)
Back Extension Machine	Reverse Hypers	Back Extensions
Incline Bench Sit-Ups	Pulldown Abs	Incline Bench Sit-ups

WEEK 3

DAY 1	DAY 2	DAY 3
3 sets of 15 reps each:	**3 sets of 15 reps each:**	**3 sets of 15 reps each:**
Box Squat (Dumbbell)	Machine Leg Press	Conventional Deadlift
Bench Press (Barbell)	Smith Machine Push-up (lower bar)	Close Grip Bench Press
Seated Cable Row (V-Grip)	Smith Machine Inverted Row (Wide Grip, Lower Bar)	Seated Cable Row (V-grip)
Overhead Press (Seated, Barbell)	Lat Pulldown (Wide Grip)	Overhead Press (Barbell, Close Grip)
Bench Press (Incline Bench, Wide Grip)	Overhead Press (Seated, Dumbell, Parallel Grip)	Lat Pulldown (Close Grip)
Incline Bench Sit-up	Planks: 30 seconds	Back Extensions
Back Extensions	Side Plank: 30 seconds	Incline Bench Sit-ups

WEEK 4		
DAY 1	DAY 2	DAY 3
3 sets of 10 reps each: Bench Press (Barbell) Seated Cable Row (V-Grip) Box Squat (Dumbbell) Lat Pulldowns (Wide Grip) Back Extensions Incline Bench Sit-Up	**3 sets of 10 reps each:** Smith Machine Push-up (Lower Bar) Smith Machine Inverted Row (lower bar) Machine Leg Press Assisted Pull-Up (Parallel Grip) Overhead Press (Standing, Barbell) Planks: 30 seconds Side Plank: 30 seconds	**3 sets of 10 reps each:** Seated Cable Row (Close Grip) Close Grip Bench Press Dumbbell Squat Overhead Press (Barbell, Close Grip) Lat Pulldown (Close Grip) Back Extensions Incline Bench Sit-Up

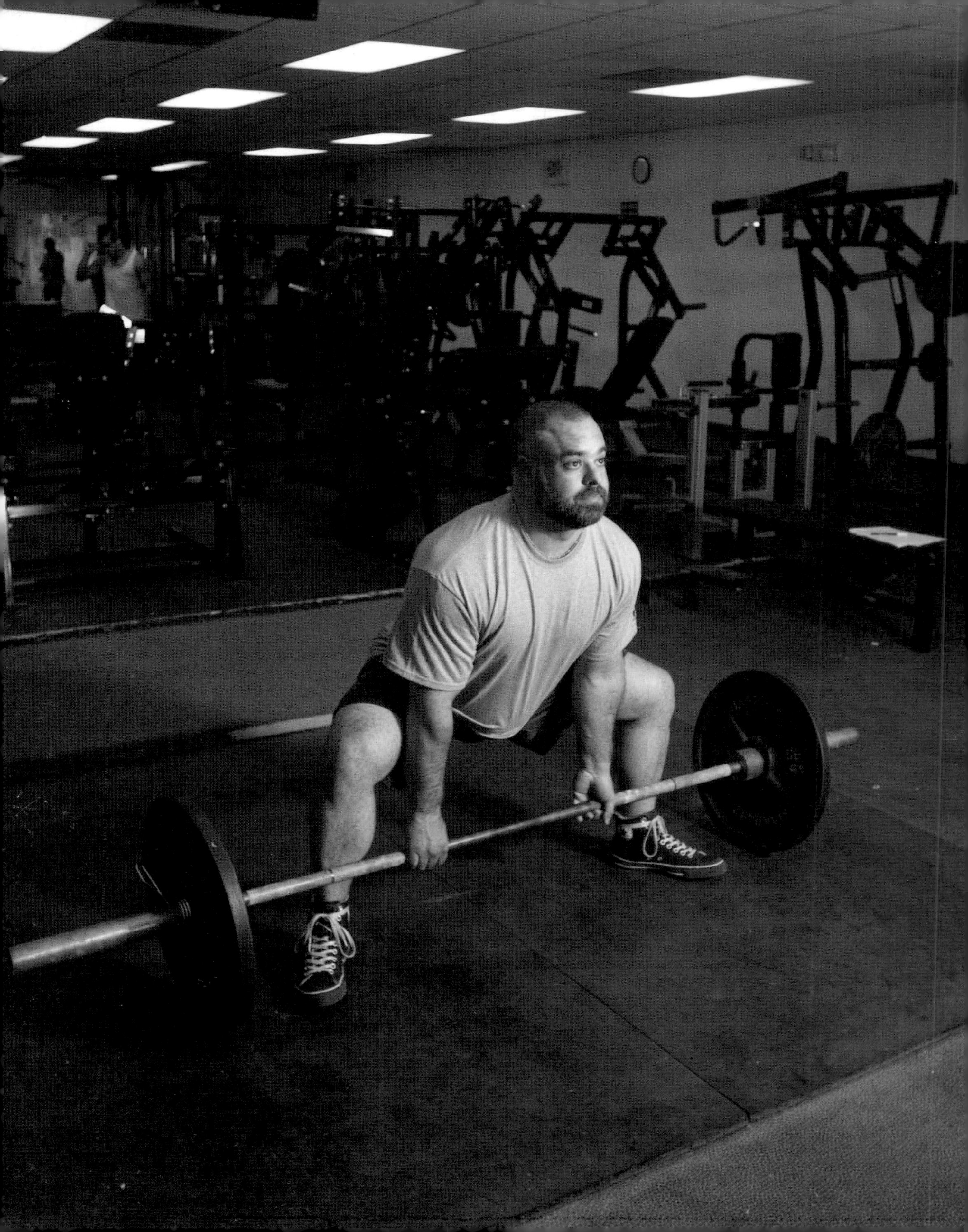

BEGINNER CYCLE

The beginner cycle is similar to the Introductory Cycle, with a few key differences:

MORE COMPLEX MOVEMENTS: While the Introductory cycle is primarily machine-based, the Beginner cycle introduces more complex free-weight movements that will be an integral part of the strength cycles to follow. Since the intensity will remain relatively low, the Beginner cycle will allow you the opportunity to practice these lifts with lower weights, reducing the chance of injury.

FEWER EXERCISES: Free weight exercises tend to be more fatiguing than machine-based exercises, even at the same weight. This is because with no pulley/cam system to keep the weight fixed, you need to work harder to maintain your technique. Since you'll be working harder on each exercise, you will not need as many of them to get the same payoff.

You'll notice that all of the programs included in this book call for training 3 days per week. The exact days are up to you, but I would recommend having at least one rest day in between each training day to allow recovery. A schedule like Monday, Wednesday, and Friday in the gym with Tuesday, Thursday, Saturday, and Sunday off is a typical schedule.

On the days where you are prescribed 15 reps of each exercise, you should have the weight at about 60 percent to 65 percent of your 1 rep max. On the days where you are prescribed 10 reps, you should use a weight around 70 percent to 75 percent.

Rest for about a minute in between sets. You can take a bit more time if you are having trouble recovering between sets, but try to limit it to three minutes at most.

If you do not know what your 1 rep max is, this is no problem. As long as you are getting the prescribed number of reps, but wouldn't be able to do much more, you are right in the range you need to be in. Since there is an inverse relationship between resistance and repetitions, you should be able to handle more weight on the 10 rep days, as opposed to the 15 rep days.

WEEK 1

DAY 1	DAY 2	DAY 3
3 sets of 15 reps each:	**3 sets of 15 reps each:**	**3 sets of 15 reps each:**
Box Squat (Barbell)	Machine Leg Press (45 degrees)	Deadlift (Barbell)
Dumbbell Bench Press	Push-Up (From Floor)	Dumbbell Bench Press (Parallel Grp)
Chest-Supported Row	Smith Machine Inverted Row (lower bar)	Chest-Supported Row (Parallel Grip)
Straight Leg Deadlift (Barbell)	Stability Ball Sit-Ups	Dumbbell Overhead Press
Dumbbell Overhead Press (Seated)	Reverse Hypers	Lat Pulldown (Reverse Grip)
Lat Pulldown (V-Grip)	Side Plank: 45 seconds	Straight Leg Deadlift (Dumbbells)
Incline Bench Sit-Up		Pulldown Abs

WEEK 2

DAY 1	DAY 2	DAY 3
3 sets of 10 reps each:	**3 sets of 10 reps each:**	**3 sets of 10 reps each:**
Dumbbell Overhead Press (Seated)	Full Range Push-up	Dumbbell Bench Press (Parallel Grip)
Lat Pulldown (V-Grip)	Smith Machine Inverted Row (Lower Bar)	Lat Pulldown (Reverse Grip)
Box Squat (Barbell)	Machine Leg Press (45 degrees)	Deadlift (Barbell)
Dumbbell Bench Press	Reverse Hypers	Dumbbell Overhead Press (Seated, Parallel Grip)
Chest-Supported Row	Stability Ball Sit-Up	Chest-Supported Row (Parallel Grip)
Straight Leg Deadlift		Straight Leg Deadlift (Dumbbells)
Incline Bench Sit-Up		Incline Bench Sit-Ups

WEEK 3

DAY 1	DAY 2	DAY 3
3 sets of 15 reps each:	**3 sets of 15 reps each:**	**3 sets of 15 reps each:**
Squat (Barbell)	Hack Squat	Front Squat (Barbell)
Dumbbell Bench Press (Alternating)	Push-Up (Close Grip)	Dumbbell Bench Press (Parallel Grip, Alternating)
Standing T-bar Row	Smith Machine Inverted Row (Reverse Grip)	Bent-Over Row (Dumbbells)
Overhead Press (Standing, Barbell)	Incline Bench Sit-Ups	Dumbbell Overhead Press (Standing, Parallel Grip)
Lat Pulldowns (Wide Grip)	Planks: 45 seconds	Good Mornings (Barbell)
Incline Bench Sit-Up (Weight on Chest)		Glute-Ham Bench Sit-Ups
Back Extensions (Holding Weight to Chest)		

WEEK 4

DAY 1	DAY 2	DAY 3
3 sets of 10 reps each:	**3 sets of 10 reps each:**	**3 sets of 10 reps each:**
Dumbbell Bench Press (Alternating)	Push-up (Close Grip)	Bent-Over Row (Dumb-bells)
Standing T-bar Row Squat (Barbell)	Smith Machine Inverted Row (Reverse Grip)	Dumbbell Bench Press (parallel grip, alternating)
Overhead Press (Stand-ing, Barbell)	Hack Squat	Front Squat (Barbell)
Lat Pulldowns	Planks: 45 Seconds	Dumbbell Overhead Press (standing, parallel grip)
Back Extensions (Holding Weights to Chest)	Side Planks: 45 Seconds	Goodmornings (barbell)
Incline Bench Sit-Up (Weights on Chest)		Glute-Ham Bench Sit-Ups

INTERMEDIATE CYCLE

Now that you have completed the Introductory and Beginner cycles, it's time to get down to the meat and potatoes portion of your training. At this point, you've built up enough physical preparedness to start a true strength program.

Since your goal has changed, and you are now focusing on strength more than general conditioning, as in the first two programs, you'll notice a few distinct changes to the structure of the Intermediate cycle:

FEWER EXERCISES: This might be surprising, as most people envision themselves doing *more* training as they improve. However, in strength training, quality takes precedence over quantity. The exercise selection is limited in this cycle so that you can focus on weight and technique without being limited by fatigue.

TEST DAYS: On the test days, your goal will be to work up to a 1 rep max on the first exercise of the day. The reason is twofold. We want to reestablish your max in order to more accurately calculate your training weights as you get stronger. We also want to let you handle very heavy weights on a monthly basis to increase maximal strength.

PERCENTAGE-BASED RESISTANCE: In the Introductory and Beginner cycles, resistance is prescribed based on the desired rep-range, with room to add weight over the progression of the program. In the Intermediate cycle, weights are prescribed based on a percentage of your max. While you probably will not know your maxes yet, for now you can base your initial percentages off of your training weights from the first cycle.

Since the Intermediate cycle includes periodic testing, you will have accurate maxes in all of your lifts within a few months.

UPPER/LOWER SPLIT: Since the main movements will now be performed at a higher intensity, you'll be splitting up your program so that you are focusing on either a lower lift or an upper body lift each day. Splitting the work in this manner will ensure that you are as fresh as possible for each lift.

VARYING REP-RANGES: In the Introductory and Beginner cycles, the exercises are all performed in the same general rep-range for that day. In the Intermediate cycle, you'll notice that as you get deeper into the training session, the reps will generally increase on each subsequent exercise. While the main lift for the day will be in the 1 to 5 rep range with heavy weights, the assistance exercises will generally be in the 8 to 15 rep range. This is so that you are handling the heaviest weights while you are fresh, and then doing the lighter weights as you fatigue.

The initial heavier sets with the bigger compound movements are there to stimulate your central nervous system to gain overall strength and power, while the lighter assistance exercises are there to stimulate muscle growth.

The single most important point to remember as you get into the Intermediate cycle is that technique trumps all. Not only is solid technique critical for avoiding injury, but it can make the difference between progression and stagnation. While it might initially be possible to progress with poor technique, you will eventually need to learn to perform the lifts correctly in order to continue improving.

Just like with any other skill, practice doesn't always make perfect, but it does make permanent. The longer you train with poor technique, the harder it will ultimately be to correct your mistakes, so you might as well start off performing the lifts correctly from the very beginning of your training.

You'll notice that all of the programs included in this book call for training 3 days per week. The exact days are up to you, but I would recommend having at least one rest day in between each training day to allow recovery. A schedule like Monday, Wednesday, and Friday in the gym with Tuesday, Thursday, Saturday, and Sunday off is a typical schedule.

For the main lifts, the percentages refer to the percentage of your 1 rep max. So if, for example your squat is 200 pounds and the training session calls for 75 percent, your working weight for the day would be 150 pounds. If you do not know what your 1 rep max is yet, plug in your 10 rep max for the 75 percent day, than add 5 percent each week until you test. After the test day, you will have a true percentage you can use.

For your assistance work, start with a weight that's somewhat challenging to get the prescribed sets and reps with, but not to the point where you risk a miss. Make conservative jumps in weight for subsequent weeks (5 to 10 pounds). By the last week performing that exercise, it should be difficult (but not impossible), to get all your sets and reps.

> In the Intermediate cycle, some exercises will be written as an expression, with the weight first, followed by the number of sets, followed by the number of repetitions in each set. For example, 3 sets of 5 repetitions with 135 pounds would be expressed as "135 x 3 x 5."

CYCLE 1: WEEK 1

In the Intermediate cycle, some exercises will be written as an expression, with the weight first, followed by the number of sets, followed by the number of repetitions in each set. For example, 3 sets of 5 repetitions with 135 pounds would be expressed as "135 x 3 x 5."

DAY 1	DAY 2	DAY 3
Box Squat (Barbell) 75% x 3 x 5	Bench Press (Barbell) 75% x 3 x 5	Conventional Deadlift (Dumbbell) 75% x 3 x 5
Straight Leg Deadlift (Barbell) 4 x 8	Bent-Over Row (Barbell) 4 x 8	Cable Pull-through 4 x 10
Back Extension 4 x 10	Lying Triceps Extension (Dumbbells) 4 x 10	Reverse Hyper 4 x 10
Pulldown Abs 4 x 10	Shoulder Raise (lateral) 4 x 10	Incline Bench Sit-Ups 4 x 10

CYCLE 1: WEEK 2

In the Intermediate cycle, some exercises will be written as an expression, with the weight first, followed by the number of sets, followed by the number of repetitions in each set. For example, 3 sets of 5 repetitions with 135 pounds would be expressed as "135 x 3 x 5."

DAY 1	DAY 2	DAY 3
Box Squat (Barbell) 80% x 3 x 5	Bench Press (Barbell) 80% x 3 x 5	Conventional Deadlift (Barbell) 80% x 3 x 5
Straight Leg Deadlift (Barbell) 4 x 8	Bent-Over Row (Barbell) 4 x 8	Cable Pull-through 4 x 10
Back Extension 4 x 10	Lying Triceps Extension (Dumbbells) 4 x 10	Reverse-Hyper 4 x 10
Pulldown Abs 4 x 10	Shoulder Raise (Lateral) 4 x 10	Incline Bench Sit-Up 4 x 10

CYCLE 1: WEEK 3

In the Intermediate cycle, some exercises will be written as an expression, with the weight first, followed by the number of sets, followed by the number of repetitions in each set. For example, 3 sets of 5 repetitions with 135 pounds would be expressed as "135 x 3 x 5."

DAY 1	DAY 2	DAY 3
Box Squat (Barbell) 85% x 3 x 5	Bench Press (Barbell) 85% x 3 x 5	Conventional Deadlift (Barbell) 85% x 3 x 5
Straight Leg Deadlift (Barbell) 4 x 8	Bent-over Row (Barbell) 4 x 8	Cable Pull-through 4 x 10
Back Extension 4 x 10	Lying Triceps Extension (Dumbbells) 4 x 10	Reverse Hyper 4 x 10
Pulldown Abs 4 x 10	Shoulder Raise (Lateral) 4 x 10	Incline Bench Sit-Up 4 x 10

CYCLE 1: WEEK 4

In the Intermediate cycle, some exercises will be written as an expression, with the weight first, followed by the number of sets, followed by the number of repetitions in each set. For example, 3 sets of 5 repetitions with 135 pounds would be expressed as "135 x 3 x 5."

DAY 1	DAY 2	DAY 3
Box Squat (Barbell) 100% x 1	Bench Press (Barbell) 100% x 1	Conventional Deadlift (Barbell) 100% x 1
Straight Leg Deadlift (Barbell) 4 x 8	Bent-over Row (Barbell) 4 x 8	Cable Pull-through 4 x 10
Back Extension 4 x 10	Lying Triceps Extension (Dumbbells) 4 x 10	Reverse Hyper 4 x 10
Pulldown Abs 4 x 10	Shoulder Raise (lateral) 4 x 10	Incline Bench Sit-Up 4 x 10

CYCLE 2: WEEK 1

In the Intermediate cycle, some exercises will be written as an expression, with the weight first, followed by the number of sets, followed by the number of repetitions in each set. For example, 3 sets of 5 repetitions with 135 pounds would be expressed as "135 x 3 x 5."

DAY 1	DAY 2	DAY 3
Barbell Squat 75% x 3 x 5 Goodmorning 4 x 8 Glute-Ham Raise 4 x 10 Planks 4 x 30 seconds	Floor Press (Barbell) 75% x 3 x 5 Chest-supported row 4 x 8 Triceps Pushdowns (Cable) 4 x 10 Face Pulls (Cable) 4 x10	Sumo Deadlift 75% x 3 x 5 Leg Press 4 x 8 Back Extensions (Holding Weight to Chest) 4 x 10 Spread-Eagle Sit-Ups 4 x 10

CYCLE 2: WEEK 2

In the Intermediate cycle, some exercises will be written as an expression, with the weight first, followed by the number of sets, followed by the number of repetitions in each set. For example, 3 sets of 5 repetitions with 135 pounds would be expressed as "135 x 3 x 5."

DAY 1	DAY 2	DAY 3
Barbell Squat 80% x 3 x 5 Goodmorning 4 x 8 Glute-Ham Raise 4 x 10 Planks 4 x 45 Seconds	Floor Press (Barbell) 80% x 3 x 5 Chest Supported Row 4 x 8 Triceps Pushdowns (Cable) 4 x 10 Face Pulls (Cable) 4 x10	Sumo Deadlift 80% x 3 x 5 Machine Leg Press 4 x 8 Back Extensions (Holding Weight to Chest) 4 x 10 Spread Eagle Sit-Ups 4 x 10

CYCLE 2: WEEK 3

In the Intermediate cycle, some exercises will be written as an expression, with the weight first, followed by the number of sets, followed by the number of repetitions in each set. For example, 3 sets of 5 repetitions with 135 pounds would be expressed as "135 x 3 x 5."

DAY 1	DAY 2	DAY 3
Barbell Squat 85% x 3 x 5 Goodmorning 4 x 8 Glute-Ham Raise 4 x 10 Planks 4 x 60 Seconds	Floor Press (Barbell) 85% x 3 x 5 Chest Supported Row 4 x 8 Triceps Pushdowns (Cable) 4 x 10 Face Pulls (Cable) 4 x10	Sumo Deadlift 85% x 3 x 5 Leg Press 4 x 8 Back Extensions (Holding Weights to Chest) 4 x 10 Spread Eagle Sit-Ups 4 x 10

CYCLE 2: WEEK 4

In the Intermediate cycle, some exercises will be written as an expression, with the weight first, followed by the number of sets, followed by the number of repetitions in each set. For example, 3 sets of 5 repetitions with 135 pounds would be expressed as "135 x 3 x 5."

DAY 1	DAY 2	DAY 3
Barbell Squat 100% x 1 Goodmorning 4 x 8 Glute-Ham Raise 4 x 10 Planks 4 x 90 Seconds	Floor Press (Barbell) 100% x 1 Chest Supported Row 4 x 8 Triceps Pushdowns (Cable) 4 x 10 Face Pulls (Cable) 4 x10	Sumo Deadlift 100% x 1 Leg Press 4 x 8 Back Extension (Holding Weights to Chest) 4 x 10 Spread Eagle Sit-Ups 4 x 10

CYCLE 3: WEEK 1

In the Intermediate cycle, some exercises will be written as an expression, with the weight first, followed by the number of sets, followed by the number of repetitions in each set. For example, 3 sets of 5 repetitions with 135 pounds would be expressed as "135 x 3 x 5."

DAY 1	DAY 2	DAY 3
Front Squat 75% x 3 x 5	Overhead Press (Barbell) 75% x 3 x 5	Deficit Deadlift (Dumbbell) 75% x 3 x 5
Zercher Squat 4 x 8	Lat Pulldowns 4 x 8	Bent-Over Rows (Barbell) 4 x 8
Straight Leg Deadlift 4 x 10	Lying Triceps Extensions (Barbell) 4 x 10	Reverse Hypers 4 x 10
Glute-Ham Bench Sit-Ups 4 x 10	Shoulder Raises (Reverse Fly) 4 x 10	Planks 4 x 30 sec

CYCLE 3: WEEK 2

In the Intermediate cycle, some exercises will be written as an expression, with the weight first, followed by the number of sets, followed by the number of repetitions in each set. For example, 3 sets of 5 repetitions with 135 pounds would be expressed as "135 x 3 x 5."

DAY 1	DAY 2	DAY 3
Front Squat 80% x 3 x 5 Zercher Squat 4 x 8 Straight Leg Deadlift (Dumbbell) 4 x 10 Glute-Ham Bench Sit-Ups 4 x 10	Overhead Press (Barbell) 80% x 3 x 5 Lat Pulldowns 4 x 8 Lying Triceps Extensions (Barbell) 4 x 10 Shoulder Raises (Reverse Fly) 4 x 10	Deficit Deadlift (Barbell) 80% x 3 x 5 Bent over Row (Barbell) 4 x 8 Reverse Hypers 4 x 10 Planks 4 x 45 sec

CYCLE 3: WEEK 3

In the Intermediate cycle, some exercises will be written as an expression, with the weight first, followed by the number of sets, followed by the number of repetitions in each set. For example, 3 sets of 5 repetitions with 135 pounds would be expressed as "135 x 3 x 5."

DAY 1	DAY 2	DAY 3
Front Squat (Barbell) 85% x 3 x 5	Overhead Press (Barbell) 85% x 3 x 5	Deficit Deadlift (Barbell) 85% x 3 x 5
Zercher Squat 4 x 8	Lat Pulldowns 4 x 8	Bent-Over Row (Barbell) 4 x 8
Straight Leg Deadlift (Barbell) 4 x 10	Lying Triceps Extensions (Barbell) 4 x 10	Reverse Hypers 4 x 10
Glute-Ham Bench Sit-Ups 4 x 10	Shoulder Raises (Reverse Fly) 4 x 10	Planks 4 x 60 sec

CYCLE 3: WEEK 4

In the Intermediate cycle, some exercises will be written as an expression, with the weight first, followed by the number of sets, followed by the number of repetitions in each set. For example, 3 sets of 5 repetitions with 135 pounds would be expressed as "135 x 3 x 5."

DAY 1	DAY 2	DAY 3
Front Squat (Barbell) 100% x 1	Overhead Press (Barbell) 100% x 1	Deficit Deadlift (Barbell) 100% x 1
Zercher Squat 4 x 8	Lat Pulldowns 4 x 8	Bent-Over Row (Barbell) 4 x 8
Straight Leg Deadlift (Dumbbell) 4 x 10	Lying Triceps Extensions (Barbell) 4 x 10	Reverse Hypers 4 x 10
Glute-Ham Bench Sit-Ups 4 x 10	Shoulder Raises (Reverse Fly) 4 x 10	Planks 4 x 90 seconds

MOVING FORWARD

By now you have just completed your first macrocycle of the program. Congrats!

Now what? Since strength programming is cyclical in nature, your next move would be to go back to the same Intermediate cycle you started with, and complete the 12-week program again. This time however, you will have concrete 1-rep-maxes to program off of, which will make your percentages even more accurate, and thus more effective.

Not only that, but after 3 months of dedicated training, you should be significantly stronger than you were before, so the work-weights should be higher than they were during the first go-around. Higher training weights will result in higher 1 rep maxes on the test days, and thus, higher training weights for the following cycle and so on.

Theoretically, you could follow this plan indefinitely and make continual progress, but unfortunately, theory doesn't always hold up in the gym, and it's common to require a few tweaks along the way in order to progress optimally. Sometimes, this will mean increasing or decreasing volume. Or, it can mean selecting more difficult assistance exercises.

Whatever the case may be, when progress stalls, resist the urge to make drastic changes. Instead, make small changes, one at a time, so that you can get a better idea of what works and what does not.

Please note that one bad test day is *not* necessarily an indication that the program isn't working for you. There are lots of reasons to miss a weight that have nothing to do with your program. It could be an undiagnosed technical mistake, or it could be your lifestyle outside of the gym (if stress levels are too high, you're not getting enough rest, not sleeping enough, etc.). Sometimes you just have a bad day. They suck, but they happen, and most of the time they don't mean anything more than that you just had a bad day.

In the event you lift less than the previous test day, do not lower your percentages for the next cycle (as long as you have been training consistently). Your all-time pr is still your pr, and unless the lower test weight is due to an injury or layoff, it's not necessarily an indication that you need to change anything.

If you do find yourself in a significant plateau (if you have not made any progress for two or more months in a row), then it's time to make some changes.

If you've been at it for more than 9 months or so, it could be very likely that your increased strength gains have made the prescribed volume too high. If that is the case, before adjusting the programming yourself, try out the Advanced cycle. But before you go changing things up, please note that most of my clients do make consistent progress on the Intermediate cycle for a year or more before needing to make any changes at all.

Perhaps the single most important rule of training is, "if it ain't broke, don't fix it." As long as a training program is working, you shouldn't change anything at all.

ADVANCED CYCLE

By the time you're ready to start the Advanced cycle, you should have about a year of dedicated training under your belt. While a year of training won't actually qualify you as "advanced" in any athletic discipline (unless you were exceptionally gifted), you will probably be strong enough at this point to take advantage of some of the changes that the Advanced cycle offers.

Truly "advanced" weight trainers generally will not use a pre-designed program at all, or at least not in its entirety. Most advanced lifters design their own programming, or heavily modify pre-existing ones to their own unique needs.

RE-INTRODUCTION OF THE BEGINNER CYCLE: Wait, what? That's right, in order to keep moving forward, you are going to take a step back for 4 weeks, every 4 months. While this may be a surprising change to a program labeled "Advanced," this type of deload is pretty common among pro-strength athletes. The stronger you become, the greater the toll your training takes on your body.

While beginner and intermediate strength trainers can usually move from one macro-cycle right on to the next, more advanced athletes will need to back off for a few weeks in order to give their bodies more time to heal. At professional powerlifting meets, where everyone is strong, the winners tend to be the ones who are the healthiest, and thus able to perform at their best.

Following each 12-week macro-cycle, you will go back to the Beginner cycle for one month before going back to Cycle 1: Week 1 of the Advanced cycle.

HIGHER TRAINING INTENSITIES: With the exception of the test days, the training intensity on the Intermediate cycle tops out at 85 percent on week 3. On the Advanced cycle, you'll go up to 90 percent on week 3, but you will also drop to 3 sets of 1.

VARYING MAIN LIFT VOLUME: In the Intermediate cycle, the main lift volume remains static at 3 sets of 15 for 3 weeks, followed by one test day. On the Advanced cycle, your volume waves up, starting at 25 total reps on the main exercise in week 1, down to 9 total reps in week 3, finishing with a 1 rep max for week 4. You'll also notice that the main lift volume even varies occasionally within the week. On week 3, the deadlift is reduced to 3 singles rather than 3 triples like the two previous days. This is so that you do not burn yourself out with 90 percent on the deadlift a few days before testing the squat.

Since the rep range will vary, so will your rest intervals. For sets in the 1-5 rep range, rest for about 5 minutes between sets. For assistance movements which will remain in the higher rep ranges, go back to the 1-3 minute range for rest periods.

You'll notice that all of the programs included in this book call for training 3 days per week. The exact days are up to you, but I would recommend having at least one rest day in between each training day to allow recovery. A schedule like Monday, Wednesday, and Friday in the gym with Tuesday, Thursday, Saturday, and Sunday off is a typical schedule.

For the main lifts, the percentages refer to the percentage of your 1 rep max. So if, for example your squat is 200 pounds and the training session calls for 75 percent, your working weight for the day would be 150 pounds. If you do not know what your 1 rep max is yet, plug in your 10 rep max for the 75 percent day, then add 5 percent each week until you test. After the test day, you will have a true percentage you can use.

For your assistance work, start with a weight that's somewhat challenging to get the prescribed sets and reps with, but not to the point where you risk a miss. Make conservative jumps in weight for subsequent weeks (5 to 10 pounds). By the last week, when performing that exercise, it should be difficult (but not impossible), to get all your sets and reps.

In the Advanced cycle, some exercises will be written as an expression, with the weight first, followed by the number of sets, followed by the number of repetitions in each set. For example, 3 sets of 5 repetitions with 135 pounds would be expressed as "135 x 3 x 5."

"Most advanced lifters design their own programming, or heavily modify pre-existing ones to their own unique needs."

CYCLE 1: WEEK 1

In the Advanced cycle, some exercises will be written as an expression, with the weight first, followed by the number of sets, followed by the number of repetitions in each set. For example, 3 sets of 5 repetitions with 135 pounds would be expressed as "135 x 3 x 5."

DAY 1	DAY 2	DAY 3
Box Squat (Barbell) 65% x 5 x 5	Bench Press (Barbell) 65% x 5 x 5	Conventional Deadlift (Barbell) 65% x 5 x 5
Straight Leg Deadlift (Barbell) 4 x 8	Bent-Over Row (Dumbbell) 4 x 8	Straight Leg Deadlift (Dumbbell) 4 x 10
Back Extension 4 x 10	Lying Triceps extension (Dumbbell) 4 x 10	Reverse Hyper 4 x 10
Pulldown Abs 4 x 10	Shoulder Raise (Lateral) 4 x 10	Incline Bench Sit-Up 4 x 10

CYCLE 1: WEEK 2

In the Advanced cycle, some exercises will be written as an expression, with the weight first, followed by the number of sets, followed by the number of repetitions in each set. For example, 3 sets of 5 repetitions with 135 pounds would be expressed as "135 x 3 x 5."

DAY 1	DAY 2	DAY 3
Box Squat (Barbell) 80% x 5 x 3 Straight Leg Deadlift (Barbell) 4 x 8 Back Extension 4 x 10 Pulldown Abs 4 x 10	Bench Press (Barbell) 80% x 5 x 3 Bent-Over Row (Dumbbell) 4 x 8 Triceps Extension (Dumbbell) 4 x 10 Shoulder Raise (Lateral) 4 x 10	Conventional Deadlift (Barbell) 80% x 5 x 3 Straight Leg Deadlift (Dumbbell) 4 x 10 Reverse Hyper 4 x 10 Incline Bench Sit-Up 4 x 10

CYCLE 1: WEEK 3

In the Advanced cycle, some exercises will be written as an expression, with the weight first, followed by the number of sets, followed by the number of repetitions in each set. For example, 3 sets of 5 repetitions with 135 pounds would be expressed as "135 x 3 x 5."

DAY 1	DAY 2	DAY 3
Box Squat (Barbell) 90% x 3 x 3	Bench Press (Barbell) 90% x 3 x 3	Conventional Deadlift (Barbell) 90% x 3 x 1
Straight Leg Deadlift (Barbell) 4 x 8	Bent-Over Row (Dumbbell) 4 x 8	Straight Leg Deadlift (Dumbbell) 4 x 10
Back Extension 4 x 10	Triceps Extension (Dumbbell) 4 x 10	Reverse Hyper 4 x 10
Pulldown Abs 4 x 10	Shoulder Raise (Lateral) 4 x 10	Incline Bench Sit-Up 4 x 10

CYCLE 1: WEEK 4

In the Advanced cycle, some exercises will be written as an expression, with the weight first, followed by the number of sets, followed by the number of repetitions in each set. For example, 3 sets of 5 repetitions with 135 pounds would be expressed as "135 x 3 x 5."

DAY 1	DAY 2	DAY 3
Box Squat (Barbell) 100% x 1 Straight Leg Deadlift (Barbell) 4 x 8 Back Extension 4 x 10 Pulldown Abs 4 x 10	Bench Press (Barbell) 100% x 1 Bent-Over Row (Dumbbell) 4 x 8 Triceps Extension (Dumbbell) 4 x 10 Shoulder Raise (Lateral) 4 x 10	Conventional Deadlift (Barbell) 100% x 1 Straight Leg Deadlift (Dumbbell) 4 x 10 Reverse Hyper 4 x 10 Incline Bench Sit-Up 4 x 10

CYCLE 2: WEEK 1

In the Advanced cycle, some exercises will be written as an expression, with the weight first, followed by the number of sets, followed by the number of repetitions in each set. For example, 3 sets of 5 repetitions with 135 pounds would be expressed as "135 x 3 x 5."

DAY 1	DAY 2	DAY 3
Barbell Squat 65% x 5 x 5	Floor Press (Barbell) 65% x 5 x 5	Sumo Deadlift 65% x 5 x 5
Goodmorning 4 x 8	Standing T-bar row 4 x 8	Machine Leg Press 4 x 8
Glute-Ham Raise 4 x 10	Triceps Pushdowns (Cable) 4 x 10	Bent-Over Rows (Barbell) 4 x 10
Glute-Ham Bench Sit-Up 4 x 10	Face Pulls (Cable) 4 x10	Spread Eagle Sit-Ups 4 x 10

CYCLE 2: WEEK 2

In the Advanced cycle, some exercises will be written as an expression, with the weight first, followed by the number of sets, followed by the number of repetitions in each set. For example, 3 sets of 5 repetitions with 135 pounds would be expressed as "135 x 3 x 5."

DAY 1	DAY 2	DAY 3
Barbell Squat 80% x 5 x 3	Floor Press (Barbell) 80% x 5 x 3	Sumo Deadlift 80% x 5 x 3
Goodmorning 4 x 8	Standing T-bar row 4 x 8	Machine Leg Press 4 x 8
Glute-Ham Raise 4 x 10	Triceps Pushdowns (Cable) 4 x 10	Bent-Over Rows (Barbell) 4 x 10
Glute-Ham Bench Sit-Ups 4 x 10	Face Pulls (Cable) 4 x10	Spread Eagle Sit-Ups 4 x 10

CYCLE 2: WEEK 3

In the Advanced cycle, some exercises will be written as an expression, with the weight first, followed by the number of sets, followed by the number of repetitions in each set. For example, 3 sets of 5 repetitions with 135 pounds would be expressed as "135 x 3 x 5."

DAY 1	DAY 2	DAY 3
Barbell Squat 90% x 3 x 3 Goodmorning 4 x 8 Glute-Ham Raise 4 x 10 Glute-Ham Bench Sit-Ups 4 x 10	Floor Press 90% x 3 x 3 Standing T-bar Row 4 x 8 Triceps Pushdowns (Cable) 4 x 10 Face Pulls (Cable) 4 x10	Sumo Deadlift 90% x 3 x 1 Machine Leg Press 4 x 8 Bent-Over Rows (Barbell) 4 x 10 Spread Eagle Sit-Ups 4 x 10

CYCLE 2: WEEK 4

In the Advanced cycle, some exercises will be written as an expression, with the weight first, followed by the number of sets, followed by the number of repetitions in each set. For example, 3 sets of 5 repetitions with 135 pounds would be expressed as "135 x 3 x 5."

DAY 1	DAY 2	DAY 3
Barbell Squat 100% x 1	Floor Press (Barbell) 100% x 1	Sumo Deadlift 100% x 1
Goodmorning 4 x 8	Standing T-bar Row 4 x 8	Machine Leg Press 4 x 8
Glute-Ham raise 4 x 10	Triceps Pushdowns (Cable) 4 x 10	Bent-Over Rows (Barbell) 4 x 10
Glute-Ham Bench Sit-Ups 4 x 10	Face Pulls (Cable) 4 x10	Spread Eagle Sit-Ups 4 x 10

CYCLE 3: WEEK 1

In the Advanced cycle, some exercises will be written as an expression, with the weight first, followed by the number of sets, followed by the number of repetitions in each set. For example, 3 sets of 5 repetitions with 135 pounds would be expressed as "135 x 3 x 5."

DAY 1	DAY 2	DAY 3
Front Squat 65% x 5 x 5	Overhead Press (Barbell) 65% x 5 x 5	Deficit Deadlift (Barbell) 65% x 5 x 5
Zercher Squat 4 x 8	Lat Pulldowns 4 x 8	Straight Leg Deadlift (Barbell) 4 x 8
Straight Leg Deadlift (Dumbbell) 4 x 10	Lying Triceps Extensions (Barbell) 4 x 10	Back Extensions 4 x 10
Incline Bench Sit-Ups 4 x 10	Shoulder Raises (Reverse Fly) 4 x 10	Planks 4 x 30 seconds

CYCLE 3: WEEK 2

In the Advanced cycle, some exercises will be written as an expression, with the weight first, followed by the number of sets, followed by the number of repetitions in each set. For example, 3 sets of 5 repetitions with 135 pounds would be expressed as "135 x 3 x 5."

DAY 1	DAY 2	DAY 3
Front Squat 80% x 5 x 3	Overhead Press (Barbell) 80% x 5 x 3	Deficit Deadlift (Barbell) 80% x 5 x 3
Zercher Squat 4 x 8	Lat Pulldowns 4 x 8	Straight Leg Deadlift (Barbell) 4 x 8
Straight Leg Deadlift (Dumbbell) 4 x 10	Lying Triceps Extensions (Barbell) 4 x 10	Back Extensions 4 x 10
Incline Bench Sit-Ups 4 x 10	Shoulder Raises (Reverse Fly) 4 x 10	Planks 4 x 45 seconds

CYCLE 3: WEEK 3

In the Advanced cycle, some exercises will be written as an expression, with the weight first, followed by the number of sets, followed by the number of repetitions in each set. For example, 3 sets of 5 repetitions with 135 pounds would be expressed as "135 x 3 x 5."

DAY 1	DAY 2	DAY 3
Front Squat 90% x 3 x 3	Overhead Press (Barbell) 90% x 3 x 3	Deficit Deadlift (Barbell) 90% x 3 x 1
Zercher Squat 4 x 8	Lat Pulldowns 4 x 8	Straight Leg Deadlift (Barbell) 4 x 8
Straight Leg Deadlift (Dumbbell) 4 x 10	Lying Triceps Extensions (Barbell) 4 x 10	Back Extensions 4 x 10
Glute-Ham Bench Sit-Ups 4 x 10	Shoulder Raises (Reverse Fly) 4 x 10	Planks 4 x 60 seconds

CYCLE 3: WEEK 4

In the Advanced cycle, some exercises will be written as an expression, with the weight first, followed by the number of sets, followed by the number of repetitions in each set. For example, 3 sets of 5 repetitions with 135 pounds would be expressed as "135 x 3 x 5."

DAY 1	DAY 2	DAY 3
Front Squat 100% x 1 Zercher Squat 4 x 8 Straight Leg Deadlift (Dumbbell) 4 x 10 Glute-Ham Bench Sit-Ups 4 x 10	Overhead Press (Barbell) 100% x 1 Lat Pulldowns 4 x 8 Lying Triceps Extensions (Barbell) 4 x 10 Shoulder Raises (Reverse Fly) 4 x 10	Deficit Deadlift (Barbell) 100% x 1 Straight Leg Deadlifts (Barbell) 4 x 8 Back Extensions 4 x 10 Planks 4 x 90 seconds

CREATING YOUR OWN PROGRAM

The best option for most novice strength trainers is to follow a pre-designed program like the ones in this book, or a program written for them by a qualified coach. There are just so many variables to an effective program that unless you have either an academic or sound practical background (or ideally both), you can waste months, if not years, trying to write a program for yourself.

However, as you mature as an athlete, your needs will become more individualized, and it might make more sense to start adjusting your programming, if not creating one from scratch. Usually by this time, your years (not months or weeks) under the bar have given you a much deeper understanding of the training process.

In most cases, the transition from following programs to designing them is gradual. Few athletes wake up one day and decide to abandon their pre-designed program and start from scratch. Usually, this switch occurs as the result of years of tinkering with and tweaking their existing programming, until it no longer resembles what they started with.

Incidentally, this is how most professional strength athletes learned to program for themselves and others.

The reason learning to program can be tricky, is that "correct" programming will vary based on the goal and the athlete. Even two athletes in the same sport might need seemingly different programs to address their specific needs.

If you've been following the programs in this book for at least a year, you've probably already figured out a few tweaks to make them work better for you. If you're going on 2 or more years, you may have made substantial changes, and be considering more.

This chapter is not so much a "how to," but a collection of principles to keep in mind as you continue to adjust and refine your training program. Despite the differences in various program templates, they all follow the same "rules" in order to keep you progressing.

ESSENTIAL ELEMENTS OF STRENGTH PROGRAMMING

For a program to be effective, there are a number of elements that must be present, regardless of the actual set-up and implementation. If you read any popular strength programs, you will see these same principles at work, no matter how dissimilar the programs seem to be.

Think of these elements as the skeleton of all programs and make sure to include them in yours.

Goal Setting

The most critical component of designing a program is goal setting. If you think of a program as a road-map, the goal is your destination.

I am a big proponent of having both short-term and long-term goals. By "short-term," I'm referring to goals you would work toward over the course of the macro-cycle, or every 12 to 16 weeks. By "long-term," I mean goals that you will keep in mind throughout the duration of your lifting career.

In order to help you settle on an appropriate short-term goal, I always recommend using the S.M.A.R.T. goal format.

Specific

Measurable

Attainable

Realistic

Time-bound

SPECIFIC: Before designing a program, you should know what specifically you are trying to accomplish. Broad goals like "get stronger" or "gain muscle" are good to motivate you in making the decision to start training, but they don't really help you put the nuts and bolts together. Instead of setting a broad goal like "get stronger," figure out how much you want to improve in the basic lifts, and work backward from there.

MEASURABLE: Setting measurable goals in training is usually pretty easy because progress is measured in reps, pounds, and kilos. Some people also like to rely on the mirror to gauge progress, but this is a tough way to quantify progress unless you have a very well-trained eye. Additionally, it is difficult to judge your own appearance because of your emotional connection to the result. In lifting, if your weights are improving, you know beyond a shadow of a doubt that you are improving.

ATTAINABLE: It's great to have lofty goals, but sometimes people set a goal for themselves without even taking the time to consider whether their goal is possible, even under the best of circumstances. I'll never forget the relatively untrained guy who walked into the gym, claiming he was going to deadlift 1,000 pounds. So far, only two men in history have ever accomplished this, and both were extraordinarily talented lifters. In cases like this, a little self-consciousness can be a good thing.

REALISTIC: This is similar to the "attainable" attribute, but I define it a bit differently in terms of goal setting. For a goal to be attainable, it must be something that is within your genetic makeup to be able to accomplish. A *realistic* goal is one that you are *willing* to work toward. For example, you might be physically capable of squatting 800 pounds one day. While this goal is *attainable,* it may not be *realistic* when you consider what sacrifices it would take to get there. Pick a goal that you can realistically imagine yourself working toward without making sacrifices you are unwilling or unable to make.

TIME-BOUND: Goals tend to work best when bound to a specific date or time frame because it keeps motivation high and encourages structure in order to accomplish them. One of the reasons competitive lifters make more progress than noncompetitive lifters is that their contest schedules give them specific dates to focus on and work toward. While time-bound goals can help keep you motivated, they can also improve patience. For example, if you establish that you have 12 weeks to add 20 pounds to your squat, you will be less inclined to go all-out on day 1 and risk injury.

Evaluation

In order to put together a sensible program for any athletic goal, you must first know your current level of conditioning. To do this, your training program must include some sort of evaluation process.

To borrow the roadmap analogy from the goal setting section, think of evaluation as your GPS, which is constantly updating you as to your progress. Most personal trainers and coaches use some sort of evaluative process to tell them if an athletes or clients are on track to hit their goals. You should do the same when programming for yourself.

The key here is to be as objective as possible. The more honest you are with yourself about your current strength level, the better prepared you'll be to address whatever might be holding you back.

In the case of strength programming, the simplest evaluative tools are the weights themselves. Your program should include periodic "testing" so that you can track your progress, as well as calculate the correct percentages for your training weights. Depending on the style of programming and your level of experience, you might test yourself anywhere from monthly to a couple of times per year. Most competitive lifters rarely test at all in training, and save their heaviest efforts for competition.

In the Intermediate and Advanced cycles, the monthly "test week" serves as both an evaluation and a training stimulus. On a linear periodization-based program, you would wait every 12 to 16 weeks to test, which is still frequent enough to gauge progress year in and year out.

The evaluative process is another reason why competitive lifters tend to progress faster. Competition is the ultimate setting to test strength because the athlete is being held to a uniform standard set by the judges. Improvement from meet to meet means a tangible gain in strength.

Progression

Unless your body is consistently challenged to perform more than before, progress will stagnate. This progression can include intensity, volume, or frequency. While progression is necessary over the course of the program, remember that we're speaking long-term here. While it's great to aspire to daily improvements, remember that the longer someone trains, the harder it will be for them to make gains from one workout to the next. In fact, strength athletes will start reducing their training intensity weeks before a competition to prevent burnout.

Instead of going "all out" in each training session, the goal should to be to make small, conservative improvements over the course of the training cycle.

You will notice that in the training cycles in this book, exercises are never performed for more than a month or so. This is because linear progress in a single exercise is not possible in the long term. For example, adding 10 pounds to your bench press in a month is not an unreasonable goal at all. To continue at that rate would mean improving by 120 pounds in a year, which is attainable for some people, but not for most. Fast forward 10 years and you would be looking at a 1,200-pound gain which has so far never been accomplished. As you become more in tune with your body, you will know when you can push and when you can't.

Overload

Overload goes hand in hand with progression. In fact, strength programming is often referred to a "progressive overload." Overload means that you are exposing your body to tasks that it is not yet able to perform. This is why exercises are performed with the goal of momentary muscular failure. This does not, however, mean that you should ever attempt a weight that you can only get three reps with when the goal is ten.

As with progression, beginners can sometimes handle more overload than experienced exercisers. This is because the nervous system of a beginner is not being taxed to the extent that an experienced exerciser's is. The stronger you get, the more taxing training is to the nervous system. For experienced lifters, a true overload is used sparingly and is used only at the end of either the meso-cycle or the macro-cycle.

Specificity

Specificity is a critically important factor in program design, although the term is often misunderstood by well-meaning, but misinformed, coaches.

The term "sport specific" has been floating around the commercial fitness and strength/conditioning industries for over a decade, but it is often interpreted to mean that the exercises used in training must perfectly replicate the skills of the sport. An example would be a golfer performing a swinging motion while holding a weighted cable.

The term "sport specific" is also often used interchangeably with "functional training," which often (and inexplicably) calls for athletes to perform exercises standing or sitting on unstable surfaces, like mats and stability balls while lifting a fraction of what they could with their feet on the floor.

With regard to training, specificity simply means that the program is written for the goal of the user. If your goal is to gain as much muscle as possible, a powerlifting-based program will help, but not as much as a program designed specifically for bodybuilding. Likewise, if your goal is improved strength and power, a bodybuilding-based program will be better than nothing, but not as helpful as a program based around the Olympic lifts or power lifts.

Balance

When I say that a program must be balanced, I do not mean the type of balance that a tightrope walker would display, but rather balance in terms of training your entire body in a way that maintains balance between muscle groups.

Muscles do not function independently of each other. Most have an agonist/antagonist relationship with at least one other muscle group. For example, when the quadriceps muscle contracts to extend the knee joint, the hamstrings (knee flexor) allow themselves to be lengthened in order to allow the knee joint to extend without resistance.

When a muscle group becomes too strong in relation to its antagonist, an imbalance develops, which can hinder performance and contribute to injury. You can see muscle imbalances like this in weight rooms across the country. When trainees (usually young men) spend too much of their time with pressing movements, like the bench press, they begin to take on a stoop-shouldered appearance, as the pecs and anterior deltoids overpower the muscles of the upper back.

Not only do these guys increase their risk of shoulder injury, but they also limit their progress in the bench press which they are trying so hard to build. When the body senses a muscular imbalance, it will limit force production in the agonist muscle to protect the antagonist muscle from being overpowered and injured.

Another common example of muscle imbalance would be tight hip flexors contributing to lower back pain. The hip/trunk flexion associated in most abdominal exercises will cause tight hip flexors if not balanced out by hip/trunk extension. Internal rotation of the shoulder, common in throwing movements, can cause rotator cuff pain if not accompanied by external rotation. Train the body as a single entity, not a collection of parts.

So if you want a big bench press, train your upper back hard, and if you want strong abdominals, train your lower back/hip extensors. For that matter, whenever you perform any movement with resistance, be sure to include an opposite movement in the same plane to avoid imbalances.

The one exception to this rule is with squatting movements because, other than leg lifts, there really isn't an opposite movement for you to work. This is because our lower bodies are designed for strong hip extension for movements like running and jumping, but only need hip flexion to return the legs to the start position.

Recovery

Recovery is an important and often overlooked aspect of exercise programming. Always keep in mind that training should be considered a stress to the body, and that much like more serious forms of trauma, this stress must be recovered from. There are two types of recovery that we want to include in any training program. They include passive recovery and active recovery.

Passive recovery means days where no training is scheduled, and activity is limited. Active recovery means taking advantage of training and techniques geared toward healing the soft tissues and nervous system.

You'll notice that almost all strength training programs, including those included in this book, have a few "off days" each week. For most people, I've found it particularly effective to train every other day or so. If you do need to train consecutive days, it's a good idea to adjust the intensity so that you are not training heavy on consecutive days.

In most cases, you can perform either active or passive recovery on your off days. Active recovery is usually better, as long as you keep any training to a low enough intensity that it doesn't affect your programmed training sessions. Keep the resistance at about 30 percent to 40 percent. The goal here is to improve circulation and pump blood into the muscles.

Compound movements are superior for strength gain, but light, single joint exercises are great for recovery. Cable and elastic band resistance is particularly effective. A good rule of thumb is that if anything you do makes you sore, then it's too intense. Other active recovery techniques can include stretching, massage, low intensity cardio, contrast showers, and yoga.

Periodization

The whole concept of programming is based on the knowledge that an organism (in this case, us) will not progress indefinitely if given the same stimulus (in this case, lifting weights). While your program is your plan to accomplish your goal, periodization is the method that determines how that plan will look. There are several forms of periodization, and they all accomplish the same objective: regulating the delicate balance between volume, load, and frequency in order to facilitate continued progress.

If you want to be able to develop programs for yourself or others, you must first decide which method of periodization you would prefer to use and why.

LINEAR PERIODIZATION: The simplest of all the periodization models, linear periodization is the easiest form of periodization to plan and follow. While not generally regarded as the most effective by experts in strength and conditioning, it *does* work and can be a good introduction to program design for your first go-around as your own coach.

The basic concept is simple. Start the program with low intensity load on the main lifts, performed with high volume, gradually transitioning to low volume and high intensity. To give a more practical example, a lifter training for a bigger squat might start the macro-cycle with weights in the 55 percent to 65 percent range, performed for 10 to 15 reps per set. Over the course of the 12 to 16 week program, the intensity would gradually move up to just over 100 percent (assuming a *pr* is made), for one repetition.

The meso-cycles are usually broken up into phases labeled "hypertrophy," "strength," "power," and "peak," although there is little substantial change from one phase to the next, other than approximately a 5 percent increase in intensity. On a graph (see below), the volume and intensities can be represented by two unbroken lines spanning the entire macro-cycle.

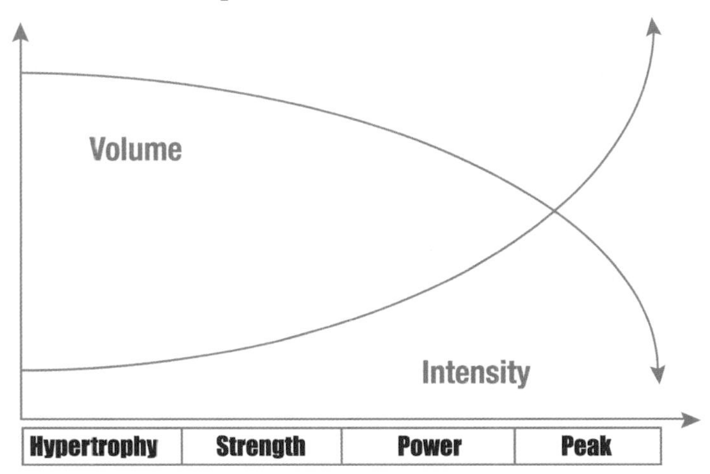

UNDULATING PERIODIZATION: Undulating periodization is a system of non-linear periodization that builds intensity in a wave over the course of the meso-cycle, then drops back down and builds back up over the next meso-cycle.

For a reference, the Intermediate and Advanced cycles included in this book use an undulating periodization scheme.

While linear periodization is a great introduction to the idea of long-term periodized programming, it does have a few drawbacks, which may make undulating periodization a more attractive choice.

The first issue with linear periodization is that you spend the majority of your maro-cycle using sub-maximal loads, which means you will only see a tangible strength gain in the last few weeks of your program. For competitive lifters who only need to be at their strongest on the day of the meet, this is really no big deal.

For the recreational lifter however, waiting 12 to16 weeks to make a personal record in a lift can be a little disheartening, especially when you are close to the beginning of your career and enthusiasm is at its highest. With an undulating periodization scheme, you have the opportunity to work at high intensity multiple times throughout the training cycle, which can be more gratifying and keeps your motivation high.

Undulating periodization will also keep you stronger throughout the year, which is a big advantage if you are using lifting to prepare for another sport.

In the Intermediate and Advanced cycles, the exercises vary from one month to the next in order to expose you to a wide variety of exercises and limit boredom, but you do not necessarily need to do this when designing your own program. If you want, you can keep the same main lifts for the program, and change only the volume and intensity.

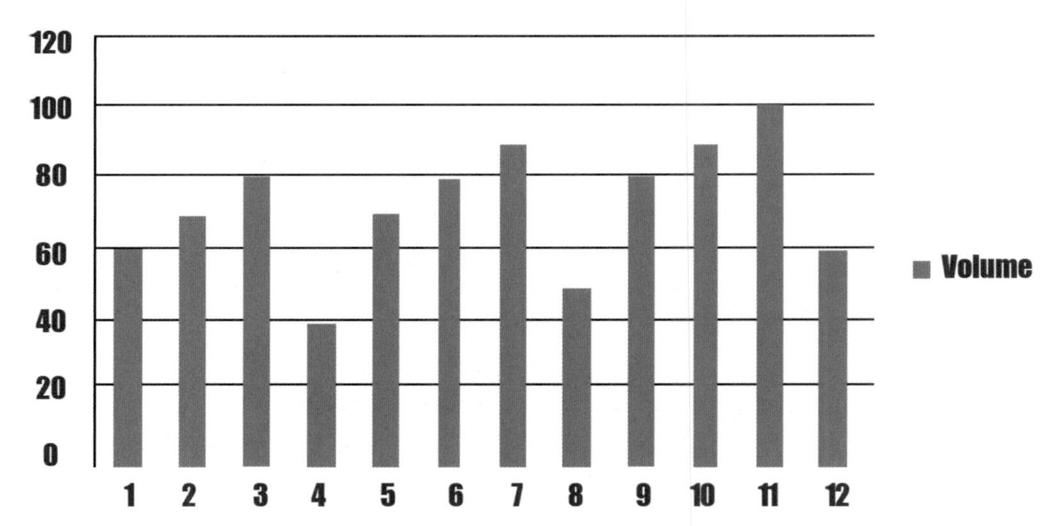

Prilepin's Chart

Based on the research of Soviet sports scientist A. S. Prilepin, Prilepin's chart is a set of guidelines that coaches and lifters use to help with the design of training programs. Essentially, what Prilepin did was to analyze the training of elite-level weight lifters to figure out the optimal relationship between volume and intensity.

His findings are the result of years of researching the best strength athletes of his era, and the chart is exceptionally accurate to this day.

% of Max	Reps Per Set	Volume of Reps		
		Low	Medium	High
50-55	3 to 6	12 to 18	18 to 24	24 to 30
55-65	3 to 6	12 to 18	18 to 24	24 to 30
60-65	3 to 6	10 to 18	18 to 24	24 to 30
65-70	3 to 5	8 to 15	12 to 20	20 to 24
70-75	3 to 6	7 to 15	12 to 20	20 to 24
75-80	2 to 4	6 to 12	12 to 18	18 to 21
85-90	2 to 4	5 to 10	10 to 15	15 to 18
85-90	2 to 3	3 to 7	8 to 12	12 to 15
90+	1 to 2	1 to 4	4 to 7	8 to 10

HOW TO READ THE CHART:

The left-most column represents your training weight, expressed as a percentage of your 1 rep max.

The next column gives you the ideal range of repetitions per set.

The next three columns give you your ideal total number of repetitions, with the medium column being the optimal range for most applications.

For example, let's say you want to figure out the optimal volume for 85 percent of your max squat. According to the chart, you will want to keep the reps between 2 and 4 reps per set, with an optimal range of 8 to 15 reps per training session. This would make any of the following set/rep schemes appropriate:

5 sets of 3 = 15
3 sets of 3 = 9
4 sets of 3 =12
3 sets of 4 = 12
5 sets of 2 = 10
2 sets of 5 =10

Most programs would use either 3 x 3 or 5 x 3, because for some reason, you just don't see a whole lot of programs using sets of 2 or 4. (I'm not sure what the reason for this is, probably just habit, but according to Prilepin, there's really no reason not to.)

A few considerations when using Prilepin's chart:

RECOVERY: If you are participating in another sport in addition to your lifting, or have a stressful schedule that makes recovery difficult, stick to the low range for rep-volume. Remember that the athletes on whom this chart was based were the thoroughbreds of Olympic weight lifting, and had few responsibilities other than their training, not to mention superior genetics.

TIME UNDER TENSION: Due to their explosive nature, the Olympic lifts (the snatch and the clean and jerk) place the athlete under tension for less time than the power lifts. So a set of three squats at 85 percent takes more straining than a set of 3 snatches at the same percentage. Taking into account that the chart was designed with weight lifters in mind, rather than powerlifters, it would probably be a good idea to stick to the low range for volume when you get to 90 percent and above.

According to the chart, the upper range of volume would be 8 to 10 total reps for 90 percent and above. Any experienced powerlifter will tell you that 10 reps at over 90 percent is a *ton* of work. The low end of 1 to 4 reps should be plenty.

LIFTER EXPERIENCE: Percentage-based training works because we can generally expect a lifter to be capable of a certain number of reps at a given percentage of their 1-rep-max. As you've probably noticed in the programming section as well as in Prilepin's chart, there is an inverse relationship between intensity and volume. This is common knowledge in training, but what is not commonly known is that this relationship will vary based on the experience level of the athlete.

For example, a novice athlete can usually be expected to perform between 10 and 15 reps with 75 percent of their max. On the other hand, an experienced powerlifter might only be able to complete 8 reps or so, although the total weight will be much heavier. This is because powerlifters have conditioned their nervous system to fire as much muscle tissue as possible for one big strain, yet they might not have the short-term muscular endurance for higher repetitions.

Bodybuilders, by contrast, generally use lower intensities with higher repetitions, and may be capable of much more reps at a given percentage than a true strength athlete would be.

Most regular lifters will fall somewhere in between these two examples—just be aware that predictions of repetitions, while a good guideline, are not set in stone, so you'll need to pay attention to trends in your training to figure out where you fall on this spectrum.

INJURY PREVENTION & MAINTENANCE

Injury prevention focuses on two key ingredients: proper exercise technique and progressively increasing load over time. If you focus on these two key elements, your likelihood of experiencing an injury related to performing an exercise is minimized, if not eliminated.

You may have heard fellow "gym rats" saying they were so sore from their workout earlier in the week. Delayed onset muscle soreness is a normal process of a strength-building program, particularly a new one. Muscle soreness can last for 24 to 96 hours. Active recovery (such as walking), getting adequate sleep, drinking water, and stretching are several ways to facilitate muscle recovery.

As professional trainers, we have provided hundreds, if not thousands, of clients with evidence-based strength programs over the years. We know from our experience, and from feedback from clients of all levels, that being strong and healthy can and *should* go together.

Injury prevention and strength maintenance should go hand in hand because strength training must be done with consistency, and with consistency comes adaptation and progression in your program.

Even with the greatest program design, every person has their *weak spots* which may affect your ability to perform a key exercise with perfect technique and form so that you can maximize strength gains and reduce the likelihood of injury. (For example, tight hips and ankles may cause knee pain and prevent proper range of motion during the squat.)

In the guidance provided within this chapter, we will focus on the main lifts that utilize our strength program philosophy of push, pull, lift, press, and extend. Several supplementary lifts that tend to be more popular will be included as well.

The lift will be listed followed by common limitation that most people experience, even professional trainers and competitive athletes. Immediately below each list of limitation are two suggested exercises that can be done to mitigate the stability or mobility you are lacking, thereby creating a better overall strength experience. Please keep in mind: t*here is no substitute for actually performing the lifts*, especially the main lifts.

THE MOBILITY MYTH

Undeniably, mobility is an important component of strength training. When the execution of a lift is inhibited by either weakness or inflexibility, the athlete is at a significantly greater risk of injury. For example, when the hamstrings are too tight, a lifter trying to break parallel in the squat may be placing excessive load on the lower back. Additionally, various forms of mobility training alleviate symptoms of existing injuries and can also help speed recovery.

For these reasons, it is not uncommon to see most athletes spend the first 20 minutes (often more) of their training sessions on the floor, using bands, rubber bands, foam rollers, lacrosse balls, and other tools to methodically stretch and massage their hips, backs, shoulders, and other muscle groups, before even looking at a barbell.

Having come from the era when athletes did little, if any, stretching before training, I have to wonder, isn't this overkill? Especially when so many of these athletes really aren't handling all that much weight to begin with?

I realize I'm bucking a very popular trend here, but I have some pretty sensible reasons to do so.

Sometimes, the very mobility regimen that these athletes are using to avoid injury might be *increasing* the likelihood of an injury. When you consistently perform a particular athletic skill or exercise, your body will go through a number of adaptations in order to perform the skill as efficiently as possible. Sometimes, this means certain muscles will become tighter over time.

Usually, athletes are encouraged to address this tightness with stretching drills or soft tissue work, but optimal mobility for a particular sport doesn't always mean maximum mobility. As long as an athlete is able to demonstrate the range of motion necessary to perform the skill he or she is required to (such as breaking parallel in the squat), does it really make sense to strive for more?

In some cases, too much mobility can actually *increase* the risk of an injury because the muscles required to stabilize the working joints (such as the hips, spine, and shoulders) are unable to maintain sufficient tightness throughout the lift.

If strength athletes tend to be tighter than most athletes, does it not stand to reason that this may be because their sport *demands* they be tighter?

There are also some compelling reasons why too much mobility work, especially when performed before lifting, can hinder performance.

Stretching and soft tissue work increase flexibility (at least in the short term) because they inhibit the stretch reflex, which in turn diminishes power. For example, try throwing a baseball with a typical wind-up, and then without. Although it is counter to popular opinion on mobility, strength athletes *want* a certain amount of tightness because the natural elasticity of the tight muscles will aid in the production of force under heavy weights.

Of course, there are exceptions to this philosophy, most notably pain. If you are experiencing pain due to muscle tightness or imbalance, then sensible mobility work becomes absolutely essential.

Likewise, if you are unable to perform certain lifts or exercises throughout the full range of motion without sacrificing technique, then increasing flexibility actually takes precedence over training the lift because until you are able to execute the lift properly, training it will force you to practice a mistake and will only hinder long-term progress.

As with any exercise, the importance of mobility training is a question of context.

MOBILITY VERSUS STABILITY

Functional training has stormed the general public with a fury over the last decade with popular training methodologies such as TRX, P90X, Insanity®, and Crossfit. These programs all have their own pros and cons in their respective space, but the average person looking to enhance their overall fitness often has no idea where to start. The underpinning of the functional training methodology can trace part of its roots back to the concept of mobility versus stability.

In the medical community, mobility refers to range of motion around a joint. In the athletic communities, mobility often refers to an approach to training such as movement-based warm-ups.

Stability is the ability to maintain your position in space when force acts upon your body. For example, while performing a walking lunge you can keep your body upright and your knee straight with gravity pulling you down. In recent years, training tools such as BOSU balls® have been used to enhance the response of your nervous system by constantly challenging you to maintain your position. Unfortunately, there's very little transfer of BOSU-ball® skills to real life, as opposed to performing an overhead press or walking lunge.

Generally speaking, you must have

stability before mobility. In real-world terms, stability refers to the execution of an exercise with proper technique, producing greater force than the dumbbell or barbell is placing on you. Once you overcome a given resistance and are stable, you can advance in that movement. This is called progressive overload. Get strong and the rest will take care of itself.

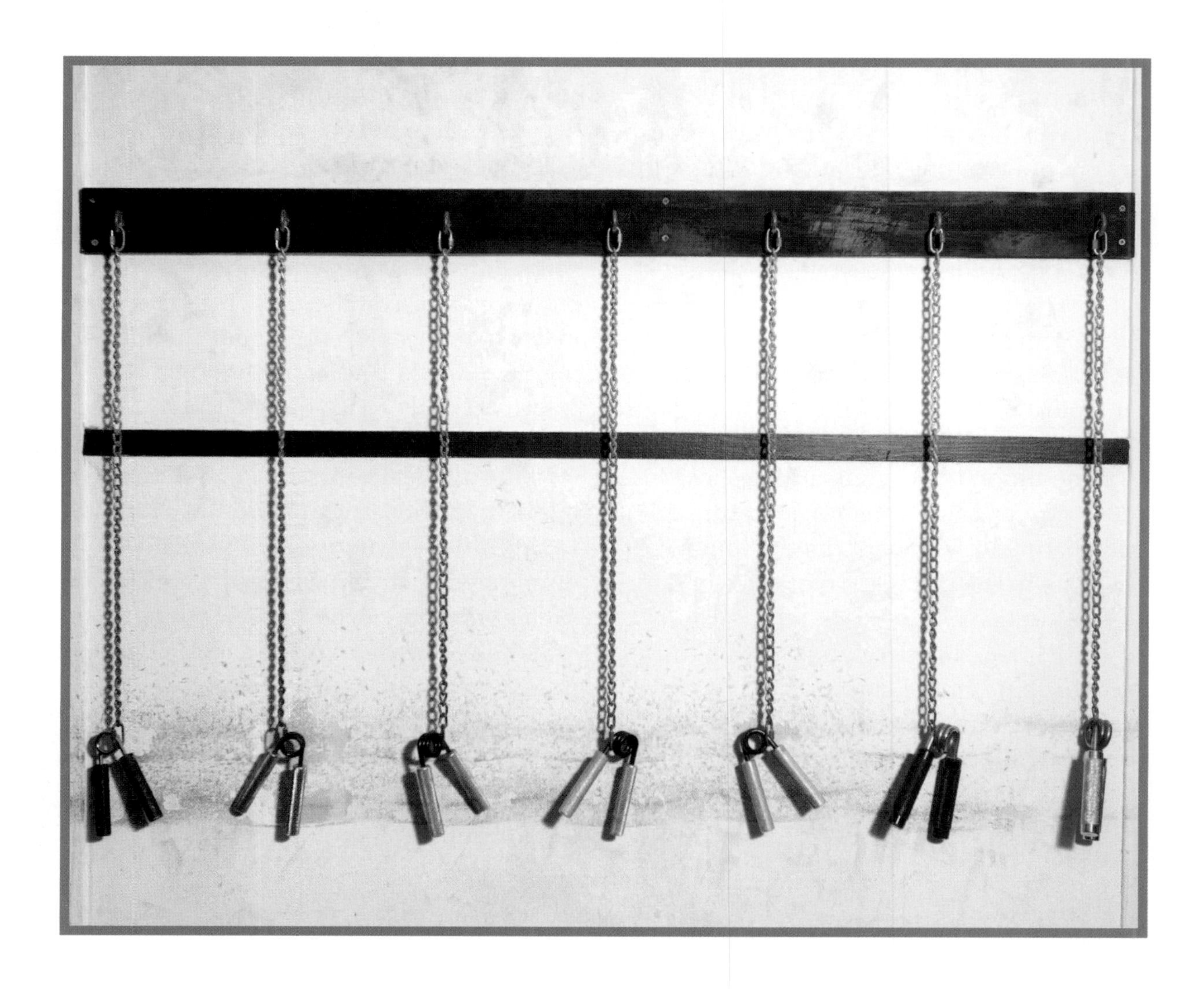

INJURY PREVENTION EXERCISES BY BODY AREA

In the following pages, you will find an in-depth description of preventative exercises grouped by body region: upper body, hip girdle, and lower body. As professional trainers, we have trained literally thousands of clients during our combined of 40 years of experience. One important fact to remember is that *every person's body is unique.* You will not need to refer to every injury prevention exercise, but we do encourage you to experiment prudently on body areas other than those you feel needed work in the earlier main lifts section.

There may arise times when due to immobility or injury, you simply cannot yet perform traditional exercises. In this case, you will need an exercise regimen aimed at first improving basic movement. We call this "getting into shape to get into shape."

Most of these exercises can also be used to address injuries and mobility issues that may arise just from working out.

UPPER BODY

GRIP/WRIST STRENGTH

Set-Up

Sit in a stable chair. Position a bucket in front of you with enough rice so that you can reach in to the middle of your forearm.

Execution

Begin to make "door knob" motions in the rice. You can also flatten your hand out with a straight arm or perform the alphabet in the rice.

The door motion is an asymmetrical movement, which simulates daily activities around your forearm and elbow. The flat hand version will focus on the shoulder and rotator cuff muscles.

Recovery

Gently stretch your hand and fingers after removing them from the bucket.

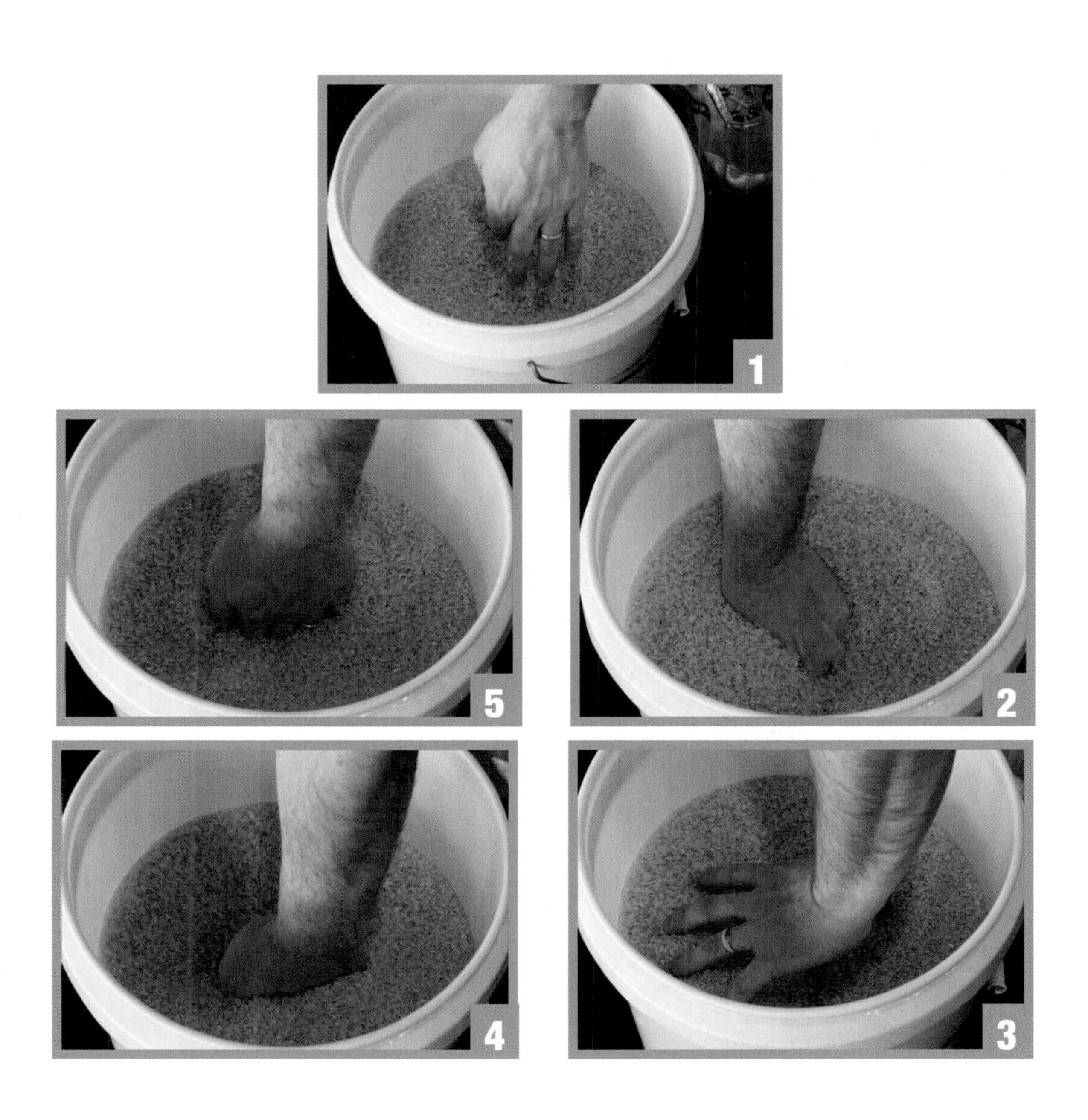
1
5
2
4
3

UPPER BODY

SHOULDER BLADE GLIDE

Set-Up

Maintain equal weight between the knees and hands. Pull the ribs “up,” engaging the stomach muscles and tightening up the horizontal corset.

Execution

Push your shoulders blades back and down. Pull your shoulder blades forward against the rib cage using the muscles around the armpits and chest.

Recovery

Find a neutral position between the push and pull movements.

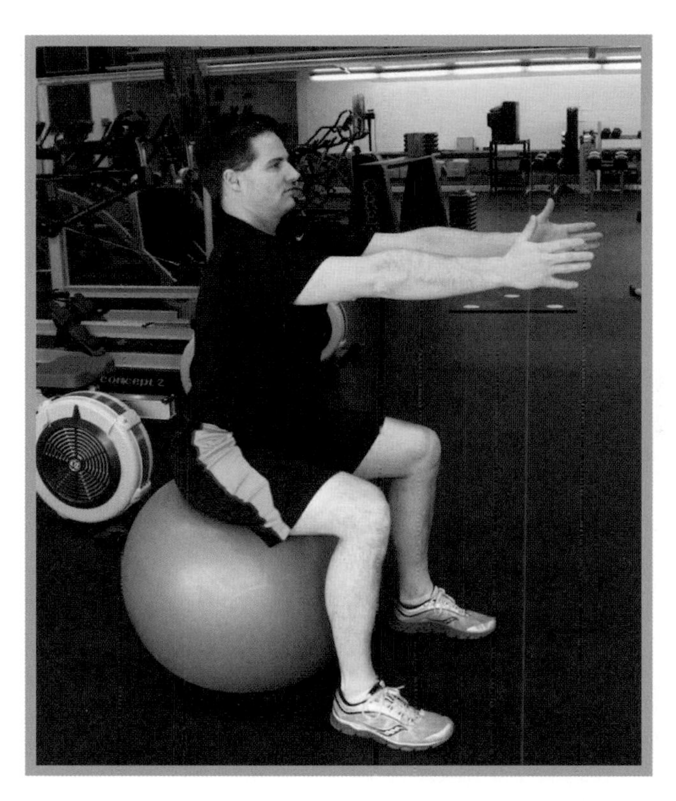
concept 2

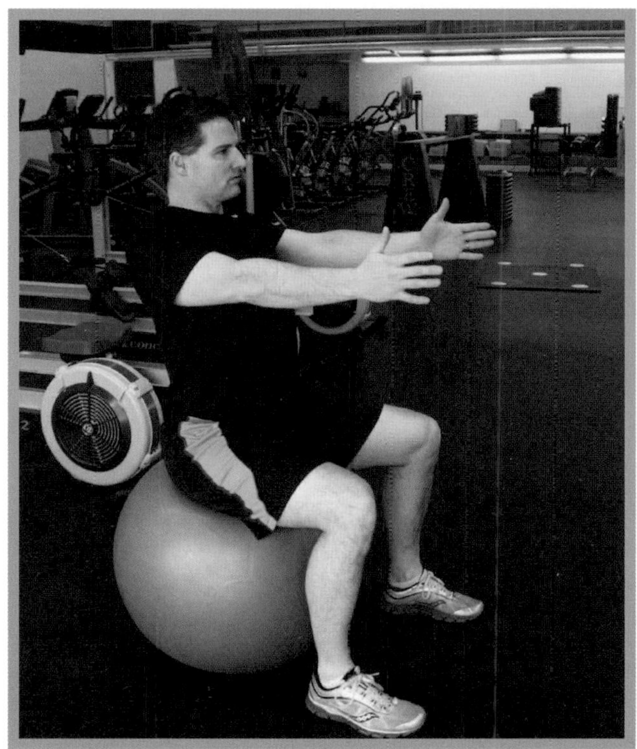

UPPER BODY

THREAD THE NEEDLE

Set-Up
Start in an all-fours position.

Execution
Reach through the mid-section of your body between the opposite side arm and hip. Keep the supporting arm slightly flexed. Focus on the "sling-system" connection between the opposite side hip and shoulder during this reaching movement, which targets the middle back

Recovery
Pull the shoulder blade back first against the ribcage wall. Pause and repeat.

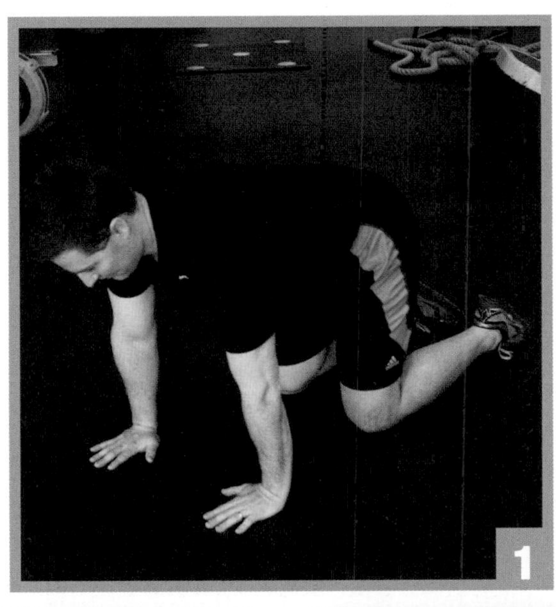
1

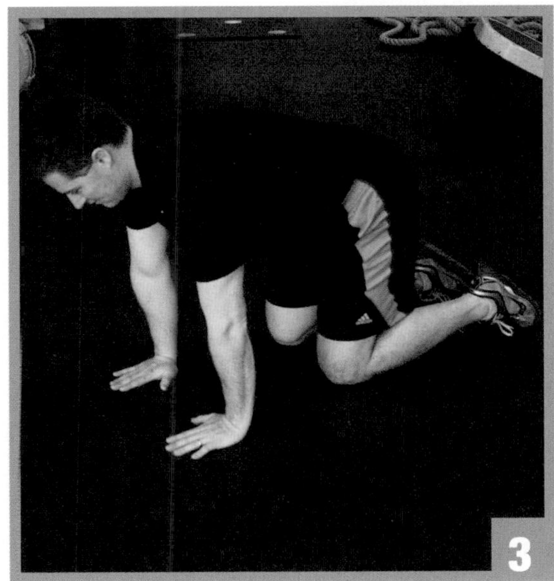
3

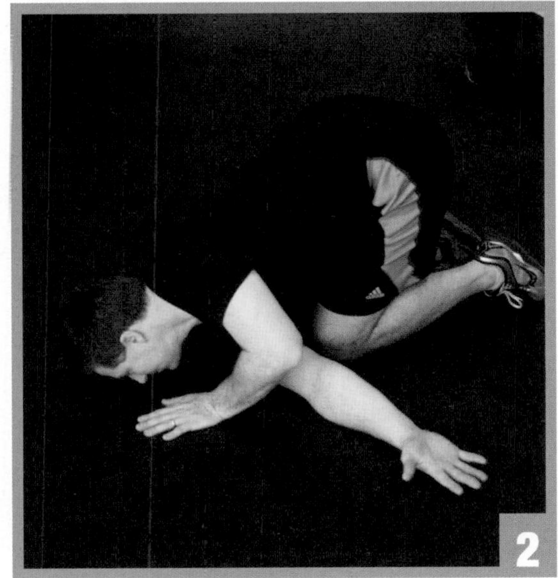
2

UPPER BODY

CAN OPENER

Set-Up
Start in an all-fours position.

Execution
Place your hand behind your head while keeping the shoulder blade against the rib-cage wall. Initiate the movement from your back and ribs. Open the shoulder girdle up, leading with the working side elbow. A rotational sensation will be felt through the ribs, stomach, and back.

Recovery
Contract the front of your body between the working side shoulder and opposite side hip.

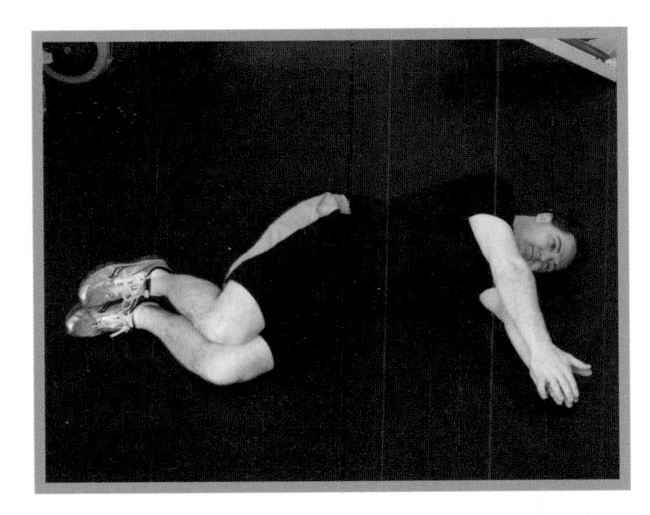

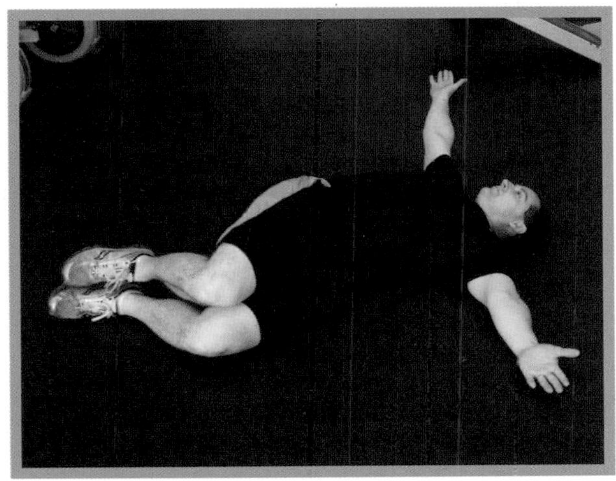

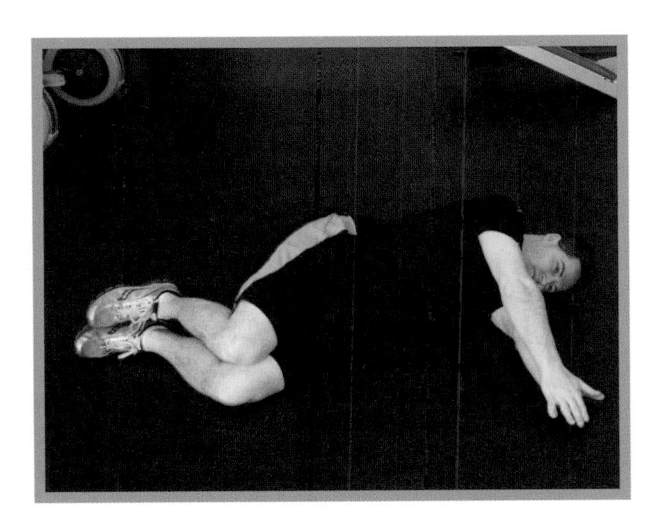

UPPER BODY

SPINAL WHIP

Set-Up

Begin in an all-fours position. Your hands should be positioned under the shoulders and your knees should be under the hips.

Execution

Arch the spine up using the stomach muscles, return to neutral starting position, and drop the hips back over the feet. Return to neutral, repeat sequence.

Recovery

Resume a neutral position between maximal upward position and downward position.

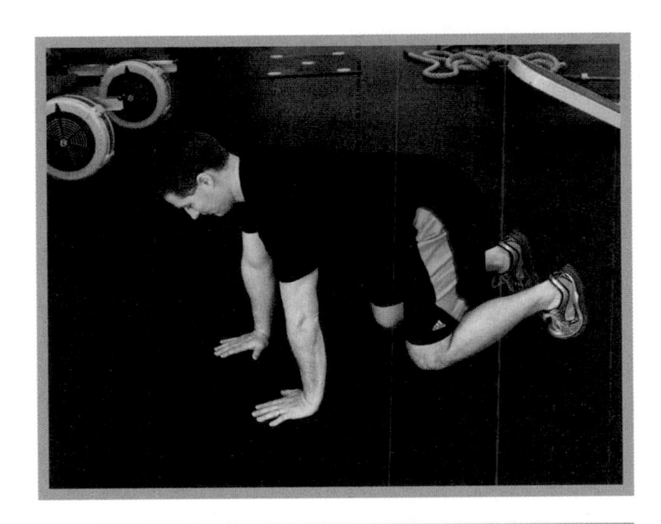

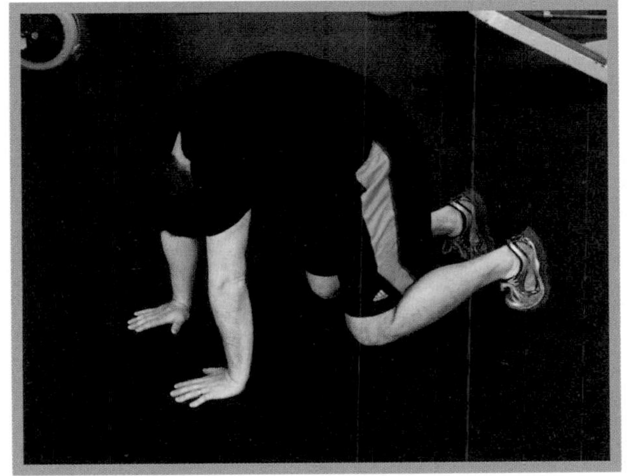

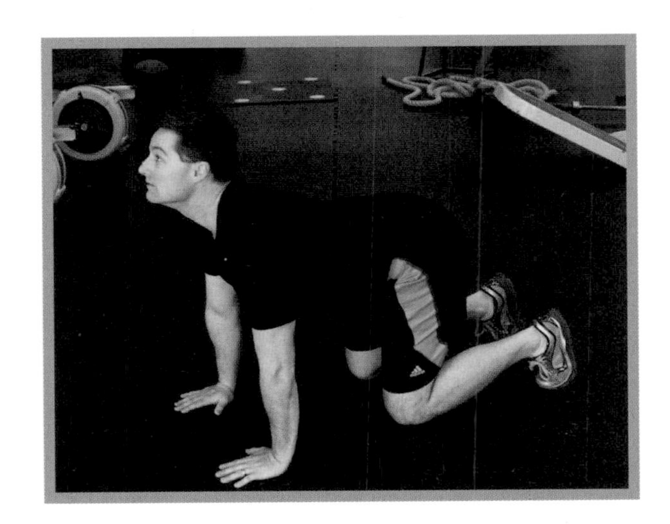

HIP GIRDLE

PHYSIOBALL GLIDES

Set-Up

Position yourself with the Physioball on your shoulders and head, with your ribs pulled into the body.

Execution

Keep the feet and shoulder girdle active. Slide side-to-side, focusing on keeping the back and hip muscles working. When sliding over to the right, tighten up the right glute. When sliding to the left, tighten up the left glute.

Recovery

Bring your hands out to the side to stabilize the body. End in the neutral position.

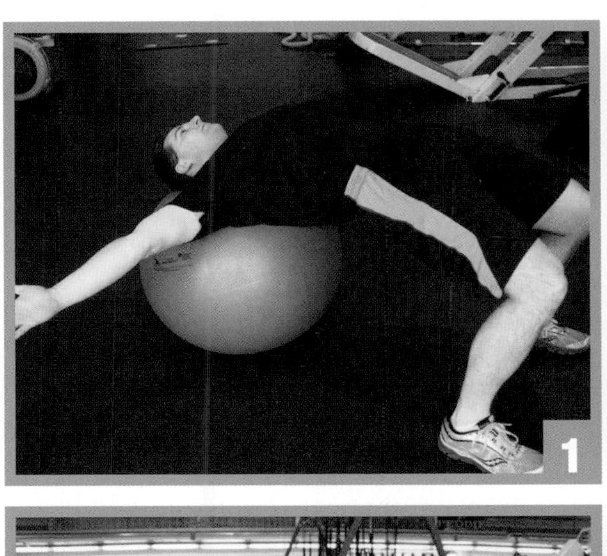
1

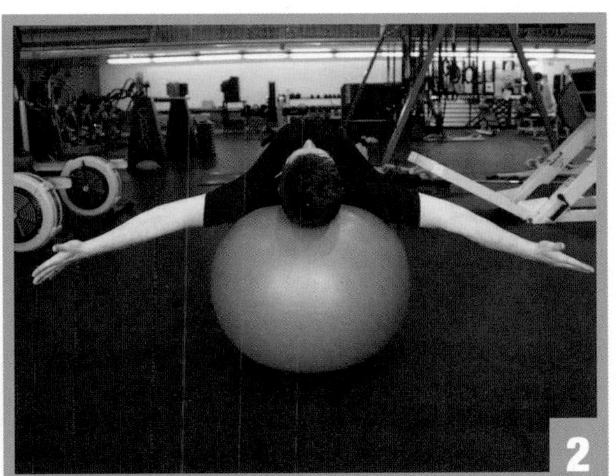
2

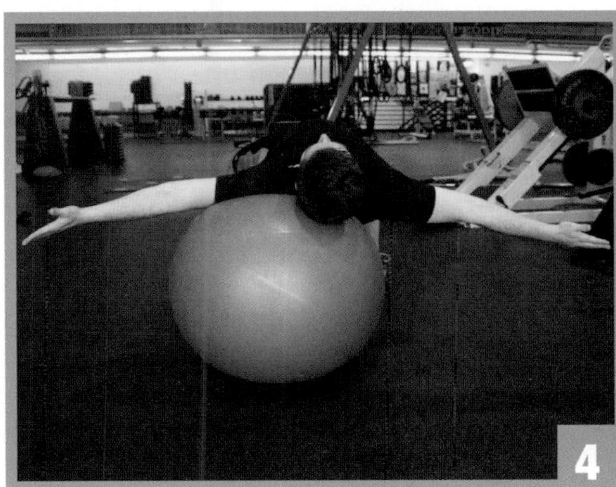
4

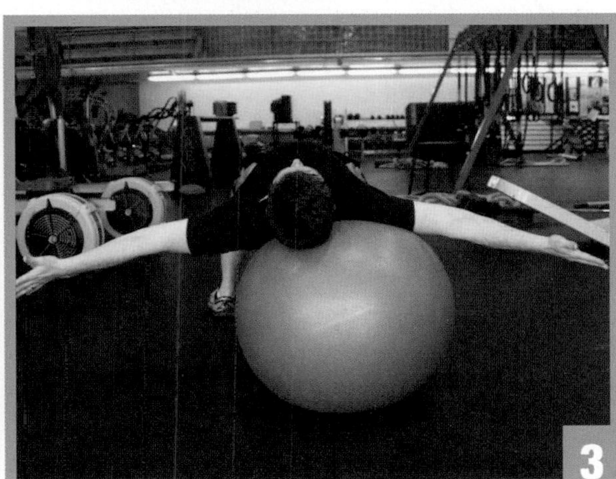
3

HIP GIRDLE

BIRD DOGS

Set-Up
Start in an all-fours position.

Execution
Keep the weight equally distributed between the knees and hands. This exercise is performed by extending the opposite side arm and leg simultaneously and holding the extended position momentarily. Imagine you are a hunting dog pointing.

Recovery
Return to an all-fours position.

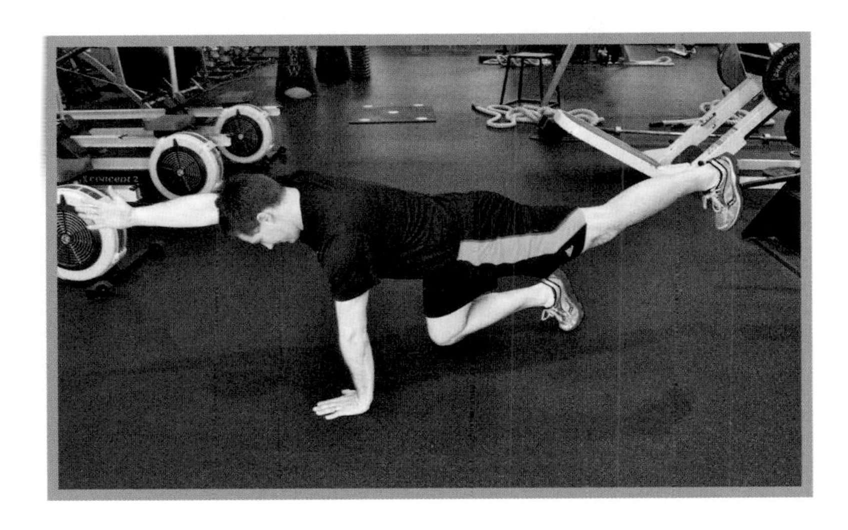

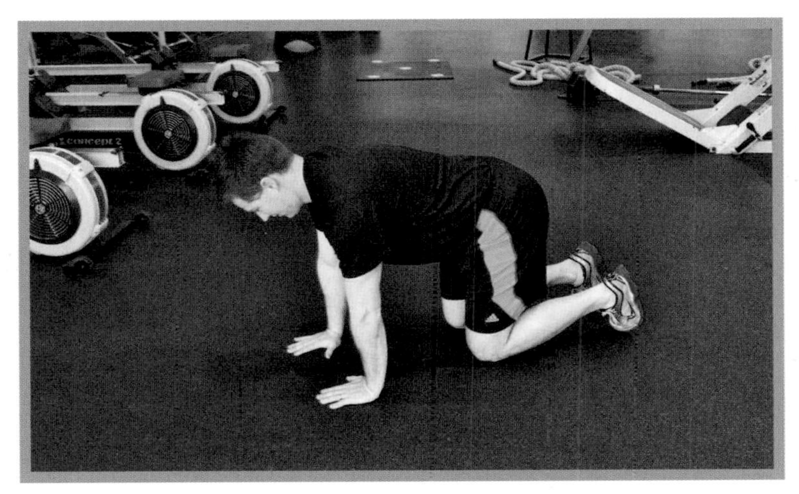

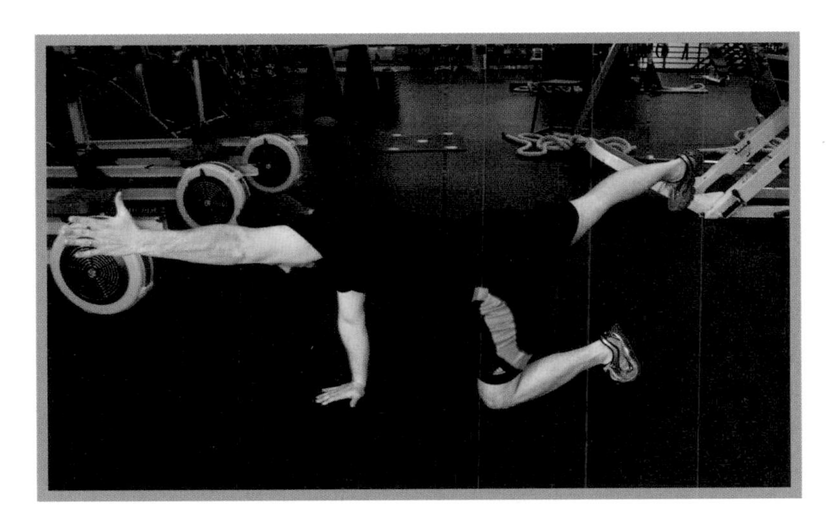

HIP GIRDLE

HIP LIFTS

Set-Up

Lie face up.

Execution

Beginning on your back, initiate the movement by pressing your heels into the floor. Push your hips up, using the backs of your legs. Your arms should remain along the sides of your body. Keep your shoulders and neck relaxed. For the single leg variation, keep the working side knee over the hips during this exercise.

Recovery

Return to the floor, starting with your shoulders and ending with your hips.

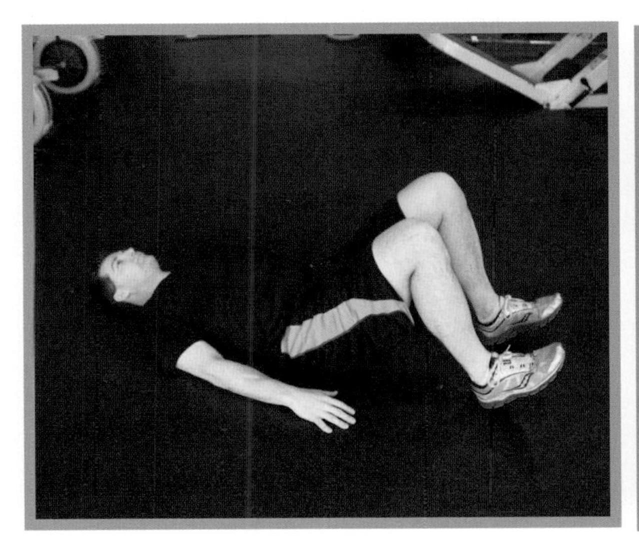

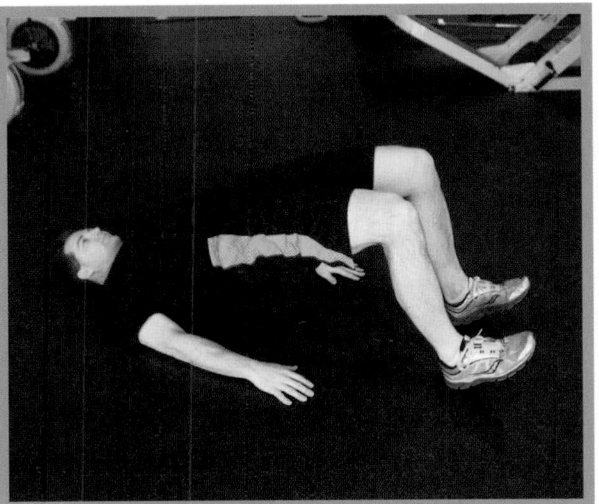

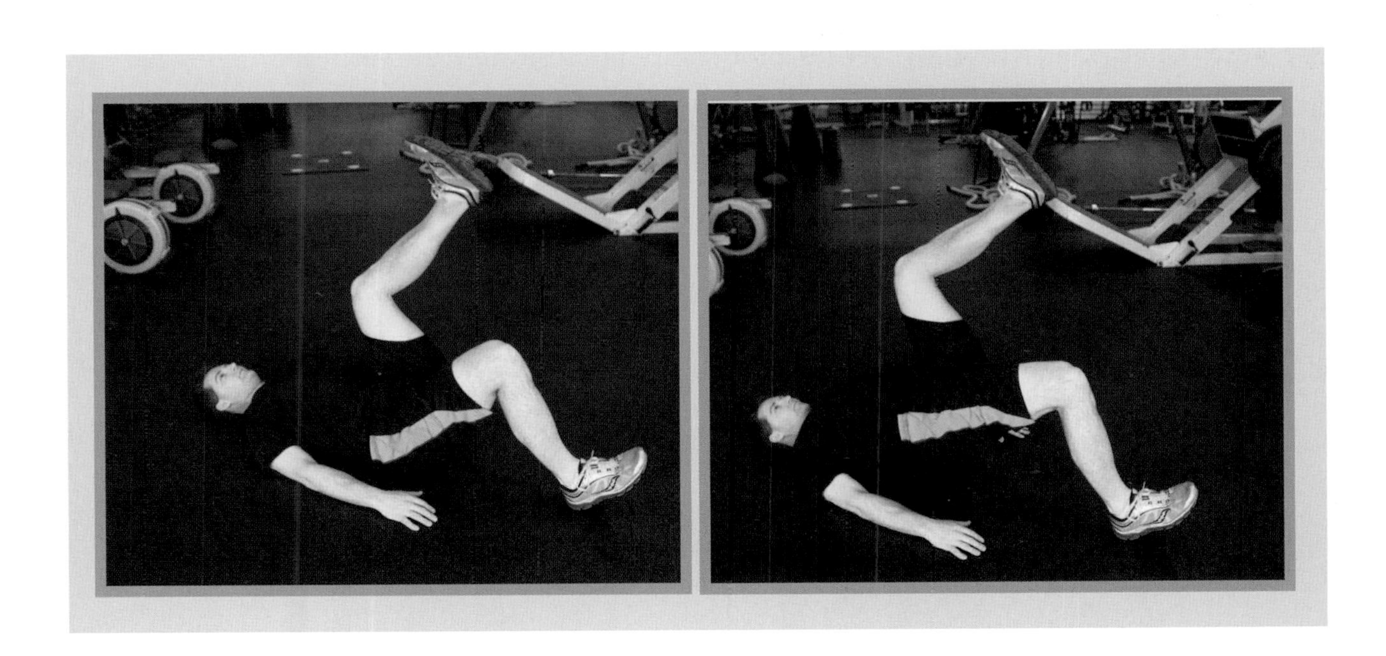

HIP GIRDLE

BACK EXTENSIONS

Set-Up

Position your body face down with the Physioball on the front of your hips. Gently press the feet into the wall and slightly extend the knees. You should feel the back, hips, and legs isometrically contracting before holding the exercise for time.

Execution

After completing the proper set-up, proceed to move through the various progressive sequences as tolerated.

Recovery

Release the lower back by decreasing the pressure on your feet.

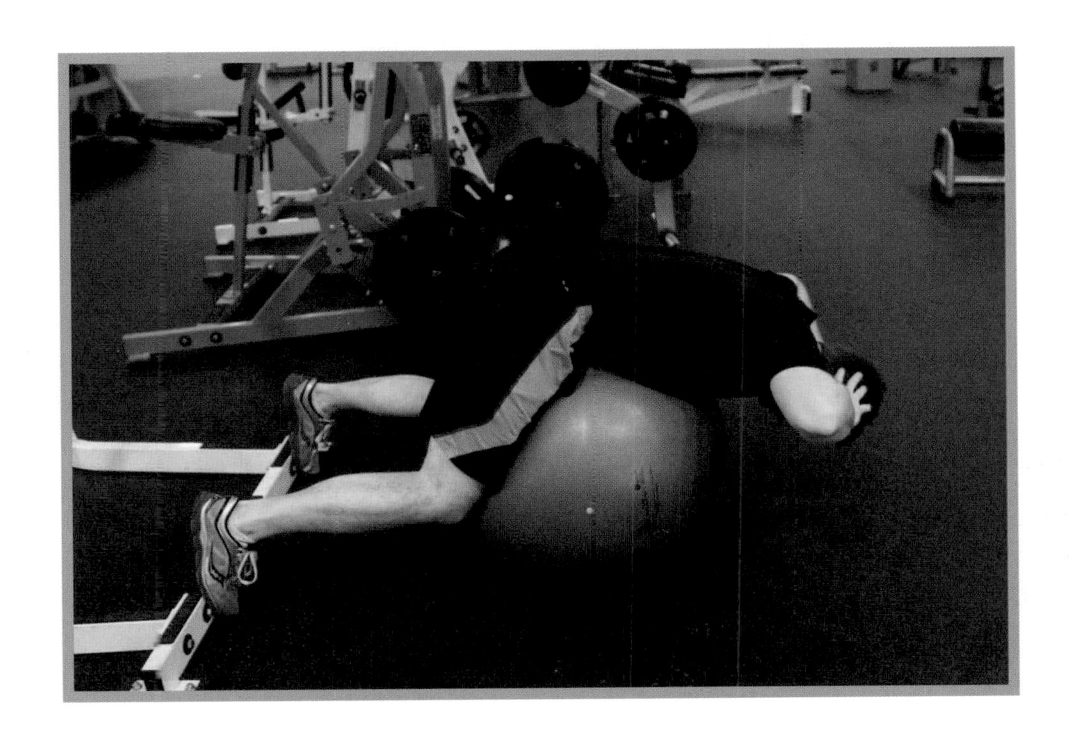

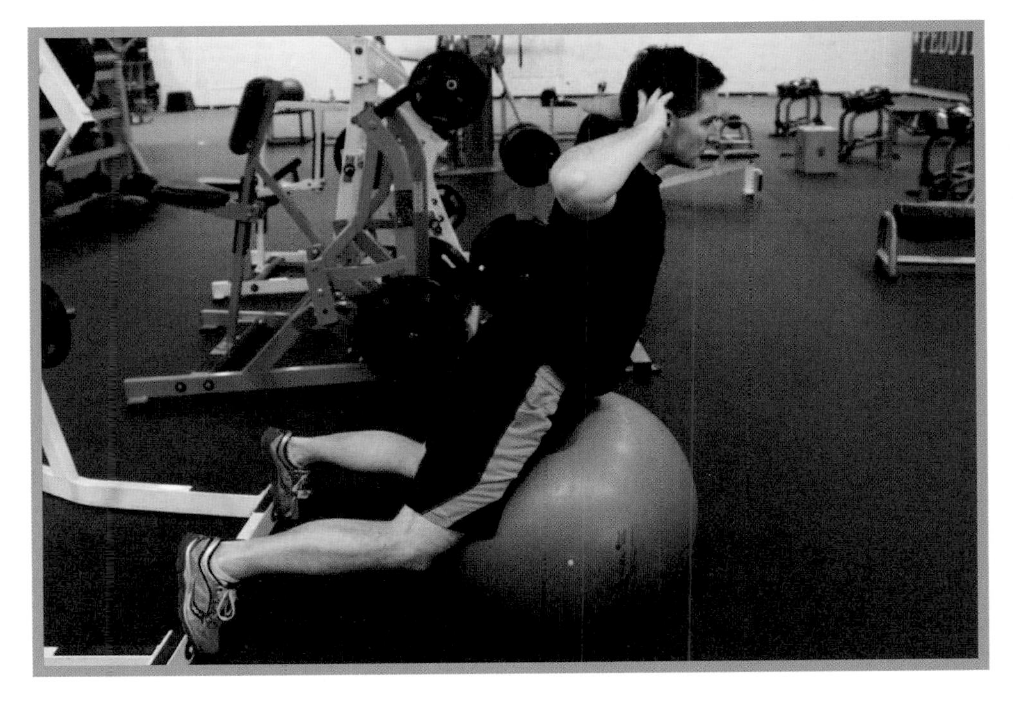

HIP GIRDLE

REVERSE HIP EXTENSIONS

Set-Up

Position your body face down, with your hands flat on the floor.

Execution

Tighten up your lower back and hips prior to lifting your lower body up. Press your heels upwards using the back of your lower body. Progress from using one leg to using both legs.

Recovery

Return your knees to the starting position.

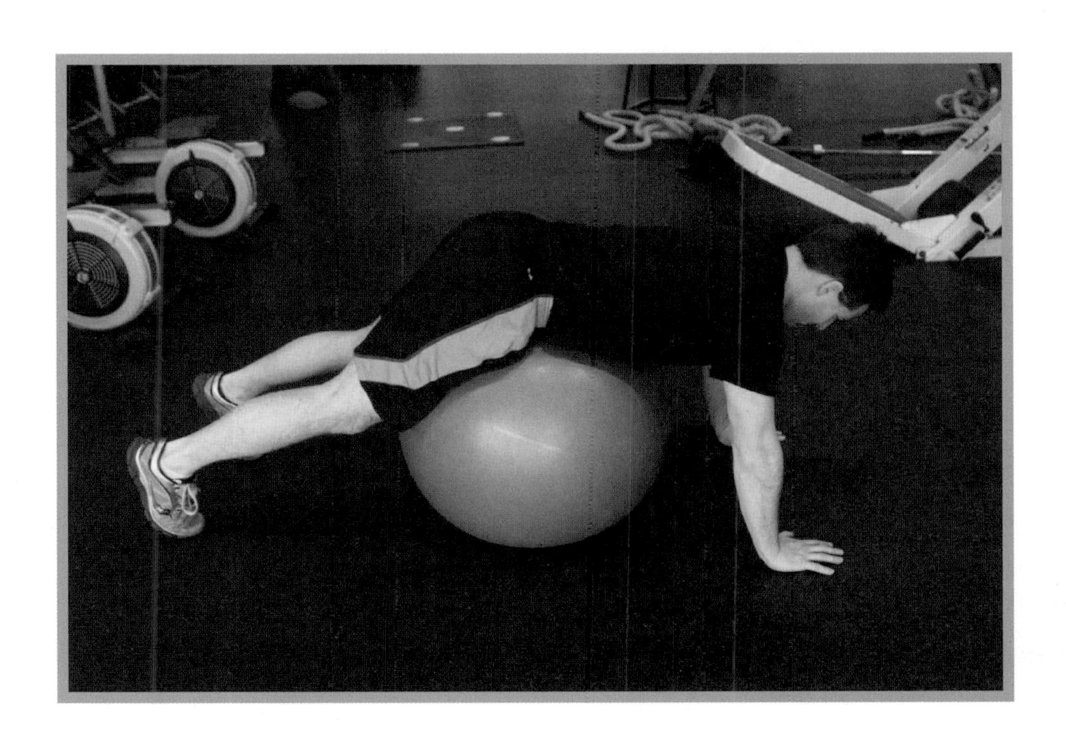

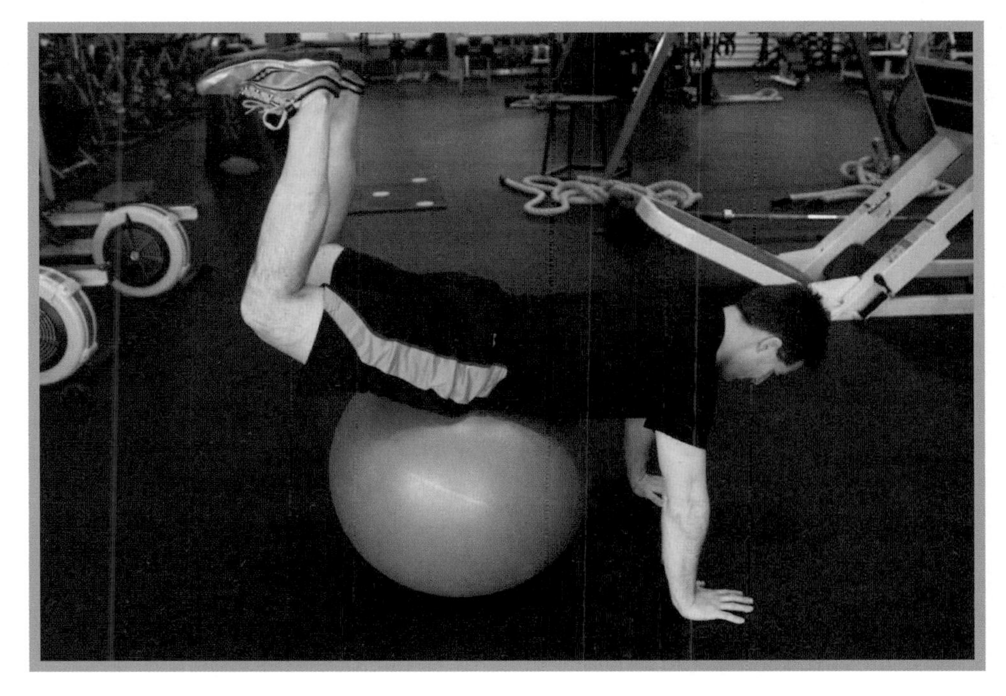

LOWER BODY

SUPERMAN

Set-Up

Position your body face down on a massage table or similar elevated flat surface. Rotate your head to the most comfortable side.

Execution

Lift the working side arm up and slightly out to the side of the shoulder.

Recovery

Return your arm to the starting position.

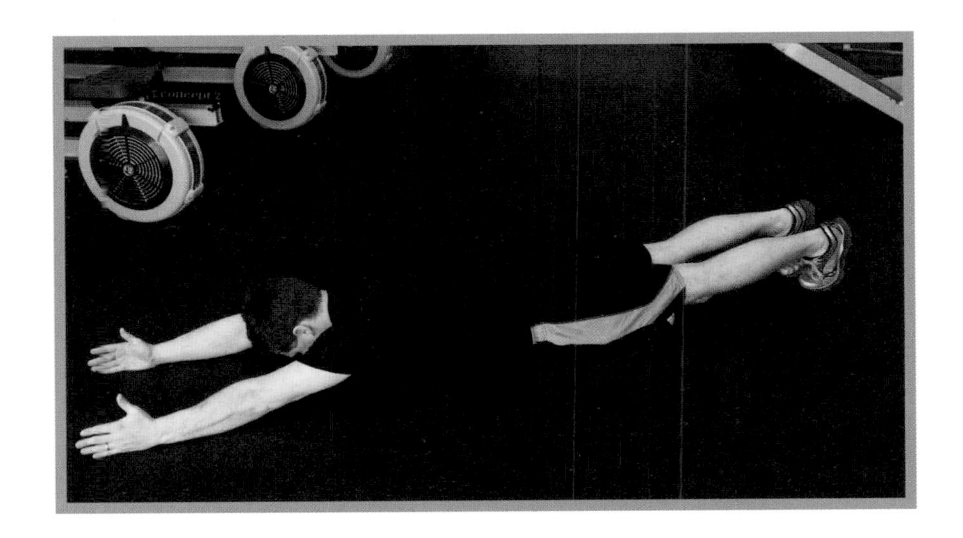

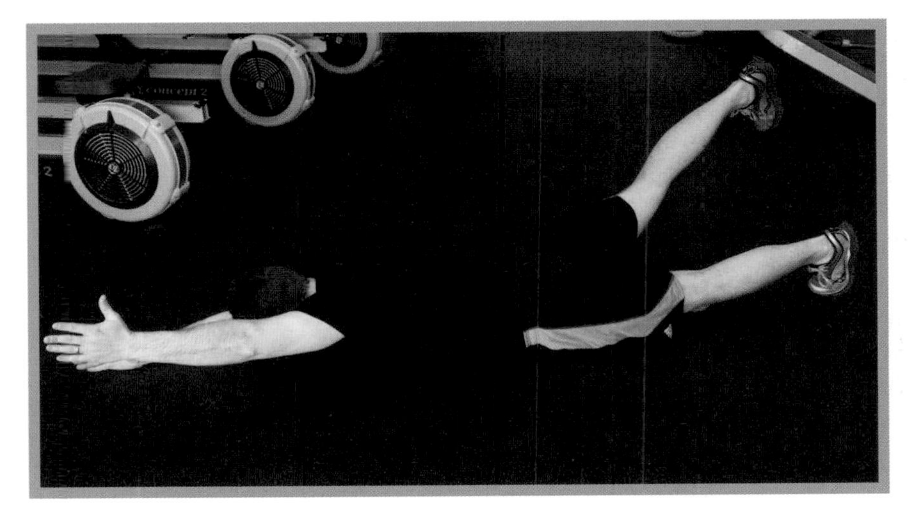

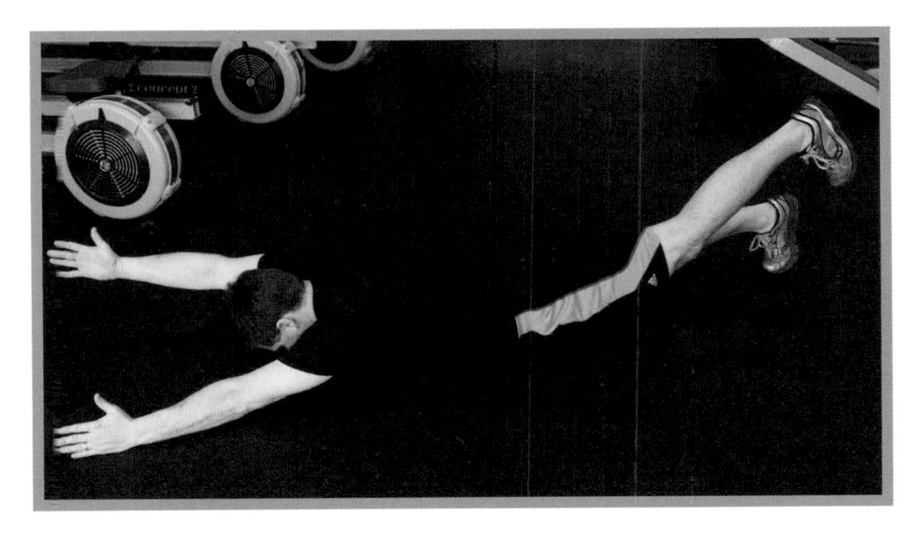

LOWER BODY

ACTIVE HAMSTRING RELEASE

Set-Up

Position your body face up with one leg straight on the wall and with the hip pushed into the wall. Form a 90-degree angle at the hip, if possible. If the hips or lower back pops up, place a soft rolled-up towel under the pelvis.

Execution

Feel the pressure from your straight leg against the wall. Draw the opposite side leg down, keeping the hips stable and the back neutral. Place a towel under your head if tension is felt in the neck or upper back.

Recovery

Lie on your back with the working leg resting on the ground.

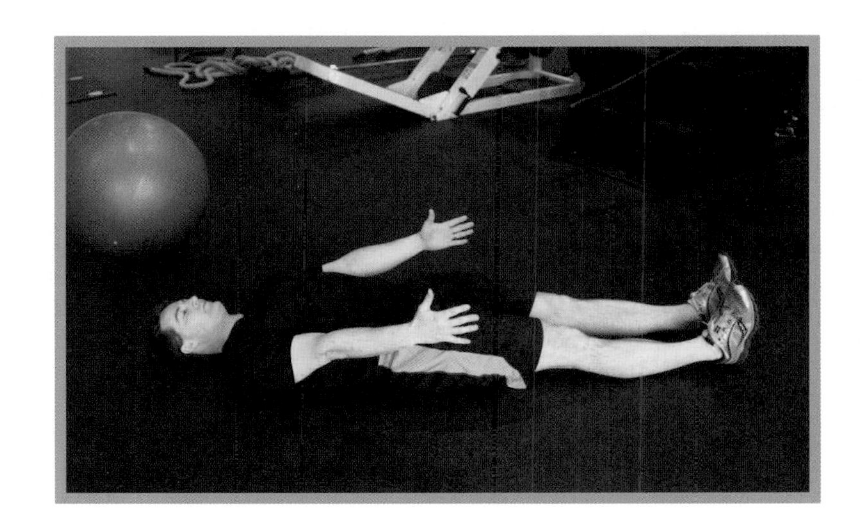

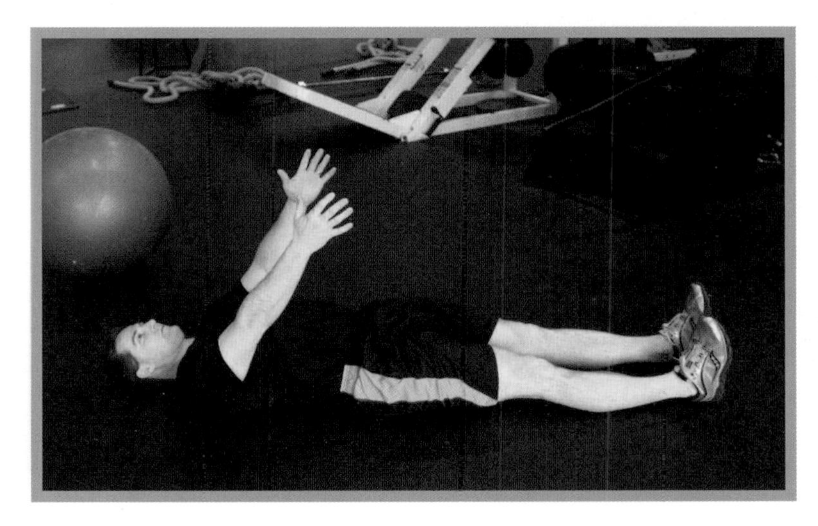

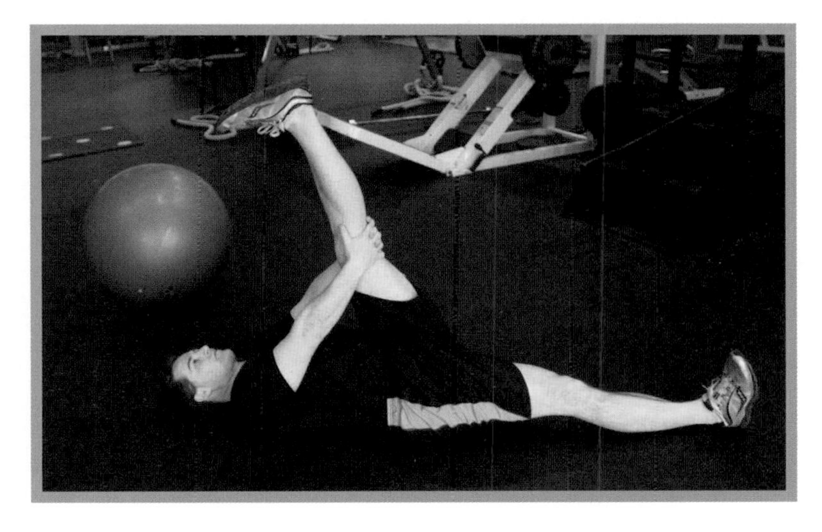

LOWER BODY

QUAD STRETCH

Set-Up
Stand upright with both feet together. Use a machine or any other fixed object to steady your balance during this stretch.

Execution
Reach back and hold your ankle, pulling it toward your glutes. Tighten the back of your hip to deepen the stretch.

Recovery
Relax and let go of your ankle.

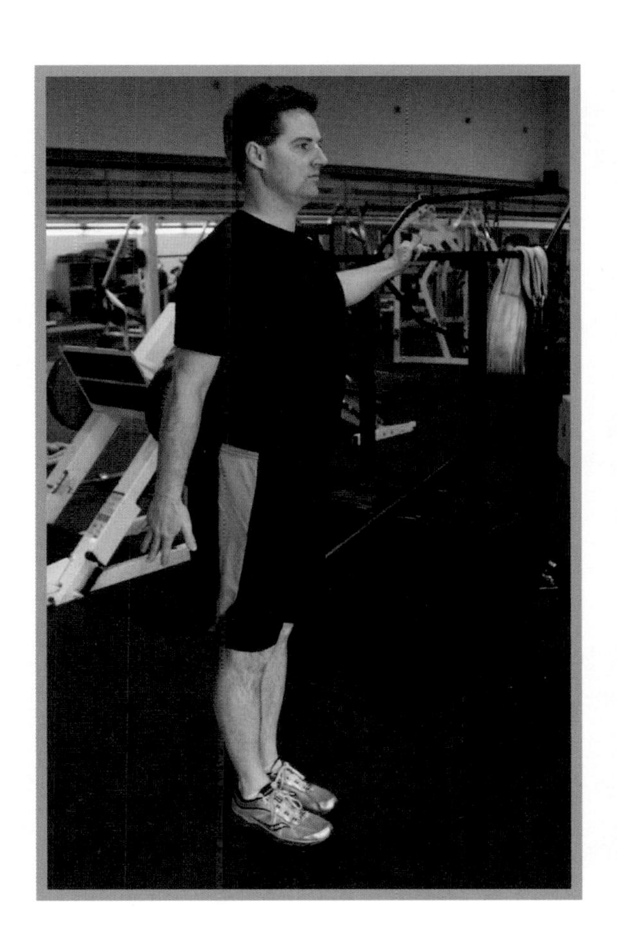

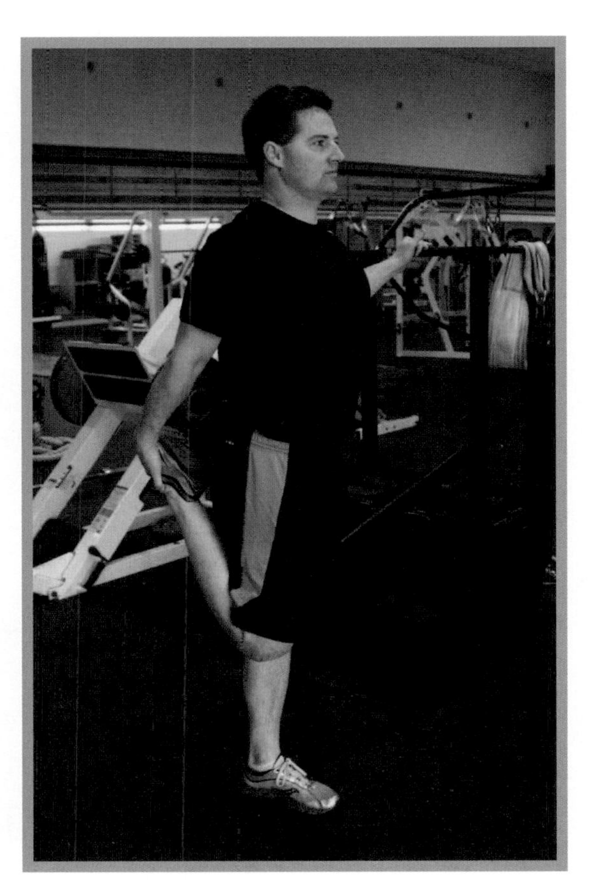

LOWER BODY

KNEELING HIP FLEXOR

Set-Up

Position one foot forward and one foot back. For the side with the foot in the back, place the knee on the ground. Position your hands behind your head or straight in the air.

Execution

Push your hips forward, keeping your lower back neutral. Upon reaching the furthest forward point, flex your upper body to the side.

Recovery

Return your upper body to the neutral position and return your hips to the starting position.

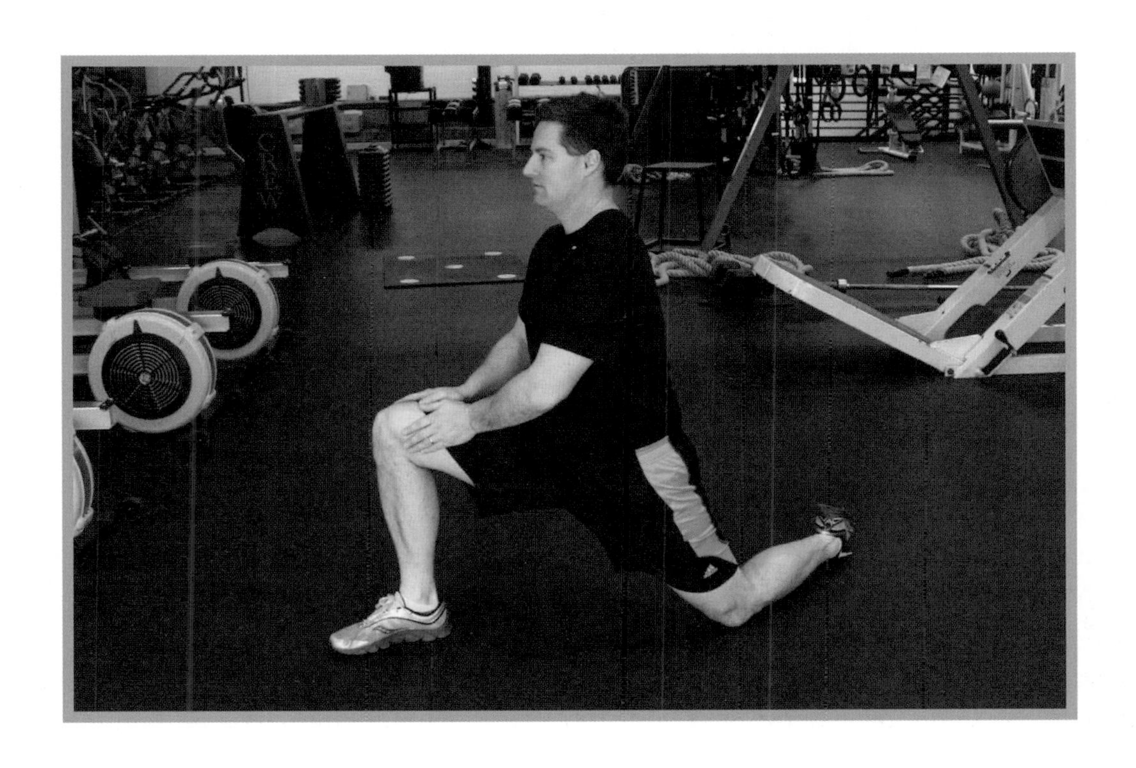

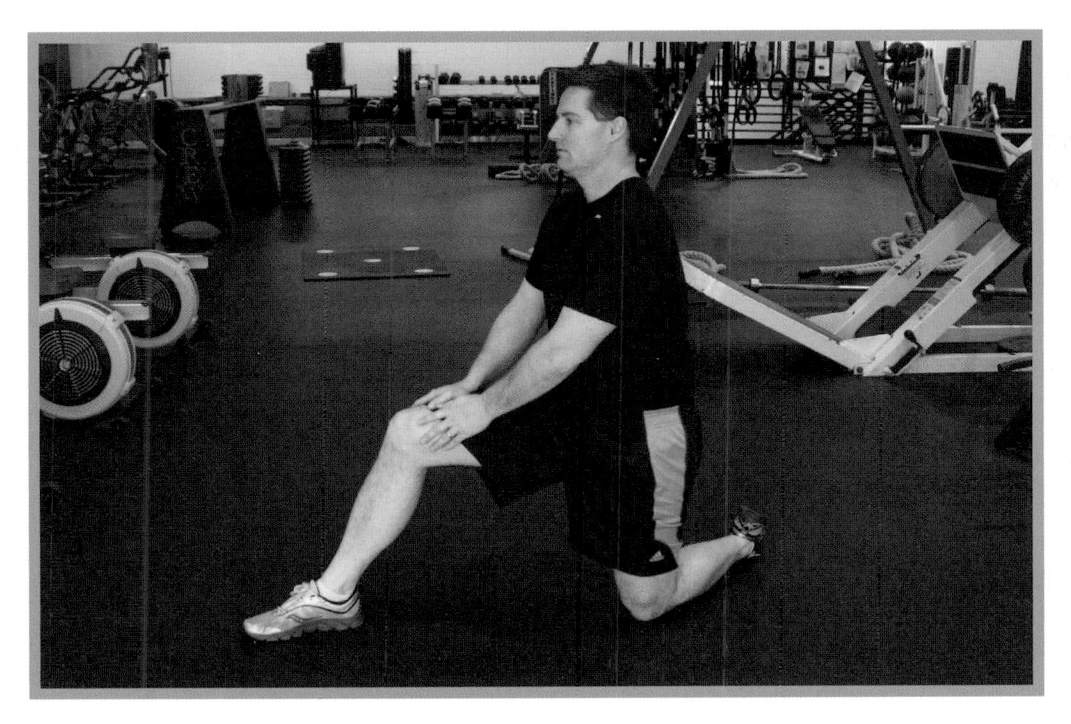

LOWER BODY

CHEST/LAT OPENER

Set-Up

Lie face down on your stomach. Your hands and elbows should be positioned close to your body.

Execution

Press the hands into the ground, breathe out, then extend the body up and out.

Recovery

Relax the back and hips.

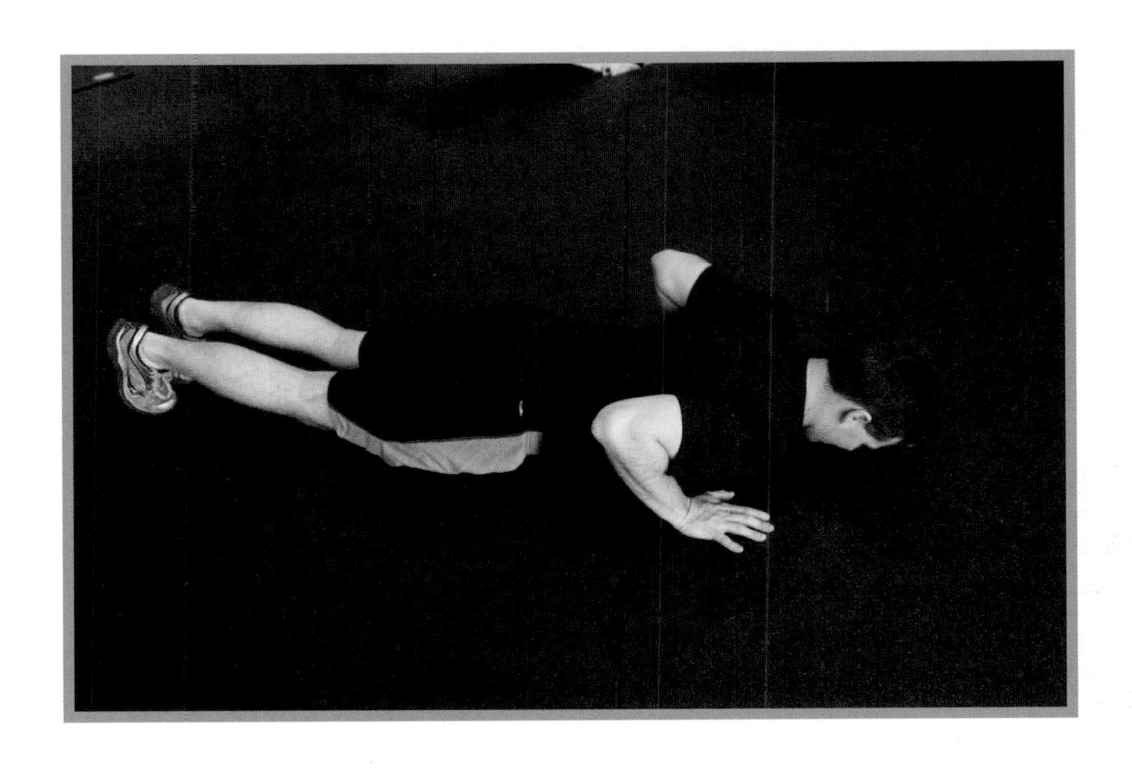

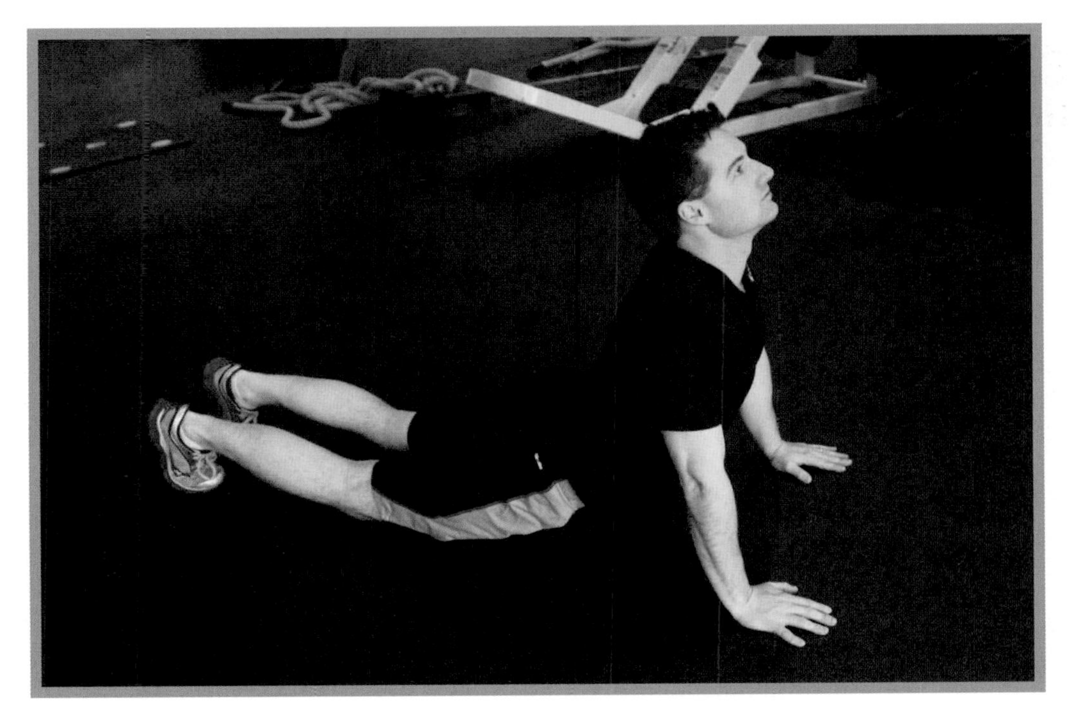

LOWER BODY

LATERAL PLANK

Set-Up

Align the elbow and shoulder, while keeping the spine neutral between the hips and shoulders.

Execution

Cue the side stomach muscles between the shoulder and hip to pull toward the ceiling. You will feel this exercise in the hip, obliques, and rib cage.

Recovery

Release your ribs and return to the floor.

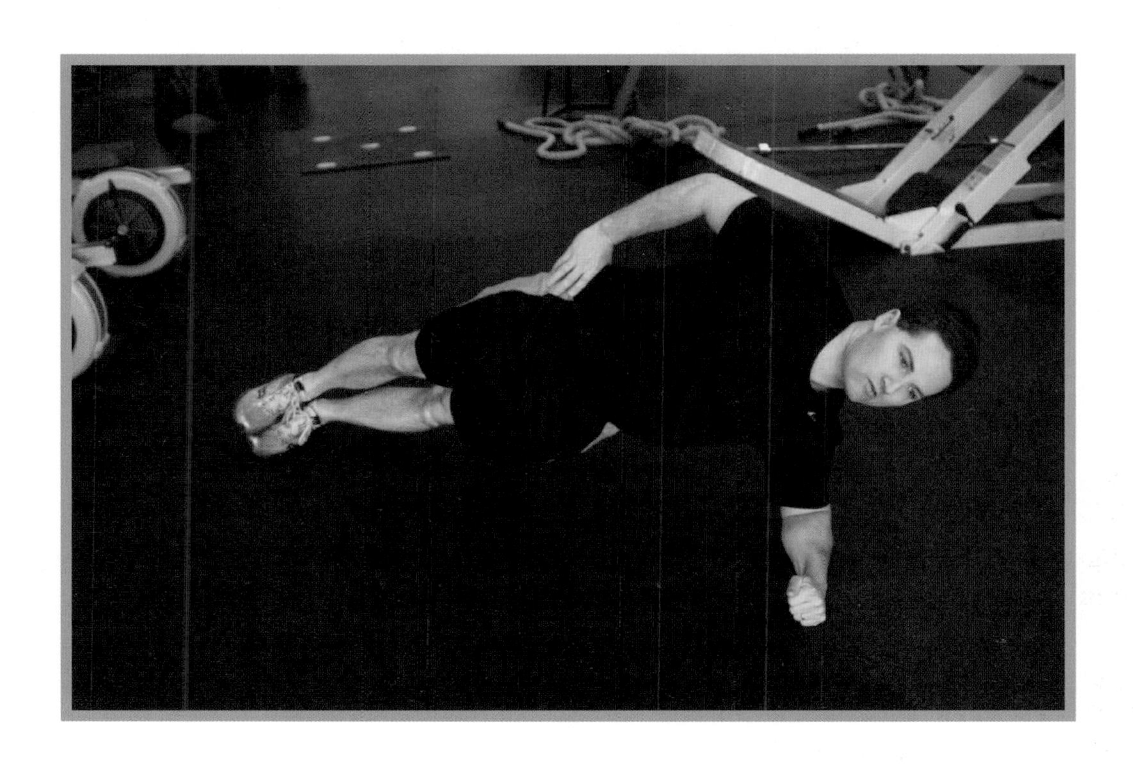

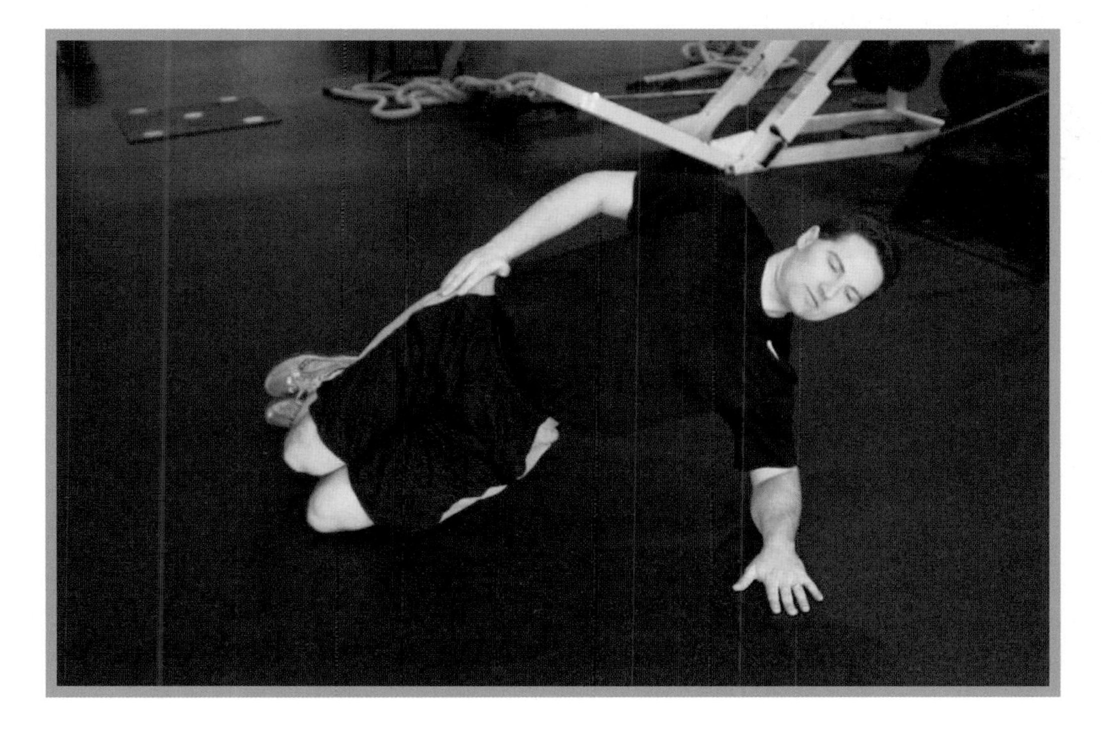

LOWER BODY

TOWEL TOE PULLS

Set-Up

Sit toward the end of a chair. Position a large towel on the floor straight out in front of you. Make sure you are not wearing any shoes or socks; this is a bare toe exercise.

Execution

Begin pulling the towel into the arches of your feet. Feel this exercise in the feet and ankles. To make it more difficult, perform one foot at a time or add light weights at the furthest point on the towel.

Recovery

Rest between sets as needed, or for approximately 1 minute. Lengthen the towel back out to the original starting position. Stretch the toes and arches of the feet between each set.

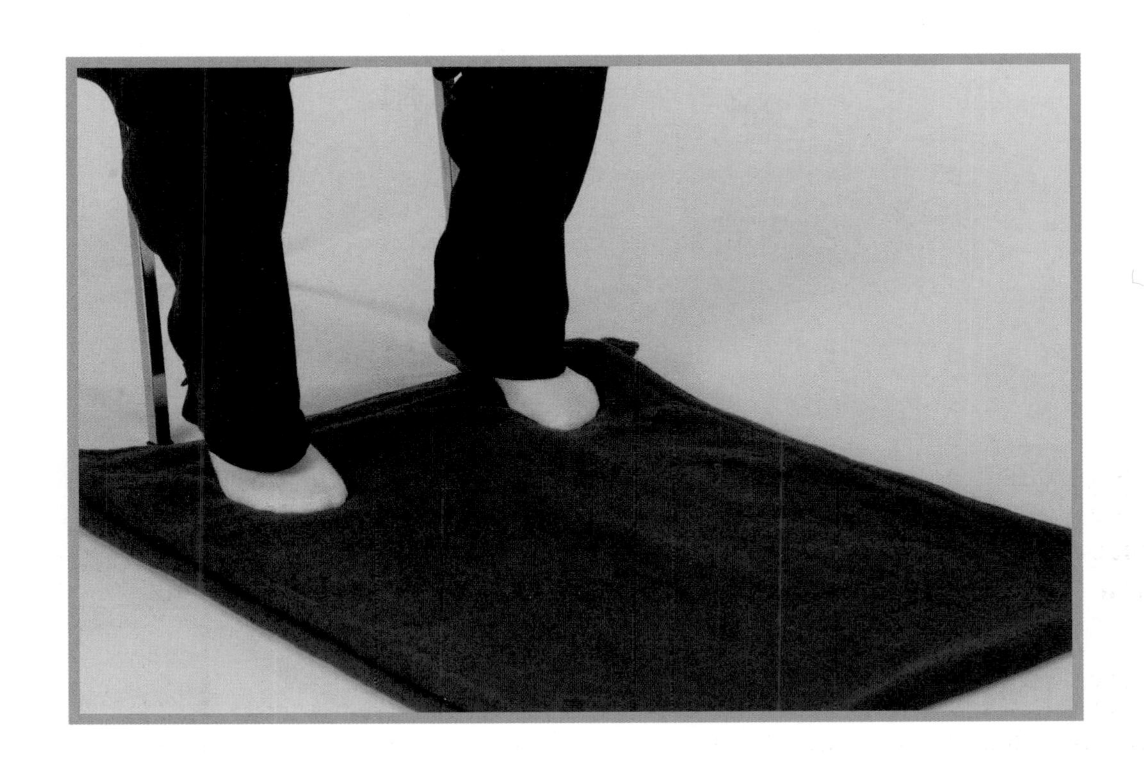

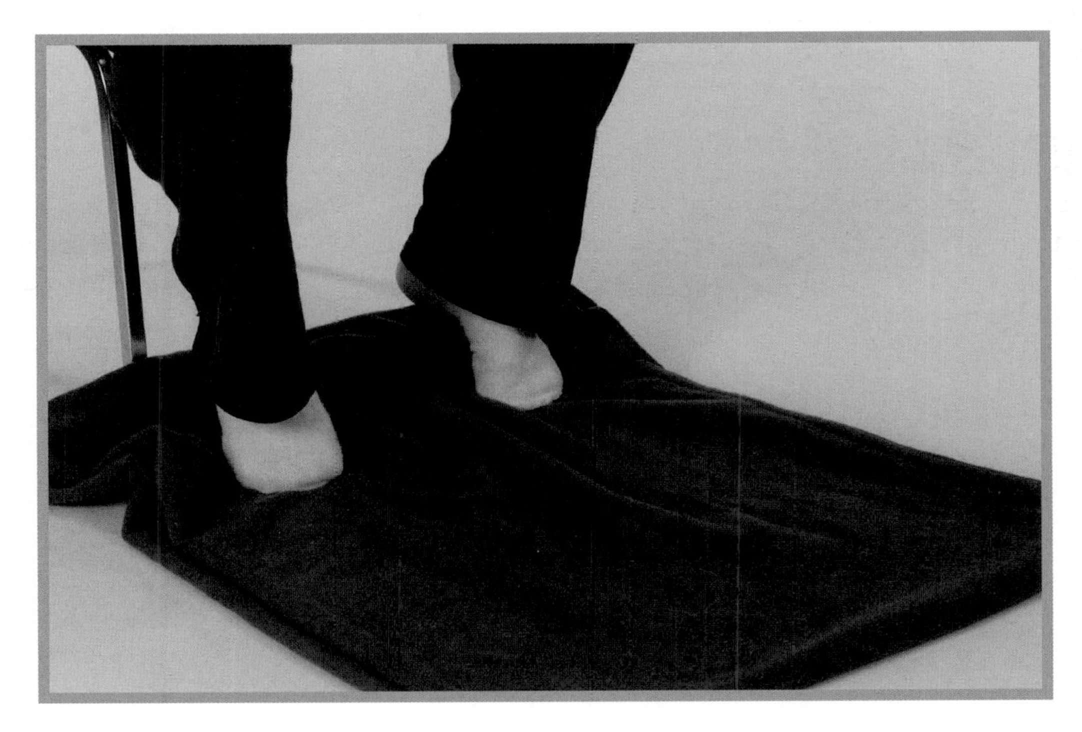

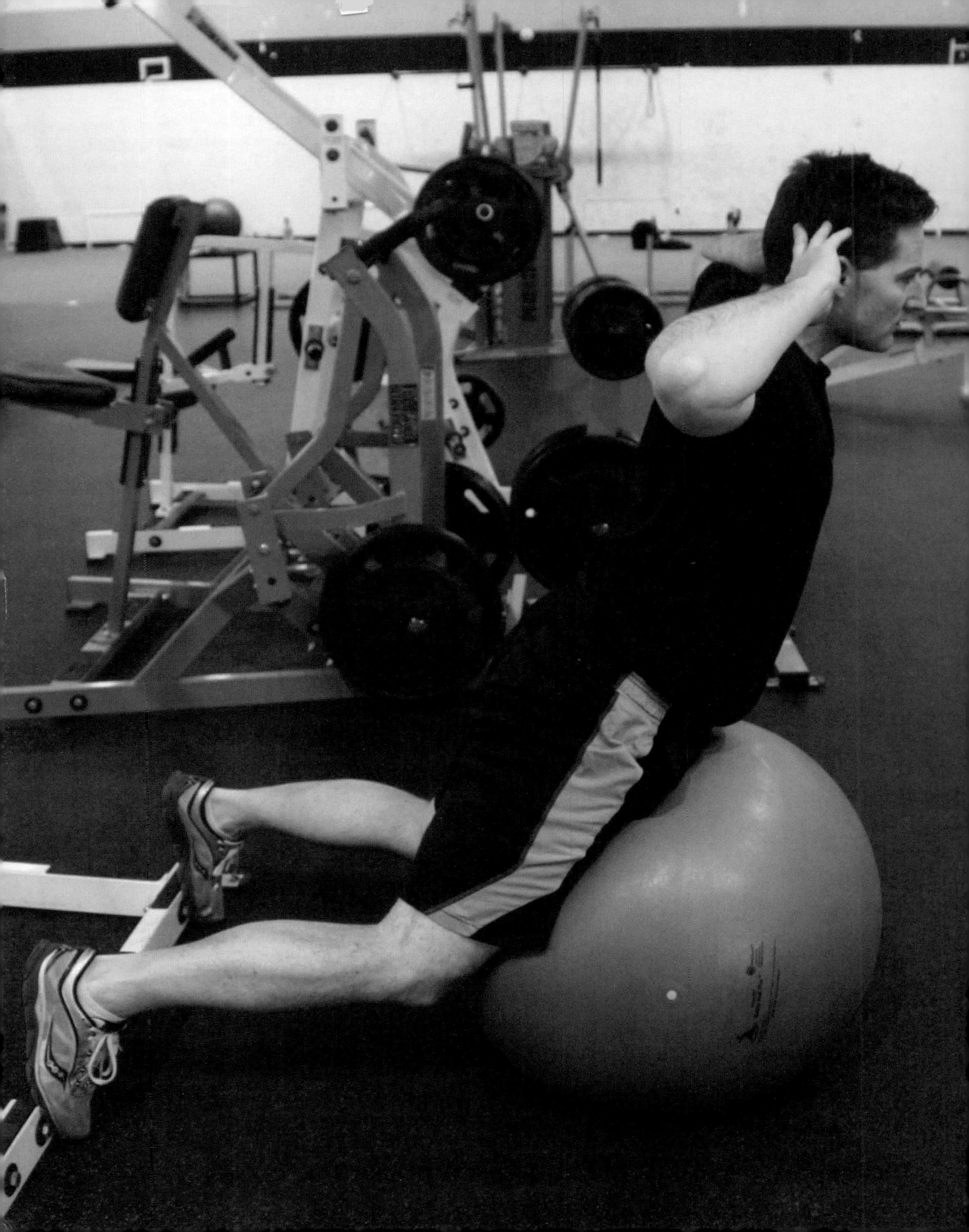

INJURY PREVENTION WORKOUTS

MAIN LIFTS: LOWER BODY

BARBELL SQUAT

Primary Limitations: Flexibility in shoulders, hips, and ankles; Strength in back and hips

EXERCISE 1: Can Opener (page 240)

EXERCISE 2: Back Extensions (page 250)

BOX SQUAT

Primary Limitations: Strength in hip girdle

EXERCISE: Physioball Glides (page 244)

FRONT SQUAT

Primary Limitations: Flexibility in shoulder girdle and wrist; Weak extensor chain: back and hamstrings

EXERCISE 1: Back Extensions (page 250)

EXERCISE 2: Active Hamstring Release (page 256)

DUMBBELL SQUAT

Primary Limitations: Flexibility in hip and ankles; Strength in middle back

EXERCISE 1: Kneeling Hip Flexor with Trunk Flex (page 260)

EXERCISE 2: Chest/Lat Opener (page 262)

DEADLIFT

Primary Limitations: Extensor chain strength: back of the body; Shoulder girdle instability

EXERCISE 1: Back Extensions (page 250)

EXERCISE 2: Reverse Hip Extensions (page 252)

SUMO DEADLIFT

Primary Limitations: Flexibility in the hip and groin; Shoulder girdle instability

EXERCISE 1: Kneeling Hip Flexor (page 260)

EXERCISE 2: Superman (page 254)

DEFICIT DEADLIFT

Primary Limitation: Weakness in hip girdle and back

EXERCISE 1: Reverse Hip Extensions (page 252)

EXERCISE 2: Lateral Plank (page 264)

PIN PULL

Primary Limitations: Poor posture; Tight hip girdle

EXERCISE 1: Bird Dogs (page 246)

EXERCISE 2: Active Hamstring Release (page 256)

MAIN LIFTS: UPPER BODY

BENCH PRESS

Primary Limitations: Weakness in shoulder girdle; Weakness in upper extremities

EXERCISE 1: Bird Dogs (page 246)

EXERCISE 2: Grip/Wrist Strength (page 234)

FLOOR PRESS

Primary Limitation: Inability to relax hip girdle

EXERCISE: Active Hamstring Release (page 256)

BOARD PRESS

Primary Limitation: Weakness in arms and shoulder girdle

EXERCISE: Push-ups: Place a folded towel on the ground. Perform push-ups to towel.

INCLINE BENCH PRESS

Primary Limitation: Instability in shoulder girdle

EXERCISE 1: Shoulder Blade Glide (page 236)

EXERCISE 2: Can Opener (page 240)

BARBELL OVERHEAD PRESS

Primary Limitation: Instability in back and shoulders

EXERCISE: Lateral Plank (page 264)

SUPPLEMENTARY EXERCISES: LOWER BODY

STRAIGHT LEG DEADLIFT

Primary Limitation: Weakness in lower back and hip girdle

EXERCISE 1: Reverse Hip Extensions (page 252)

EXERCISE 2: Active Hamstring Release (page 256)

GLUTE-HAM RAISE

Primary Limitation: Weakness in extensor chain: back of body

EXERCISE 1: Superman (page 254)

EXERCISE 2: Lateral Plank (page 264)

REVERSE HYPEREXTENSIONS

Primary Limitations: Weak back; Tight hamstrings

EXERCISE: Reverse Hip Extensions (page 252)

BACK EXTENSIONS

Primary Limitations: Weak general back muscles; Tight/overactive hamstrings

EXERCISE 1: Active Hamstring Release (page 256)

EXERCISE 2: Superman (page 254)

SUPPLEMENTARY EXERCISES: UPPER BODY

DUMBBELL BENCH PRESS

Primary Limitation: Weakness in shoulder girdle

EXERCISE: Bird Dogs (page 246)

DUMBBELL OVERHEAD PRESS

(also see Barbell Overhead Press, page 272)

Primary Limitation: Instability in back and shoulder girdle

EXERCISE: Lateral Plank (page 264)

BENT OVER ROWS

Primary Limitations: Flexibility in back of body hamstrings; Weakness in back and hips

EXERCISE 1: Active Hamstring Release (page 256)

EXERCISE 2: Reverse Hip Extensions (page 252)

SEATED CABLE ROWS

Primary Limitations: Instability in shoulder girdle; Weakness in back

EXERCISE: Back Extensions (page 250)

PULLDOWN

Primary Limitation: Limitation or restriction in back muscles
EXERCISE 1: Lateral Plank (page 264)
EXERCISE 2: Shoulder Blade Glide (page 236)

PULL-UPS

Primary Limitations: Weakness in upper body; Grip strength
EXERCISE: Grip/Wrist Strength (page 234)

TRICEPS PUSHDOWNS

Primary Limitation: Weakness in upper extremities and shoulder girdle
EXERCISE 1: Lateral Plank (page 264)
EXERCISE 2: Grip/Wrist Strength (page 234)

SHOULDER RAISES

Primary Limitation: Weakness in shoulder girdle
EXERCISE: Lateral Plank (page 264)

BICEPS CURLS

Primary Limitation: Upper body strength, including grip strength
EXERCISE: Grip/Wrist Strength (page 234)

PLANKS: ABDOMINALS

Primary Limitation: Discomfort in lower back
EXERCISE: Lateral Plank (page 264)

FINAL WORDS

The information provided in this book should give you everything you need to successfully start strength training, but please understand there is a whole lot more to the experience than this or any book can truly prepare you for.

Henry Rollins once said, "Knowledge without mileage is B.S." and I can't think of any better embodiment of this sentiment in regards to training. Over the course of your training career, you'll learn far more under the bar than you will from any book, seminar, or website.

Strength training is a marathon, not a sprint. Greatness isn't achieved overnight, rather it adds up over countless small prs over the course of a lifetime. If you take one lesson to heart from this entire book, it's this: *Enjoy the process.*